FAMILY HEALTH FOR POPULATION HEALTH

FAMILY HEALTH FOR POPULATION HEALTH

An Interdisciplinary Approach to Person-Centered Care, Education, Research, and Policy

ROSEMARY W. EUSTACE

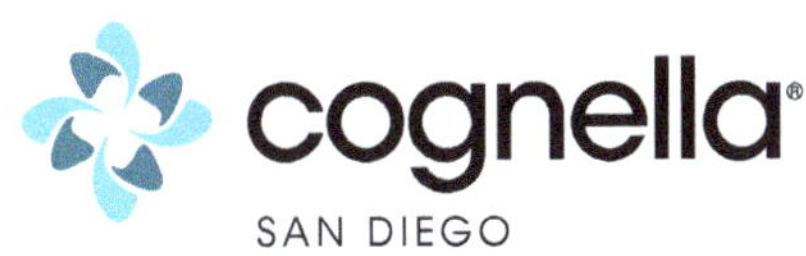

Bassim Hamadeh, CEO and Publisher
Amanda Martin, Executive Publisher
Zoe Flores, Project Editor
Jeanine Rees, Production Editor
Emely Villavicencio, Senior Graphic Designer
JoHannah McDonald, Licensing Coordinator
Natalie Piccotti, Director of Marketing
Kassie Graves, Senior Vice President, Editorial
Alia Bales, Director, Project Editorial and Production

Printed in the United States of America.

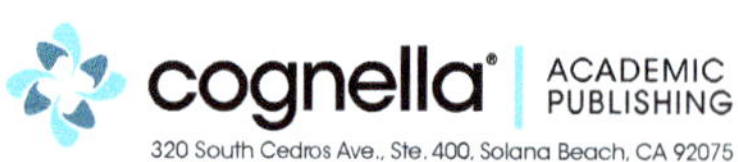

Brief Contents

Preface xv

PART I FOUNDATIONAL CONCEPTS FOR FAMILY HEALTH PRACTICE 1

CHAPTER 1 Introduction to Family Health in the Context of Health Care 3

CHAPTER 2 The Importance of Family Health Theories in Health Care 25

CHAPTER 3 Social Determinants of Family Health 57

CHAPTER 4 Patient and Family Engagement, and Levels of Professional Involvement in Family Health Care 73

PART II GENERALIST ENTRY-LEVEL FAMILY HEALTH CARE COMPETENCIES ACROSS MULTIPLE DISCIPLINE 93

CHAPTER 5 Levels of Health Care Workers' Involvement in Family Health Care 95

CHAPTER 6 Family Assessment in Family Health Care 123

CHAPTER 7 Person-Centered Relationships and Communication in Family Health Care 147

CHAPTER 8 Intersectorial and Multisectorial Approaches and Family Health Care 167

CHAPTER 9 Evidence-Based Family-Level Interventions in Family Health Care 181

CHAPTER 10 Advocating for Evidence-Based Person- and Family-Centered Health Policies, Programs and Practices 207

PART III FAMILY HEATH PRACTICE OPPORTUNITIES 229

CHAPTER 11 Experiential Learning for 21st-Century Family Health Professionals 231

CHAPTER 12 Career in Family Health Teams 239

CHAPTER 13 The Future of Family Research in 21st-Century Health Care and Public Health System(s) 253

CHAPTER 14 The Role of Professional Organizations in Promoting Family Health 265

CHAPTER 15 Building a Family Health Professional Portfolio for 21st-Century Health Care and Public Health Systems 269

Index 275

Detailed Contents

Preface xv

PART I FOUNDATIONAL CONCEPTS FOR FAMILY HEALTH PRACTICE 1

CHAPTER 1 **Introduction to Family Health in the Context of Health Care 3**

Learning Objectives 3
Historical Context of Family Health Care and Family Science 4
What Is Family in Family Health Care? 8
Relationships Between Individual Health, Family Health, Population Health, and Public Health 11
Barriers and Facilitators to Implementation of Family-Focused Health Care 17
Conclusion 19
Suggested Websites 19
Reflection Question 19
References 19

CHAPTER 2 **The Importance of Family Health Theories in Health Care 25**

Learning Objectives 25
An Overview of Family Health Theories, Conceptual/Theoretical Frameworks, and Models 26
Terminologies in Theorizing Family Health 26
Metaparadigms 26
Person, Environment, Health, and Nursing 27
Philosophical Assumptions 28
Conceptual/Theoretical Frameworks or Models 29
Theory 30
Borrowed and Shared Theories 30
Theoretical Paradigms 31
Conceptual/Theoretical Frameworks and Theories of Family Health 31
Biomedical Perspective 31
Biopsychosocial and Systems Thinking Perspective 33
Trajectory Models 40

Stress and Coping Perspective 45
Conclusion 48
Suggested Websites 49
Suggested Readings 49
Reflection Questions 50
References 50

CHAPTER 3 Social Determinants of Family Health 57
Learning Objectives 57
Determinants of Health and SDoH Defined 58
Family Health as an Upstream Social Determinant of Health 60
Prioritizing SDoH and Social Needs in Family Health 62
Social and SDoH Needs 62
Characteristics of a Health Family and Healthy Community 63
The Role of Epidemiology in Family Health 64
Conclusion 70
Suggested Websites 70
Reflection Questions 71
References 71

CHAPTER 4 Patient and Family Engagement, and Levels of Professional Involvement in Family Health Care 73
Learning Objectives 73
The Importance of Patient and Family Engagement in Health and Health Care 74
Sample Facts on the Importance of Patient Engagement 74
Conceptual Background of Patient and Family Engagement in Health Care 76
Levels of Engagement 77
Level of the Healthcare System Engagement 77
Determinants of PFE in Health Care 79
Individual Health 79
Family Health 80
Population Health 81
Community Level 83
Public Health 83
Conclusion 85
Suggested Websites 85
Suggested Readings 86
Reflection Questions 86
References 86

PART II GENERALIST ENTRY-LEVEL FAMILY HEALTH CARE COMPETENCIES ACROSS MULTIPLE DISCIPLINE 93

CHAPTER 5 **Levels of Health Care Workers' Involvement in Family Health Care 95**

Learning Objectives 95
Global Health Care Workforce Trends as of 2024 96
Health Care Workforce in the United States in 2022 96
Fact Sheet 97
The Importance of a Diverse Health Care Workforce in Family Health and Whole Health Care Health Systems 98
The Public Health Workforce and Essential Health Services in Family Health Care 99
The Theoretical Foundations of Health Care Professional Involvement and Collaboration With Families in Whole Health Care 101
Levels of Family Health Care Professional Involvement With Families 102
Application of the LFI Framework 103
Family and Professional Roles in the LFI Frameworks 104
Collaborative and Integrated Interprofessional Family Health Care Teams 105
Interprofessional Competency Frameworks 109
Occupational Challenges and Opportunities in Building and Strengthening a Whole Health Care Workforce Within 4HEALTHS 112
Burnout and Burnout Disparities Among Health Care Providers 112
Conclusion 117
Suggested Websites 117
Suggested Readings 118
Reflection Questions 118
References 118

CHAPTER 6 **Family Assessment in Family Health Care 123**

Learning Objectives 123
Importance of Family Assessment and Intervention in Family Health Care 124
Defining Family Assessment 124
Family Assessment Tools and Models From Multidisciplinary Theoretical Perspectives 125
Family Health History, Family Genogram, and Family Ecomap for Whole Health 135
Family Health History 135
Family Health Genogram 136
Family Ecomap 138
Ethical Considerations in Family Health Assessment 138
Organizing Family Health Assessment for Holistic Whole Health Care 139
Challenges and Opportunities of Family Health Assessment Within 4HEALTH 142

Conclusion 143
Suggested Websites 144
Suggested Readings 144
Reflection Questions 144
References 144

CHAPTER 7 Person-Centered Relationships and Communication in Family Health Care 147

Learning Objectives 147
Importance of Effective Communication and Relationships in Health Care Settings 148
Therapeutic Communication Processes, Mediums and Strategies 149
Communication Model 149
Mediums of Communication 151
Person-Centered Care Communication 151
Effective Communication Strategies 152
Barriers to Person-Centered Therapeutic Communication and Relationships in Family Health Care 159
Conclusion 161
Suggested Websites 161
Reflection Questions 162
References 162

CHAPTER 8 Intersectorial and Multisectorial Approaches and Family Health Care 167

Learning Objectives 167
Definition of Intersectorial and Multisectorial Approach 168
The Role of Intersectorial and Multisectorial Approach in Family Health Care 169
Era 3.0 Health Systems Transformation Framework and Family-Centered Intersectorial and Multisectorial Perspectives 170
Factors Influencing Intersectorial, and Multisectorial Collaboration in Family Health Care 174
Barriers and Enablers 174
Barriers and Facilitators of Person and Family-Centered Intersectorial and Multi-sectorial Approach within the 4HEALTHS Contexts 175
Individual and Family Health 175
Population Health 176
Public Health 177
Conclusion 178
Suggested Websites 178
Suggested Readings 178
Reflection Question 178
References 179

CHAPTER 9 Evidence-Based Family-Level Interventions in Family Health Care 181

Learning Objectives 181
The Importance of Family-Level Interventions and Intervention Research in Family Health Care 182
Typology of Family Health Interventions in Family Health Care 183
Levels of Prevention in FHI 183
Common Risks and Protective Factors Addressed by FHIs 184
Mechanism of Actions and Delivery Modes 186
Family Outcomes 189
Adaptation and Implementation of Evidence-Based Family Health Interventions 189
Implementation of FHI 190
Efficacy and Effectiveness in FHI 197
Implementation FHI Challenges and Opportunities in Person-Centered Care Within 4HEALTH 198
Conclusion 200
Suggested Websites 200
Suggested Readings 200
Reflection Questions 201
References 201

CHAPTER 10 Advocating for Evidence-Based Person- and Family-Centered Health Policies, Programs and Practices 207

Learning Objectives 207
Definition of Policy and Health Policy 208
The Importance of a Family Perspective in Evidence-Based Policymaking 208
Advocating for Evidence-Based Family-Focused Public Health Policies, Programs, and Practices 210
Family and Family Health 212
Health Equity and Health Disparity 213
Definition of Evidence-Informed Policy Decision-Making 214
Defining the Health Policymaking Process 215
Factors Influencing the Uptake of Evidence-Based Health Policy-Making Processes Within the 4HEALTHS Context 221
Conclusion 223
Suggested Websites 223
Suggested Readings 223
Reflection Questions 224
References 224

PART III FAMILY HEATH PRACTICE OPPORTUNITIES 229

CHAPTER 11 Experiential Learning for 21st-Century Family Health Professionals 231

Learning Objectives 231
Importance of Experiential Learning in Higher Education 231
Importance of Service-Learning Programs 232
Benefits of Family-Focused SL Programs 233
Core Principle of SL Programs 233
Conclusion 235
Suggested Websites 235
Suggested Readings 235
Reflection Questions 236
References 236

CHAPTER 12 Career in Family Health Teams : A Connecting Bridge Between Individual and Population Health in 21st-Century Person-Centered Health Care and Public Health Systems 239

Learning Objectives 239
The Importance of Culturally Competent Family Health Professional Teams 239
Diverse Health Care Settings for Family Health Teams in the 21st Century 240
Essential Competencies for FHTs in Primary Care and Community-Oriented Care 241
Examples of Professional Family Health Competencies 244
WHO Self-Care Competencies 248
Conclusion 248
Suggested Readings 249
Reflection Questions 249
References 249

CHAPTER 13 The Future of Family Research in 21st-Century Health Care and Public Health System(s) : Individual and Population Health Care and Outcomes 253

Learning Objectives 253
Importance of Family Research in Health Care and Public Health in the 21st Century 253
Criteria for Family Research 256
How to Build a Program of Family Research 258
Conclusion 260
Suggested Websites 261
Suggested Readings 261
Reflection Questions 261
References 262

CHAPTER 14 The Role of Professional Organizations in Promoting Family Health 265

Learning Objectives 265
Role of Professional Associations in Family Science and Health 265
Benefits of Professional Associations 266
Conclusion 267
Suggested Websites 267
Reflection Questions 268
References 268

CHAPTER 15 Building a Family Health Professional Portfolio for 21st-Century Health Care and Public Health Systems 269

Learning Objectives 269
Importance of Qualified Family Health Teams 270
Components of a Family Health Professional Portfolio 270
Conclusion 273
Suggested Website 273
Suggested Readings 273
Reflection Question 273
References 274

Index 275

Preface

This book is designed to bring to light the role of family in health development and health care practice. While it is impossible to include everything, the book provides a foundational perspective that is vital for educators, practitioners and scholars interested in understanding and studying the role of family in health and public health care.

I grew up in a small rural mining town in a traditional extended family with eight blood-related siblings and several in and out cousins. During my early childhood and middle childhood years, I was a pretty active child who frequent the hospital for childhood illnesses. In my late teens following an off-time death of my father, I lived in informal foster homes and learned how to navigate the healthcare system both tradition and non-traditional in the hands of multiple and diverse care givers. As a teenager, I suffered severe hay related allergies that kept me awake, with on and off leg blisters that my maternal grandmother used to describe as "endwala nkulu" in her mother tongue—the haya tribe in Tanzania, which meant a "chronic illness." Until today, I wonder if my early-adulthood diabetes diagnosis of "unkown" cause was related to what my grandma saw. During my early and later life years, I have learned a lot about how families live, play, eat, pray, and age and how they influence one's health and the health of others around them.

Over the years, my nursing experience and family science background continue to facilitate my curiosity about the role of family in health care and self-care management. Unfortunately, for more than a decade as I taught family nursing and community/public health nursing, I kept struggling to choose a book that met or checked all of my boxes of what I wanted my nursing students to know about families and its role in human health development. As a result, I tapped into different sources and piecemealed content to get by. My initial curiosity led me to innovate two *family health* promotion teaching strategies with colleagues as a piecemeal solution among pre-licensure nursing students. The award-winning innovation pushed my curiosity further to consider writing my own book to shed a new light on the role of health care professionals in putting family first in their practice.

This book is written with graduate students in health care fields in mind. The book captures the essence of family and health from a health care and public health context. This book differs from other books in that it is a simple read that covers general information but yet essential issues to health care professionals that include, the meaning of family, theoretical underpinnings of family and health, social determinants of *family health*, family policy and the role of *family health* care interprofessional teams within the context of multisectoral approaches. It advocates for a clear understanding of the context of *family health* care, also described in the book as the "4HEALTH" where the family is seen as the needed bridge between individual and *population health* in the 21st Century. The book's disciplinary and interdisciplinary lenses show that *family health* and illness, and *family health* care, needs all of us to act together. Thus, the book prepares health care professionals that see themselves as part of the *family health* care team vs individual professionals.

PART I

FOUNDATIONAL CONCEPTS FOR FAMILY HEALTH PRACTICE

CHAPTER 1

Introduction to Family Health in the Context of Health Care

A healthy outside starts from the inside.

—Robert Urich

Learning Objectives

By the end of this chapter, learners will do the following:

- Examine the basic key terminologies used in *family health* care.
- Describe important historical milestones in the field of family science in health care.
- Articulate the relationship between the 4HEALTH contexts: *individual health*, *family health*, *population health*, and public health.
- Describe the settings for *family health* care.
- Discuss the barriers and facilitators for implementing *family health* care in health care settings.

Before you read on, consider the following questions:

- As a current or future health care provider, have you ever wondered …
    - ▹ how important is family to health and health care?
    - ▹ what exactly is "family" in health care?
    - ▹ been trained to study, teach, and work with families?
- What are the challenges of working with families in your practice area?

In recent years, the role of *family health* in health care has become increasing recognized, especially in the wake of successes, failures, and lessons learned from individual-focused behavioral practices in various health care settings such as hospitals, long-term care, rehabilitation care, home care, and ambulatory care (Sharby, 2005). The benefits of supportive family relationships in acute and chronic disease management and overall well-being are increasing becoming central to the maintenance of health and the prevention of diseases across the life cycle. In this chapter, I assemble evidence of *family health* care and family science, citing both historical context and contemporary examples across the globe. The relationship between what I call the "four health contexts"; namely, health, *family health, population health*, and public health are explored to create an introductory understanding of *family health* care in the context of *population health*. The challenges of implementing *family health* care are introduced to increase one's curiosity on what is known and not known in health care and what can be done to close the research and practice gaps in individual- and family-level practice.

Historical Context of Family Health Care and Family Science

It is difficult to discuss about *family health* care without reflecting on the definition of health. The mostly widely cited definition across disciplines is the World Health Organization's (WHO) long-lasting definition that has been reaffirmed: "Health is a state of complete physical, mental and social well-being and not merely the absence of disease or infirmity" (para. 1). The definition reflects the holistic view that encompasses the different medical and nonmedical determinants of health. A diverse health care work force has a vital role to play in helping individuals, families, populations, and communities meet their determinants to achieve the highest attainable standard of health. Interests in *family health* as a determinant of individual- and family-level health outcomes has grown in the last decade, especially in advancing the science of minority and at-risk populations. Scholars have called on efforts to incorporate interventions and models that move beyond individual-level factors to family-level factors (Sharby, 2005). The inclusion of family-level factors in health care incorporates a biopsychosocial model of care beyond the traditional biomedical, disease-focused approach (Engel, 1977). Family-level factors encompass "collective measures of *family health* behaviors and processes or pathways or performing interventions with multiple family members" (National Institute of Health, 2021, para. 4).

There is no single definition of *family health* in the family and health literature (Anderson & Tomlinson, 1992). According to Hanson (2005), *family health* is a "dynamic changing state of well-being, which includes the biological, psychological, spiritual, sociological, and cultural factors of individual members and the completely family systems" (p. 7). In the *family health* model, family nurse scientist, Sharon Denham (2002) describes *family health* "as the ways in which the household, as a whole, engages in daily activities to promote the well-being of its members and is emotionally invested in the maintenance of health over time" (p. 62). The focus of *family health* care is on *family-based relational* and *preventative* acts contributing to health outcomes and health equity (Ellis et al., 2023).

From a historical perspective, *family health* care can be examined from various examples of early pioneering *family health* work in societies to seminal initiatives, reports, and empirical *patient- and family-centered care and family science* since the pre-industrial era. Table 1.1 provides some examples from around the globe. This list is not exhaustive, but it provides a summary of important milestones of recognizing *family health* as an important component of *population health* and public health. Historically, *family health* care took place in home environments, with women playing a significant role in caring for the sick and healthy family members. Pioneers in public health nursing and social work visited homes to empower vulnerable individuals and their families to better their health and social lives. During the pre- and postindustrial eras, families dealing with mental health issues also received help from therapist and counselors. In Indigenous communities, traditional witchcrafts, religious leaders, and tribal leaders also performed the healing practices in the context of family. Likewise, some Indigenous people and communities continue to preserve customary laws that govern consanguineous marriages to either guarantee wealth or prevent genetic risks (Hamamy et al., 2011). During inpatient hospitalization, the patient and family took passive roles, with health care professionals making all decisions.

TABLE 1.1 **Historical Context of *Family Health* Care**

Year	Organization/Initiatives	Goal
Before the 1800s	Pre-industrial era	Family members cared for their sick with women assuming the *family health* care role.
1893	Henry Street Settlement	Public health nurse Lillian Wald founded the Henry Street Settlement in 1893 to provide nursing services to the indigent citizens of New York.
Early, 1920s, 50s, and 60s	Marriage counseling and family therapy movement	1920s: Movement on family centered on schizophrenia, development of professional social work with at-risk populations: mothers and children 1950s: Development of professional social work 1960s: The marriage counseling movement
1978	World Health Organization	1978: "Report on Health And The Family: Studies on The Demography of Family Life Cycles and Their Health Implications" 2002: "Published the Report on The *Family Health* Nurse: Context, Conceptual Framework, and Curriculum To Introduce A New Type of Nurse, The *Family Health* Nurse, Who Will Make A Key Contribution Within A Multidisciplinary Team of Health Care Professionals" 2005: "The WHO Patients for Patients Safety (PFPS)" Programme was established in London. Its vision was to engage, empower, encourage, and facilitate patients and families to build and/or participate in a global network advocating for and partnering with health professionals and policymakers to make health care services safer, more integrated and people centered. 2013: "The Family as Center of Health Development" report. The report highlighted the role of the family in promoting and protecting health in southeast Asia. 2022: "WHO promotes Self Care Interventions for Hand Well-being"

1980s	Medical family therapy	Medical family therapy emerged to address the gap in the healthcare system between biological and psychosocial health (Tyndall et al., 2014).
1987	National Council for Family Relationships (NCFR)	NCFR TaskForce on the Development of the Family Discipline officially endorsed the field of family science.
1988	International Family Nursing Association (IFNA) (informal)	Informal networks of family nurses, hosted by universities in various countries including Canada, Chile, Japan, Thailand, and the United States, took place to discuss family research, interventions, and policy, as well as to share strategies for teaching family nursing to undergraduate and graduate nurses.
1992	Institute of Patient- and Family-Centered Care (IPFCC)	A nonprofit organization, IPFCC was founded as an essential leader to advance the understanding and practice of patient- and family-centered care
1994	United Nations Population Funds	The Cairo International Conference on Population and Development (ICPD) Programme of Action made a call to action to foster men and women as equal partners in *family health*. Men's involvement was emphasized in responsible parenthood and sexual and reproductive behavior, including family planning; prenatal and maternal child health; prevention of sexually transmitted diseases, including HIV; prevention of unwanted and high-risk pregnancies; shared control and contribution to family income, children's education, health, and nutrition; recognition and promotion of the equal value of children of both sexes.
2001a	Institute of Medicine (IOM) report	Published the report *Crossing the quality chasm: A new health system for the 21st century*. National Academies Press that described the importance of redesigning the American health care systems.
2001b	Institute of Medicine (IOM) report	Published the report Health and Behavior: The Interplay of Biological, Behavioral, and Societal that described the importance of family intervention research for chronic disease management among adults
2009	International Family Nursing Association (IFNA)	International Family Nursing Conference was formally established in Reykjavik, Iceland. The organization embraces a compassionate family focus on health, social justice, human dignity, and respect for all.
2011	Olso & Institute of Medicine (IOM)report	The IOM released the Towards an Integrated Science of Research on Families workshop report on the science of research on families. The purpose of the workshop was to examine the broad array methods used to understand the impact of families on children's health and development form a multidisciplinary approach.

2012	Institute of Medicine (IOM) report	The IOM report Living Well With Chronic Illness: A Call for Public Health Action, was released detailing psychosocial-, economic-, and health-related consequences of chronic illness for families and advocated for greater public health action.
2002–2022	National Institute of Health Requests for Applications (RFAs)/Program Announcements (PAs)	2002: The National Institute of Mental Health requested research application that addressed family process issues to address HIV/AIDS and/or its consequences. 2021: Initiative to advance the science of minority health and health disparities by supporting research on ***family health*** and well-being and resilience. 2022: Announcements calling for family-level research. Recently, the NIH branch of minority health initiatives called for advances research on ***family health*** and well-being and resilience in response to adverse social and environmental exposures.
2020	Healthy People 2030	Goals were set for parents and caregivers on how they can help keep the people they care for—and themselves—healthy and safe.
	Examples of seminal articles	Ellis K. R., Young, T, L., & Langford, A. T. (2023). Advancing racial health equity through family-focused interventions for chronic disease management. *Prev Chronic Dis, 20*, 220297. http://dx.doi.org/10.5888/pcd20.220297 Gilliss, C. L., Pan, W., & Davis, L. L. (2019). Family involvement in adult chronic disease care: Reviewing the systematic reviews. *Journal of Family Nursing, 25*(1), 3–27. Ruane-McAteer, E., Amin, A., Hanratty, J., Lynn, F., van Willenswaard, K. C., Reid, E., ... & Lohan, M. (2019). Interventions addressing men, masculinities and gender equality in sexual and reproductive health and rights: An evidence and gap map and systematic review of reviews. *BMJ Global Health, 4*(5), e001634. Ruane-McAteer, E., Gillespie, K., Amin, A., Aventin, Á., Robinson, M., Hanratty, J., ... & Lohan, M. (2020). Gender-transformative programming with men and boys to improve sexual and reproductive health and rights: A systematic review of intervention studies. *BMJ Global Health, 5*(10), e002997.

In today's health care environment, more patients are actively engaged in their health care by learning about their illness, the quality and appropriateness of the interventions, and the providers and life adaptations (Pomey et al., 2015). Despite the lack of a unified framework for length of stay (LoS) predictions for efficient management of cost, satisfaction, and clinical outcomes across health care settings, the need to reduce LoS continues to grow, partly in order to meet patients' preferences and health care needs outside formal settings (Stone et al., 2022). Hence, as equal partners in managing health, patients and families and their communities are expected to take active *self-care* roles that involve the ability to promote, prevent disease, maintain health, and cope with illness and disability and provide care to dependent persons with or without the support of a health worker (WHO, 2023). According to the WHO facts on self-care, an individual spends an average of less than an hour with a health care provider and 8,700 hours a year in self-care. Thus, when a family member assumes the *sick role*, the family system or its subsystem plays a critical role in self-care management within the family environment.

With advancements in medicine, a plethora of literature and initiatives describing the role of the family and health care outcomes has come into fruition. The interprofessional scientific field of family study and family relationships, family science has continued to evolve (NCFR, 2022). The study of families has advanced from studying what family demography or characterization and how to dissolve family challenges to determining why, how, where, what and when family and family relationships can effectively influence individual and *family health* outcomes. Scholars in various disciplines have made efforts to explain the terms that are useful in understanding "the family" in health care.

What Is Family in Family Health Care?

To better understand the meaning of *family health*, it is important that students, practitioners, and scholars articulate what *family* or *families* mean in their practice and/or also research studies. Similar to *family health*, the concept of family or families has had little consensus on a universal definition (Gilby & Pederson, 1982; McCarthy & Edwards, 2010; Weigel, 2008). It is an evolving concept that has been used in diverse health-oriented disciplines and sectors (Rothausen, 1999; Trost, 1990). The term household has been used in family studies, which means all the people who occupy a housing unit including the related family members and all the unrelated people (U.S. Census, 2021). In clinical practice, the most commonly used definition for charting purposes is the U.S. Census definition of family (Medalie & Cole-Kelly, 2002). However, with the evolution of complex family structures and functions and their impact on the illness type, disease stage, and life cycle stage of the patient and family across cultures, a more flexible definition that is inclusive has been warranted (Hanson, 2005, Medalie & Cole-Kelly, 2002). Some of the common definitions include the following:

> *Family* as a group of two people or more (one of whom is the householder) related by birth, marriage, or adoption and residing together; all such people (including related subfamily members) are considered as members of one family. (U.S. Census, 2021)

> *Family* is the central and important social institution for health development in which individuals are born and receive resources for their growth and development. (World Health Organization (WHO) Regional Office for South East Asia, 2013, p. 5)

> *Family* as a basic unit of understanding of how family-based life and interpersonal relationships influence individual and community well-being across the continuum from health and illness, life courses, and diverse care settings. (Berge & Everst, 2011)

> *Family* refers to "two or more individuals who depend on one another for emotional, physical and economical support. The members of the family are self-defined." (Hanson, 2005, p. 7)

> *Family* refers to "people related by marriage, birth, consanguinity or legal adoption, who share a common kitchen and financial resources on a regular basis." (Sharma, 2013, p. 307)

In the *family health* and illness cycle, family attributes can be described through multiple perspectives that include *biological* (Medalie & Cole-Kelly, 2002), *family structures*, and *family functions* (Medalie & Cole-Kelly, 2002; Weigel, 2008). The biological perspective emphasis is on the biomedical model of using the *family health history* tool for assessing health risks to determine genetic and familial disposition to illness (Wildin et al., 2021). Unfortunately, this may be difficult to conceptualize among nonblood-related family members. However, with the evolution of the field of "*precision medicine*," also known as "personalized medicine," the considerations of environmental, socioeconomic, and psychological determinants beyond pathological determinants is emphasized (Delpierre, & Lefèvre, 2023). Thus, familial-related health and illness factors can be examined beyond heredity to include the intersectionality of genes and family-related contextual variables.

The structural perspective captures increasingly and evolving diverse family forms/types and how they affect family experiences with health and health events (Sharma, 2013). Attributes for family structures include family living arrangement and marital transitions within residential and nonresidential relationships (IOM, 2011). For example, when there are infectious disease considerations, health care providers define the family structure by examining the members of the household (i.e., all members residing in the home or visiting the home; Medalie & Cole-Kelly, 2002). Some of the common family structures in the literature include the traditional nuclear family with two married parents with biological children; extended families and new arrangements that are single-parent or no-parent families; stepfamilies; blended families; cohabiting families; and adopted families. It is important to be familiar with diverse family structures and family life and how they are shaped by the history of a country and culture so that one can understand families' unique richness and complexities (Leeder, 2020; Sharma, 2013). Accounting for family attributes such as family dynamics, power structures, and the heterogeneous complex nature of families is essential for programming interventions aimed at the individual and family level (WHO, 2023). For example, family studies have demonstrated gender power dynamics (norms, roles, and relations) results in inequities and inequalities in health outcomes (Manandhar et al., 2018; Paulino et al., 2019). Although the demographic changes in family structure are important, attributes that delineate family function and processes such as family resilience, coping, caring and support are essential in clinical and prevention science (Olson et al., 2011, Weigel, 2008).

Within the functional perspective, family is considered a social institution that serves several functions, including reproduction, socializing the new generation, providing affection by promoting identity and belonging to members, providing economic support, and meeting health care needs (Leeder, 2020; Marilyn et al., 2019). The functional family definition is important in preventing and managing chronic illnesses (Medalie & Cole-Kelly, 2002). Family functioning is described as family self-efficacy in maintaining cohesive relationships, adjusting to new family routines, and communicating effectively with each other (Zhang, 2018). Constructs such as normalization have been central to the function of families during the management of chronic conditions (Knafl & Deatrick, 1986). Weiss-Laxer et al. (2020) summarized the unique family roles associated with the health care functions that include (a) *continuity*: families provide continuity through reproduction; (b) *context*: families provide a context for the development to health and health behaviors that promote health, reduce risks, and reduce vulnerability to disease onset and relapse; (c) *care and caring*: families provide a context for care and caring during health, illness appraisal, acute response to serious illnesses, adaptation to illness, and aiding in recovery and adaptation to end of life; and (d) *connections*: families provide connections to community resources and opportunities both informal and formal.

Likewise, family functions and processes can be examined from a systems perspective. In the family systems model, family members are viewed within the contexts of the family subsystems and the "whole" family system (Christie-Seely, 1981). Within this model, over time, individual positive or negative health factors influence positive or negative *family health* factors, and vice versa. For example, during a stressful health event like an illness, the family endures disruptions in its patterns and routines and is forced to adapt different coping processes to maintain functioning (Walsh & McGoldrick, 2023). For some families, the adaptation and transitions maybe difficult, while for others the process can be smooth depending on family perceptions, available resources, and the extent of the demands (Bell, 2009; Newby, 1996). Providers using a family systems approach in chronic disease management can make the inevitable family demands (stressor and strains) more manageable through a comprehensive psychosocial assessment of the changing family systems interactions over the course of the illness and the life cycle (Rolland, 2005). Friedemann (1989) articulated a system-based approach for practicing family nurses that included three levels of care: (a) the *individual level*, which addresses the family as the context of the individual care; (b) the *interpersonal level*, which addresses family subsystems as the context of care; and (c) the *family system level*, which addresses the "whole" system, including the structural and functional system components interacting with the environment as the context of nursing care. Family systems-level practice requires a holistic understanding of the complex family relationships among family system components (Friedemann, 1989). Individual-level practice is most common among health care providers and in most health care settings. Hence, as we strive to create a culture of family wellness and *population health*, it is imperative that a family system thinking approach is fostered as the benefits of supportive family relationships are increasingly becoming central to the maintenance of health and the prevention of diseases across the life cycle and diverse communities (Ellis et al., 2023; Sharby, 2005).

Relationships Between Individual Health, Family Health, Population Health, and Public Health

Family health care is best understood within the four health contexts which is indetified a correct work identified as "4HEALTHS" in this textbook. The four contexts represent *individual health*, *family health*, *population health*, and public health (see Figure 1.1). *Individual health* is described in the WHO's definition of health described earlier in the chapter. *Family health* on the other hand is defined earlier in the chapter as a dynamic state of well-being of the individual members and the family system that is influenced by the "families' interactive, developmental, functional, psychosocial, and health processes" (Denham, 2002, p. 62). *Population health* has been defined as "a cohesive, integrated and comprehensive approach to health that considers the distribution of health outcomes within a population, the *health determinants* that influence distribution of care and the policies and interventions that impact and impacted by the determinants" (Kindig & Stoddart, 2003, p. 380). Within varied care settings and disciplines, *population health* has been defined differently depending on the context and perspective. For example, family physicians and nurses define *population health* as "the health outcomes of a group of individuals (patient panel), including the distribution of such outcomes within the group" (Kindig & Stoddart, 2003, p. 380). Nurses have described *population health* as an approach that "spans the health care delivery continuum from public health prevention to disease management of populations, and describes collaborative activities with both traditional and non-traditional partnerships with affected communities, public health, industry academic, health care, local governments entities, and others for the improvement of equitable *population health* outcomes" (American Association of Colleges of Nursing [AACN], 2021, p. 33). The American Psychology Association (APA, 2022) describes *population health* as a "multi-tiered approach" that includes "(a) universal provision of preventative tools and health promotion for all people, families, and communities; (b) monitoring, anticipatory guidance, and early intervention for those with risk factors for physical, mental health, and substance-related conditions; and (c) psychosocial and mental health/substance use care for those experiencing illness and/or escalating physical health and mental distress" (p. 1).

The term *public health*, on the other hand, is defined as the science of protecting and promoting the *health* of all people and their communities using evidence-based science to give everyone a safe place to live work and play (American Public Health Association [APHA], 2023). Public health aims to prevent people from getting sick or injured in the first place. Additionally, a *population-based approach* is essential in public health as it promotes efforts that not only span in caring for the illbut also caring for healthy populations (Shahzad et al., 2019). Some of the important attributes of a population-based approach include a focus on health and wellness rather than illness, a focus on population orientation rather than individual orientation, community outreach to understand needs and solutions, addressing health disparities and social determinants of health, and inter-sectoral action and partnerships (Cohen et al., 2014).

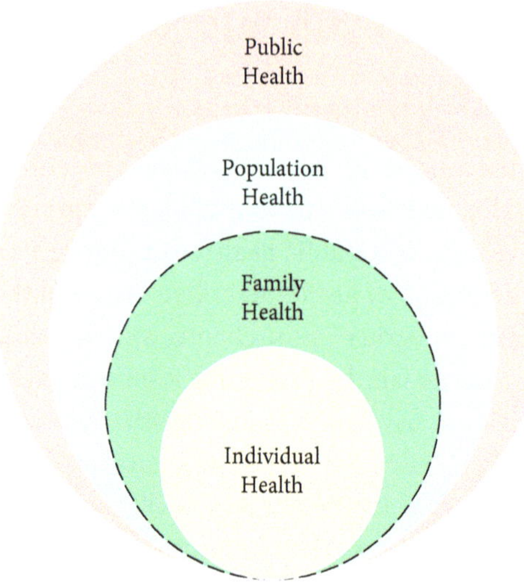

FIGURE 1.1 Interrelationship between *individual health*, *family health*, *population health*, and public health.

Hereafter, population-focused *family health* care is best understood within the larger social contexts of the community and systems within which individual and families live. Public health nurses identify individuals and families they work with as belonging to either a *population at risk*, a population with a common identified risk factor or risk exposure that poses a threat to health, or a *population of interest*, a population that is essentially healthy but could improve factors that promote or protect health (Schaffer et al., 2011). Within the population-based approach, health care providers are expected to manage care for individuals and families not in isolation but as part of a population that is defined by a health care system(s) or a community where they live, eat, work, learn, and worship. The ultimate family and *population health* goals are usually to protect and promote the health of the public at large. An example of how health care providers can intersect with the "four healths" context is health care providers providing population-based practice with patients and families (individual and *family health* focus) dealing with communicable diseases such as tuberculosis and HIV/AIDS and noncommunicable diseases (NCDs) and comorbidities such as cardiovascular disease, diabetes mellitus, and chronic lung cancer or osteoarthritis (*population health* focus) to improve health outcomes such as length of life (premature deaths from the diseases) and quality of life (self-reported psychical and mental wellness; public health focus).

According to the Minnesota Department of Health (2019), population-based public health interventions can be practiced at three levels: First is the *individual/family focus*, which focuses on changing knowledge, attitudes, beliefs, practices, and behaviors of individuals and families. This practice level is directed at individuals, alone or as part of a family, class, or group. The *community-focused* level focuses on changing community norms, attitudes, awareness, practices, and behaviors. This practice level is directed at entire populations within the community or occasionally toward target groups within those populations. The *systems-focus* level focuses on changing organizations, policies, laws, and power structures. The focus is not directly on individuals and communities but on the systems that impact health. Changing systems often impact *population health* in a more effective and lasting way than requiring change from every individual in a community.

Family-focused population-based practice is usually directed at individuals alone or a family system or family subsystem or as part of a group of families. Within the family-focused lens, it is important for *family health* practitioners and scholars to consider positive and negative determinants of *family health* to promote *family health* and address the social determinants of health and heath inequities. Equity efforts should consider efforts that are tailored inside, outside, and alongside families (Ellis et al., 2023). Efforts that are inside families target family heath history with individuals while outside efforts target the broader sociocultural and contextual factors. Alongside family efforts target community-engaged and participatory approaches. With these different approaches, it is easy to grasp the concepts of *family systems thinking* and *holism* when working from a *family health* perspective. For example, system thinking health care providers assess how family characteristics influence the health outcomes of young people by examining the multiple characteristics of the systems (holistic) within the family units and how they are dynamic and interconnected rather than examining the individual characteristic alone (Michaelson et al., 2016). This new way of thinking calls on providers to grasp the "four healths" context and population-based public health interventions at the individual/family level from a *biopsychosocial* or *ecological* health perspective (Maurice & Houeto, 2021) as opposed to the traditional biomedical perspective alone. Swannack and Appleby (2020) and Taukeni (2019) delineated the differences between the ecological model and biomedical model by focusing on different areas of disease management as summarized in Table 1.2. In other words, the "4HEALTHS" address the disease management and prevention processes and the *patient-as-a-person* process through an understanding of the *mind/body/spirit* connection (Karf, 2009).

TABLE 1.2 **Conceptualizing Disease Management Using the Ecological Model versus the Biomedical Model**

Areas of Disease Management	Biomedical Model	Ecological Model
Views on What Causes Illness	Only takes account of biological factors. All physical factors—pathogens, injury, physiological change. Example: Biological factors (chemical imbalances, bacteria, viruses and genetic predisposition)	Takes account of multiple factors—physical, social, and psychological. Example: Biological (virus), psychological (beliefs, behavior), and social (unemployment
Patient Responsibility	Individuals are regarded as victims of some external force causing internal changes. Because illness is seen as a result of biological changes beyond their control, individuals are not seen as responsible for their illness The responsibility for treatment rests with the medical profession.	Individuals should be held responsible for their health and illness because lifestyle has an influence. The focus is the whole person to be treated not just their physical illness; the patient is therefore responsible for their treatment (e.g., taking the medication or changing their behavior)
Treatment Style	Bodily interventions only. Through vaccination, surgery, chemotherapy, pharmacotherapy, and radiotherapy, all of which aim to change the physical state of the body.	Whole person themes, mind and body

Role of Psychology (Mind–Body Connection)	No relationship with physical illness. The mind and body function independently. In other words, the mind and body are separate entities. Illness may have psychological consequences, but not psychological causes (e.g., cancer may cause unhappiness, but mood is not seen as related to either the onset or progression of the cancer).	Causal influence and consequence of physical illness. The focus is on an interaction between the mind and the body. The mind and body interact. Psychological factors not only as possible consequences of illness but as contributing to it at all stages along the continuum, from healthy to being ill.

Sources: Adapted from Swannack and Appleby (2020) and Taukeni (2019)

The biopsychosocial approach has been used in nursing practice and is known as the "cure, care, and core" approach, which was originally developed by nurse theorist Lydia Halls in the 1960s (Hall, 1968). The *core* was considered as the patient receiving the *care*; the *cure* focused on the biomedical aspects, including medication administration; and reconciliation and the care can be referred to performing the noble tasks of nurturing the patient as an individual. In medical care, *care* has also been acknowledged within the establishment of a patient–doctor healing relationship. According to Suchman and Matthews (1988), a healing connection is considered a "fundamental clinical task which is coequal with diagnosis and biotechnical treatment, whether the relationship is to last 5 minutes or 50 years" (p 129). Patients in every culture need caring/healing relationships, and healers who provide this relationship are usually successful (Suchman & Mathew, 1988).

Collectively, these concepts referred to what we now call *patient-centered care*, also known as *patient- and family-centered care* (PFCC). Patient centeredness is now a global health issue and one of the important six attributes of health care quality, including safety, timeliness, effectiveness, efficiency, and equity (IOM, 2001). In the family studies and health care literature, patient- and family-centered care has been acknowledged in improving quality health care across age groups, conditions, and health care settings (Park et al., 2018). However, there continues to be debates as to what exactly constitutes a "patient" as to whether it focuses only on a patient (a person assuming the sick role) or is more inclusive of others such as person, people, or family (WHO, 2007). Some scholars have argued that the use of the term *patient-centered care* is narrow as it only focuses on the patient and does not address holistic health care and broader health challenges (WHO, 2007). In the literature, there are variety of terms and meanings for person-centered care, including *patient-centered care*, *client-centered care*, and *relationship-centered care* (HealthCare Improvement Scotland, 2021). The concept of person has been fundamental to the nursing discipline (Fawcett, 1978). Broadly, the discipline refers to persons beyond patients to include other recipients of nursing care, such as individuals, groups, families, and communities. It is important for family scholars and practitioners to understand the differences in terminology and how they are conceptualized by in diverse practice settings, populations, and disciplines.

Established in 1992, the Institute for Patient- and Family-Centered Care (IPFCC, 2022) has been the leader in advancing the practice of patient- and family-centered care in the

United States and worldwide. According to the IPFCC, patient- and family-centered care is defined as "an approach to the planning, delivery, and evaluation of health care that is grounded in mutually beneficial partnerships among health care professionals, patients, and families" (para. 1). According to the IPFCC, the following four core concepts of PFCC: (a) respecting and dignifying patients' and families' perspectives and preferences; (b) valuing and sharing information with patients and families; (c) encouraging and supporting patients and families participations in care and decision-making and; (d) collaboration among patients and families, health care practitioners, and health care leaders in in policy and program development, implementation, and evaluation and in research, facility design, and professional education. The IPFCC definition of *patient-centered care* shares common principles with other definitions such as that of the IOM (2001), "patient-centered care is providing care that is respectful of and responsive to individual patient preferences, needs, and cultural values and ensuring that patient values guide all clinical decisions" (p. 6), and that of the Health Foundation (2019), "health and social care professionals work collaboratively with people who use services" (p. 4). Likewise, when examining health and health care beyond traditional health systems (i.e., acute care), it is important to contextualize PFCC within the concepts of primary health care (PHC) and primary care (PC). These concepts play an increasingly important role in today's health care delivery systems, especially when it comes to caring for patients and families dealing with multimorbidities (Schuttner et al., 2022). By definition,

Primary health care (PHC) is a broader whole-of-society approach with three components: (a) primary care and essential public health functions as a core of *integrated health services*, (b) multisectoral policy and action, and (c) empowered people and communities. This strategy also ensures that health care is delivered in a way that is *people centered* by focusing on people's needs and respects their preferences. In addition, according to the American Psychosocial Association the integrated health care services are characterized by a high degree of collaboration and communication among a diverse groups of health professionals (e.g., physicians, nurses, psychologists, and other health professionals) to meet the needs of patient(s). This approach is unique in that it incorporates the sharing of information among team members related to patient care and the establishment of a comprehensive treatment plan to address the biological, psychological, and social needs of the patient. This approach also puts emphasis on addressing the whole person.

Primary care is a model of care that supports first-contact, accessible, continuous, comprehensive, and coordinated person-focused care. The goal of primary care is to optimize *population health* and reduce disparities by ensuring equal access to services. The core functions of primary care include (a) creating a strategic entry point for and improved access to health services (*first-contact accessibility*); (b) promoting the development of long-term personal relationships between a person and a health professional or a team of providers (*continuity*); (c) ensuring that a diverse range of promotive, protective, preventive, curative, rehabilitative, and palliative services are provided (*comprehensiveness*); organizing services and care across levels of the health system and over time (*coordination*); and (d) ensuring that people have the education and support needed to make decisions and participate in their own care (*people-centered care*).

The term patient-centered medical home (PCMH), although poorly understood inmedical literature, is also another important concept in primary (O'Dell, 2016). The Agency for Healthcare Research and Quality (AHRQ, 2022 defines PCMH as follows:

> Patient-Centered Medical Home is a promising model for organizing primary care in America by 1) providing interprofessional *comprehensive care* patient's physical and mental health care needs, including prevention and wellness, acute care, and chronic care; 2) providing *patient-centered care* that is relation-based with a focus on the whole person; 3) providing *coordinated care* across all elements of the broader health care systems; and 4) providing *quality* and *safety* by engaging in activities such as using evidence-based medicine and clinical decision-support tools.

Efforts to fund and support evidence-based patient- and family-centered care in the healthcare system have also been underway. For instance, the U.S. Patient-Centered Outcomes Research Institute (PCORI) is one of the pioneer funders and supportive organization for PFCC in the United States and abroad. The focus of the PCORI is to generate evidence that empowers patients and families to make better-informed health and health care decisions through patient-centered comparative clinical effectiveness research. Patient- and family-centered evidence from PCORI-designed interventions have been translated in acute care and beyond. One of the goals of PCORI is to put the evidence generated to work so that the findings can reach and benefit patients and families. This process includes sharing PFCC research findings (*dissemination*) and facilitating an uptake of findings in practice settings (*implementation*) to improve quality of care, health outcomes, and health care cost.

Thus, as we reimagine 21st-century medicine and health care in improving *population health* outcomes and health equity across the life span and diverse groups, it is vital that we are intentional on preparing a generation of family systems thinking health care providers with knowledge in the evidence-based practice process, as well as in the *dissemination and implementation of the evidence. Family health* practitioners should have a better understanding of how to develop, adapt and tailor population-focused *family interventions* at the primary, secondary, and tertiary *levels of prevention* to varied contexts and settings.

In disease prevention, providers should be able to identify primary prevention population-based focused family interventions that focus on actions aimed at avoiding the manifestation of a disease/condition, secondary prevention interventions that deal with early detection and early treatment of diseases/conditions, and tertiary prevention interventions that focus on dealing with limiting further negative effects from a problem and aim to keep existing problems from getting worse. In health promotion, providers should know which interventions focus on empowering individuals and families to increase self-control over their health and determinants. Skills in adapting multidisciplinary patient and family centered care health care teams that are invested in the community and community health by demonstrating strong bonds with the citizens are vital for family-level self-care initiatives. In addition, adapting health care systems that embrace multisectoral actions to increase access to community resources through referral agreements and utilizing a health-in-all policy—an approach that addresses "the determinants of health across many sectors by developing the needed leadership and governance and sustained partnerships for actions between sectors," is essential for better health outcomes (WHO, 2018, p. 2).

Barriers and Facilitators to Implementation of Family-Focused Health Care

It is important to know that efforts to improve health care today are targeted toward developing and delivering best practice interventions that can be translated to routine health care practice (Westerlund et al., 2019). With the growing number of empirical family studies, we are generating knowledge that will facilitate the uptake of family-focused interventions to improve *family health* outcomes and ultimately population outcomes. Failing to appropriately implement effective family-based interventions, guidelines, or policies severely limits the potential for patients and communities to benefit from advances in health promotion, medicine, and public health. With limited resources in health care systems, as uncovered during the COVID-19 pandemic, it is paramount that we utilize evidence-based strategies to ensure that research investments maximize health care value and improve public health. To facilitate the uptake of patient- and family-centered evidence, all family scholars and health care practitioners must have at least basic knowledge of *implementation science*, "the scientific study of methods to promote the systematic uptake of research findings and other evidence-based practices into routine practice, and, hence, to improve the quality and effectiveness of health services" (Eccles & Mittman, 2006, p 1). Curra (2020) developed a simple tool that is useful to new learners in the field of implementation in need of a brief and plain nonscientific language to key concepts in implementation science. The simple tool consists of the following elements:

- The intervention/practice/innovation (the thing)
- Effectiveness research looks at whether the thing works
- Implementation research looks at how best to help people/places do the thing
- Implementation strategies are the things we do to try to help people/places do the thing
- Main implementation outcomes are how much and how well they do the thing

The implementation field incorporates a scope broader than traditional clinical research, focusing not only on the patient level, but also on the provider, organization, and policy levels of health care (Bauer et al., 2015). Thus, understanding barriers and facilitators contributing to the implementation of family-focused interventions at multiple levels in a variety of *health care settings* is essential. Some of the recognized and acknowledged challenges of implementing PFCC models include the lack of clear definitions on who the "patient" or "family" is (e.g., patient/client/person/family/people/consumer; Costa et al., 2019); lack of comprehensive PFCC models across age groups, conditions and care settings, and few evaluation studies on the benefits of PFCC patient, caregiver, and health system outcomes (Kokorelias et al., 2019). Table 1.3 summarizes these barriers to implementation of *family health* care at different levels of influence.

TABLE 1.3 Barriers to Implementation of *Family Health* Care

Patient and Family Level	Provider Level	Organizational Level	Policy Level
Families seen as causing problems rather than as a resource Families often blame one person Logistically hard to convene family members Patients do not have relatives Patient confidentiality Patient does not want to involve family Difficult family dynamics Frustration toward services Foreign culture or language Family members' unwillingness to negotiate and participate actively in the care Intimidating behaviors toward providers Preferring to work with one provider of the other Fear of health outcomes	Clinicians focus on one disease or person Curricula in medicine and psychology focus on one person Logistically hard to convene family members Emotionally daunting to meet with more than one person Lack of role modeling Clinicians do not see system thinking as problem solving Lack of competencies and experience Attitudes inhibiting family involvement, view family members as distracters Insufficient interaction with families, competing priorities Lack of emotional support from providers Lack of explanation of medical procedures, illnesses, and treatment outcomes to patients and family Difficult communication between providers and family members. For example, using medical jargon, giving too much information to family members Discouraged to discuss issues with families Communication barriers between providers	Charts are person focused, not family focused Billing systems and codes do not recognize family problems or treatment Individual focus takes less time in day-to-day care Lack of regular measurement and feedback reporting evaluating routine Lack of training structures Lack of shared knowledge, perceptions, and practice (e.g., professional culture) Lack of strong, senior leadership commitment Lack of communication of strategic vision Lack of resources to implement new practice Lack of resources to perform family involvement Competing with other tasks Inadequate material resources, such as good beds and linens, human resources, including nurses and doctors Inadequate use of spiritual advisors Inadequate cultural and ethnic diversity Lack of private spaces for family, technology Traditional practices and work environment built on biomedical model Implementation gaps in *family health* history Lack of employee satisfaction Lack of incentives and accountability	Lack of guidelines and policies Policy restricting family presence and visits

Sources: Hansson et al. (2022); Kiwanuka et al. (2019); HealthCare Improvement Scotland (2021); Phiri et al. (2020)

Conclusion

In summary, this chapter presents important introductory information about family-focused efforts in health care. In the next chapters, more information about family systems across the life span and the social determinants of *family health* are introduced. The chapters will provide information that will facilitate a better understanding of the challenges existing and emerging in health care that may benefit from family-based strategies to improve individual and population outcomes across health care systems and communities.

Suggested Websites

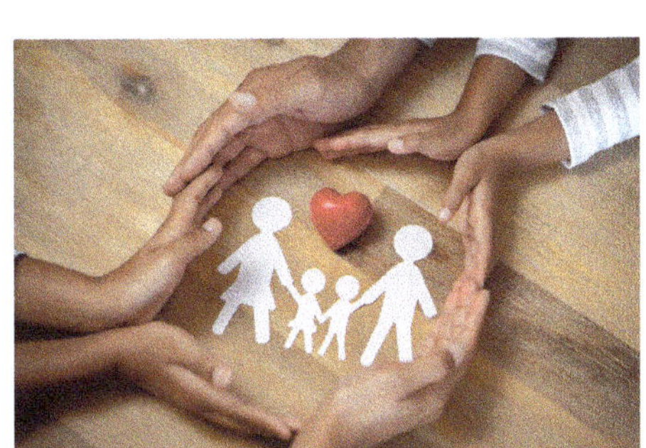

IMG 1.1

American Public Health Association: https://www.apha.org/
American Psychology Association: https://www.apa.org/
Institute of Patient-and Family-Centered Care: https://www.ipfcc.org/
International Family Nursing Association: https://internationalfamilynursing.org/
National Academy of Medicines: https://nam.edu/
National Council for Family Relationships: https://www.ncfr.org/
Patient-Centered Outcomes Research Institute: https://www.pcori.org/
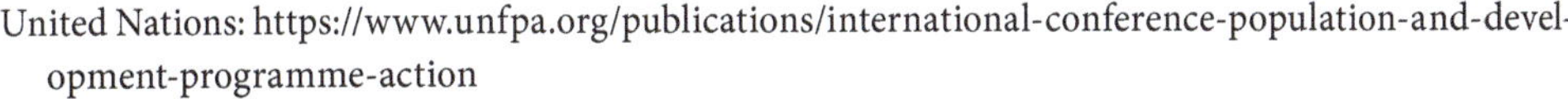
United Nations: https://www.unfpa.org/publications/international-conference-population-and-development-programme-action
World Health Organization: https://www.who.int/

Reflection Question

Think about your general family life and health care experiences and what you have learned in this chapter and reflect on these questions:

1. Why do you think *family health* is important in health care?
2. Why do you think the shift from the traditional biomedical model toward the biopsychosocial model is necessary in health care?
3. Why should *family health* care be holistic care?

References

Agency for Healthcare Research and Quality. (2022). *Defining the PCMH.* https://www.ahrq.gov/ncepcr/research/care-coordination/pcmh/define.html

Ahmad, N., Ellins, J., Krelle, H., & Lawrie, M. (2019, Nov) *Person-centered care: from ideas to action.* https://www.health.org.uk/sites/default/files/PersonCentredCareFromIdeasToAction.pdf

American Association of College of Nursing. (2021). *The Essentials: Core competenices for professional nursing education.* https://www.aacnnursing.org/Portals/0/PDFs/Publications/Essentials-2021.pdf

American Association of Colleges of Nursing (2023). *Person-centered Care.* https://www.aacnnursing.org/5b-tool-kit/themes/person-centered-care

American Psychology Association. (2022, February). *Psychology's role in advancing population health.* https://www.apa.org/about/policy/population-health-statement.pdf

American Public Health Association. (2023). *What is public health?* https://www.apha.org/What-is-public-health

Anderson, K. H., & Tomlinson, P. S. (1992). The *family health* system as an emerging paradigmatic view for nursing. *Image: The Journal of Nursing Scholarship, 24*(1), 57–63.

Bauer, M. S., Damschroder, L., Hagedorn, H., Smith, J., & Kilbourne, A. M. (2015). An introduction to implementation science for the non-specialist. *BMC psychology, 3*(1), 1–12.

Berge, J. M., & Everts, J. C. (2011). Family-based interventions targeting childhood obesity: A Meta-Analysis. *Childhood obesity, 7*(2), 110–121. https://doi.org/10.1089/chi.2011.07.02.1004.berge

Bell, J. M. (2009). Family systems nursing: Re-examined. *Journal of family nursing, 15*(2), 123–129.

Cohen, D., Huynh, T., Sebold, A., Harvey, J., Neudorf, C., & Brown, A. (2014). The *population health* approach: A qualitative study of conceptual and operational definitions for leaders in Canadian healthcare. *SAGE open medicine, 2.*

Christie-Seely, J. (1981). Teaching the family system concept in family medicine. *The Journal of Family Practice* , *13*(3), 391–401.

Curran, G. M. (2020). Implementation science made too simple: a teaching tool. *Implementation Science Communications, 1*(1), 1–3.

Delpierre, C., & Lefèvre, T. (2023). Precision and personalized medicine: What their current definition says and silences about the model of health they promote. Implication for the development of personalized health. *Frontiers in sociology, 8.* https://doi.org/10.3389/fsoc.2023.1112159

Denham, S. A. (2002). Family routines: A structural perspective for viewing *family health. Advances in Nursing Science, 24*(4), 60–74.

Eccles, M. P., & Mittman, B. S. (2006). Welcome to implementation science. *Implementation Science, 1*(1). https://doi.org/10.1186/1748-5908-1-1

Ellis, K. R., Young, T. L., & Langford, A. T. (2023). Advancing racial health equity through family-focused interventions for chronic disease management. *Prev Chronic Dis, 20.* http://doi.org/10.5888/pcd20.220297

Engel, G. L. (1977). The need for a new medical model: a challenge for biomedicine. *Science, 196*(4286), 129–136.

Fawcett, J. (1978). The "what" of theory development. *NLN Publications, 15*(1708), 17–33

Gilby, R. L., & Pederson, D. R. (1982). The development of the child's concept of the family. *Canadian Journal of Behavioural Science 14*(2), 110–121.

Friedemann, M. L. (1989). The concept of family nursing. *Journal of Advanced Nursing, 14*(3), 211–216.

Gilliss, C. L., Pan, W., & Davis, L. L. (2019). Family involvement in adult chronic disease care: Reviewing the systematic reviews. *Journal of Family Nursing, 25*(1), 3–27.

. Hall, L. E. (1968). Another view of nursing care and quality. *Maryland Nursing News, 36*(1), 2–12.

Hamamy, H., Antonarakis, S. E., Cavalli-Sforza, L. L., Temtamy, S., Romeo, G., Kate, L. P. T., Bennet, R, L., Shaw, A., Megarbane, A., Duijn, C.v., Bathija, H., Fokstuen, S. Zlotogora, J., Dermitzakis, E., Bottani, A. Dahoun, S., Morris. M.A., Arsenault, S., Aglan, M.S., ... & Bittles, A. H. (2011). Consanguineous marriages, pearls and perils: Geneva international consanguinity workshop report. *Genetics in Medicine, 13*(9), 841–847.

Hanson, S. M. H. (2005). *Family health* care nursing: an introduction. In S. M. H. Hanson, V. Gedaly-Diff & J. W. Kaakinen (Eds.), *Family health care nursing: Theory, practice and research,* (3rd Ed., pp. 3–37). F.A. Davis

Hansson, K. M., Romøren, M., Pedersen, R., Weimand, B., Hestmark, L., Norheim, I., ... & Heiervang, K. S. (2022). Barriers and facilitators when implementing family involvement for persons with psychotic disorders in community mental health centres–a nested qualitative study. *BMC Health Services Research, 22*(1), 1–16.

HealthCare Improvement Scotland. (2021) How is person-centered care understood and implemented in practice? A literature review. https://ihub.scot/media/8367/20200621-person-centred-care-review-v20.pdf

The Health Foundation. (2014). *Person-centred care made simple: What everyone should know about person-centred care. https://www.health.org.uk/sites/default/files/PersonCentredCareMadeSimple.pdf*

Institute for Patient- and Family-Centered Care. (2023). *Patient- and family-centered care.* https://www.ipfcc.org/about/pfcc.html

Institute of Medicine. (2001a). *Crossing the quality chasm: A new health system for the 21st century.* National Academies Press. https://nap.nationalacademies.org/read/10027/chapter/1

Institute of Medicine. (2001b). *Health and behavior: the interplay of biological, behavioral, and societal influences.* National Academies Press. https://nap.nationalacademies.org/read/9838/chapter/1

Institute of Medicine. (2012). *Living well with chronic illness: A call for public health action.* National Academies Press. https://nap.nationalacademies.org/read/13272/chapter/1

Karff, S. E. (2009). Recognizing the mind/body/spirit connection in medical care. *Virtual Mentor, 11*(10), 788–792. https://doi.org/10.1001/virtualmenor.2009.11.10.msocl-0910

Knafl, K. A., & Deatrick, J. A. (1986). How families manage chronic conditions: An analysis of the concept of normalization. *Research in Nursing & Health, 9*(3), 215–222.

Kindig, D., & Stoddart, G. (2003). What is *population health? American journal of public health, 93*(3), 380–383.

Kiwanuka, F., Shayan, S. J., & Tolulope, A. A. (2019). Barriers to patient and family-centred care in adult intensive care units: A systematic review. *Nursing open, 6*(3), 676–684.

Kokorelias, K. M., Gignac, M. A., Naglie, G., & Cameron, J. I. (2019). Towards a universal model of family centered care: a scoping review. *BMC health services research, 19,* 1–11.

Leeder, E. J. (2004). *The family in global perspective: A gendered journey.* SAGE.

Manandhar, M., Hawkes, S., Buse, K., Nosrati, E., & Magar, V. (2018). Gender, health and the 2030 agenda for sustainable development. *Bulletin of the World Health Organization,* 96(9), 644–653.

Maurice, A. T., & Houeto, D. S. (2021). Why public health interventions need a multidisciplinary approach to understand and address behaviors effectively? *Prev Med Epid Public Heal, 4*(2), 1–5. https://doi.org/10.31038/PEP.2021241

Marilyn, R., Friedman, B., & Vicky, R. J. (2019). *Family nursing: Research, theory, and practice.* Pearson.

McCarthy, J. R., & Edwards, R. (2010). *Key concepts in family studies.* SAGE.

Medalie, J. H., & Cole-Kelly, K. (2002). The clinical importance of defining family. *American Family Physician, 65*(7), 1277–1280.

Michaelson, V., Pickett, W., King, N., & Davison, C. (2016). Testing the theory of holism: A study of family systems and adolescent health. *Preventive medicine reports, 4,* 313–319.

Minnesota Department of Health. (2019). *Public health interventions: Applications for public health nursing practice* (2nd ed.). https://www.health.state.mn.us/communities/practice/research/phncouncil/docs/PHInterventions.pdf

National Council on Family Relations. (2022). *What Is Family Science?* https://www.ncfr.org/about/what-family-science#What

National Institutes of Health. (2021). Risk and protective factors of *family health* and family level interventions. https://grants.nih.gov/grants/guide/pa-files/PAR-21-358.html

Newby, N.M (1996). Chronic illness and the family life-cycle. *Journal of advanced nursing, 23*(4), 786–791

O'Dell M. L. (2016). What is a patient-centered medical home?. *Missouri medicine, 113*(4), 301–304.

Olson, S., Institute of Medicine, & National Research Council Committee on the Science of Research on Families. (Eds.). (2011). *Toward an Integrated Science of Research on Families: Workshop Report.* National Academies Press.

Paulino, N. A., Vázquez, M. S., & Bolúmar, F. (2019). Indigenous language and inequitable maternal health care, Guatemala, Mexico, Peru and the Plurinational State of Bolivia. *Bulletin of the World Health Organization, 97*(1), 59–67.

Phiri, P. G., Chan, C. W., & Wong, C. L. (2020). The scope of family-centred care practices, and the facilitators and barriers to implementation of family-centred care for hospitalised children and their families in developing countries: an integrative review. *Journal of Pediatric Nursing, 55*, 10–28.

Pomey, M. P., Ghadiri, D. P., Karazivan, P., Fernandez, N., & Clavel, N. (2015). Patients as partners: a qualitative study of patients' engagement in their health care. *PloS One, 10*(4), e0122499. https://doi.org/10.1371/journal.pone.0122499

Rolland, J. S. (2005). Cancer and the family: An integrative model. *Cancer: Interdisciplinary International Journal of the American Cancer Society, 104*(S11), 2584–2595.

Rothausen, T. J. (1999). "Family" in organizational research: A review and comparison of definitions and measures. *Journal of Organizational Behavior, 20*(6), 817–836.

Schoon, P. M., Porta, C. M., & Schaffer, M. A. (2018). *Population-based public health clinical manual: The Henry Street model for nurses.* Sigma.

Schuttner, L., Hockett Sherlock, S., Simons, C. E., Johnson, N. L., Wirtz, E., Ralston, J. D., ... & Sayre, G. (2022). My goals are not their goals: Barriers and facilitators to delivery of patient-centered care for patients with multimorbidity. *Journal of General Internal Medicine, 37*(16), 4189–4196.

Shahzad, M., Upshur, R., Donnelly, P., Bharmal, A., Wei, X., Feng, P., & Brown, A. D. (2019). A population-based approach to integrated healthcare delivery: A scoping review of clinical care and public health collaboration. *BMC Public Health, 19*(1), 1–15.

Sharby, N. (2005). *Health and Behavior, the Interplay of Biological, Behavioral and Societal Influences.* Committee on Health and Behavior, Institute of Medicine Research Practice and Policy Board on Neuroscience and Behavioral Health. National Academies Press.

Sharma R. (2013). The family and family structure classification redefined for the current times. *Journal of family medicine and primary care, 2*(4), 306–310. https://doi.org/10.4103/2249-4863.123774

Stone, K., Zwiggelaar, R., Jones, P., & Mac, P. N (2022). A systematic review of the prediction of hospital length of stay: Towards a unified framework. *PLOS Digit Health, 1*(4), e0000017. https://doi.org/10.1371/journal.pdig.0000017

Suchman, A. L., & Matthews, D. A. (1988). What makes the patient-doctor relationship therapeutic? Exploring the connexional dimension of medical care. *Annals of internal medicine, 108*(1), 125–130.

Swannack, M., & Appleb,y B. (2020). *Models of Health.* https://simplemed.co.uk/subjects/population-and-social-science/models-of-health

Taukeni, S. G. (Ed.). (2019). Psychology of health: Biopsychosocial approach. IntechOpen.

Trost, J. (1990). Do we mean the same by the concept of family. *Communication research, 17*(4), 431–443.

U.S Census. (2021, December). *Subject Definitions: Family.* https://www.census.gov/programs-surveys/cps/technical-documentation/subject-definitions.html#family

Walsh, F., & McGoldrick, M. (2023). A family systems perspective on loss, recovery and resilience. In P. Sutcliffe, G. Tufnell, & U. Cornish (Eds) *Working with the Dying and Bereaved* (pp. 1–26). Routledge

Weigel, D. J. (2008). The concept of family: An analysis of laypeople's views of family. *Journal of Family Issues, 29*(11), 1426–1447.

Weiss-Laxer, N. S., Crandall, A., Hughes, M. E., & Riley, A. W. (2020). Families as a cornerstone in 21st century public health: Recommendations for research, education, policy, and practice. *Frontiers in Public Health, 8*, 503.

Westerlund, A., Nilsen, P., & Sundberg, L. (2019). Implementation of implementation science knowledge: The research-practice gap paradox. *Worldviews on evidence-based nursing, 16*(5), 332.

Wildin, R. S., Messersmith, D. J., & Houwink, E. J. F. (2021). Modernizing *family health* history: Achievable strategies to reduce implementation gaps. *Journal of community genetics, 12*(3), 493–496. https://doi.org/10.1007/s12687-021-00531-6

World Health Organization. (1978). *Health and the family: Studies on the demography of family life cycles and their health implications.* https://iris.who.int/bitstream/handle/10665/40336/16937_eng.pdf

World Health Organization. (2007). *People-Centered Health Care.* https://iris.who.int/bitstream/handle/10665/207004/9789290613930_eng.pdf

World Health Organization Regional Office for South East Asia (2013). Family as centre of health development report of the regional meeting Bangkok, Thailand, 18–20 March 2013. https://iris.who.int/bitstream/handle/10665/205062/B4972.pdf?sequence

World Health Organization. (2018). *Health in All Policies as part of the primary health care agenda on multisectoral action. https://iris.who.int/bitstream/handle/10665/326463/WHO-HIS-SDS-2018.59-eng.pdf*

World Health Organization. (2023). *Self-care for health and wellbeing.* https://www.who.int/health-topics/self-care#tab=tab_1

Zhang, Y. (2018). Family functioning in the context of an adult family member with illness: A concept analysis. *Journal of clinical nursing, 27*(15–16), 3205–3224.

Figure credit

CHAPTER 2

The Importance of Family Health Theories in Health Care

The first and simplest emotion that we discover in the human mind is curiosity.

—Edmund Burke

Learning Objectives

By the end of this chapter, learners will do the following:

- Define the following basic terms used to describe *family health* theories: theory, conceptual framework/model, grand theory, and middle range theory.
- Identify and describe the use/application and limitation of the following theoretical perspectives in *family health*: biomedical, biopsychosocial, trajectory, systems, stress, and coping perspectives.
- Compare and contrast different disciplinary perspectives and their contributions to understanding families, *family health*, and *family health* care.
- Articulate the implication of family theoretical perspectives within the 4HEALTH contexts: *individual health*, *family health*, *population health*, and public health.
- Develop a personal philosophy of *family health* through a personal *family health* experience(s)/encounter(s).

Before you read on, consider the following questions:

- What do health and illness mean within the context of family and beyond?
- What are the causes of health and illness in the context of the family and beyond?
- How can the causes of health and illness be addressed within the context of the family and beyond?
- When do health and illness occur in the context of family?
- Do we need research to understand the mechanisms on heath and illness within the context of the family?
- Are theories of *family health* needed in health care?

It is apparent from the questions that *family health* and illness are complex issues. Often times when learners or laypersons hear the term *family theory* they become skeptical as to what is it all about and what it has to say about the ideologies or philosophical perspectives of family life or family issues. What is always missing is the understanding of "family theories" or "family philosophical ideas" as road maps or blueprints to explain what individuals and families experience in daily lives through seeing, feeling, hearing, smelling, and touching and how they make sense of their life choices, including health choices. In this chapter, *family health* theories, conceptual/theoretical frameworks, and models are introduced. The 4HEALTH context is discussed in relation to the conceptualization of family and *family health* beyond the the individual to the inclusion of the broader environment.

An Overview of Family Health Theories, Conceptual/ Theoretical Frameworks, and Models

Family theories are integral to *family health* care, *family health* promotion, and *family health* research. The theories are essential in how *family health* data is or should be collected, interpreted, applied, and evaluated in health care. For example, family theories help in understanding demographic, structural, relational, and transitional aspects at the family level and beyond (Burr et al., 1979; Fine & Fincham, 2013). In addition, theories provide frameworks onto which the roles of families in health care decision-making in the promotion of health, prevention of diseases, and management of diseases/illness are understood. The ultimate goal of *family health* theories is to support excellence in *family health* care. What exactly is a *family health* theory?

Terminologies in Theorizing Family Health

It is important to be familiar with different terminologies used in theory development and their essence in conceptualizing *family health* care. In this chapter, different terminologies used in theory development from the "least abstract to the most abstract, namely *metaparadigm(s), philosophy/philosophical assumption(s), conceptual/theoretical model or framework(s),* to *theory(ies)*" (Black, 2014) are discussed within the context of *family health* care.

Metaparadigms

The definition of metaparadigms has evolved over the years. In nursing, nurse theorist Jacqueline Fawcett pioneered the term *metaparadigm*. In her latest definition, she defines *metaparadigms* as "global concepts that identify the phenomena of central interest to a discipline, the global non-relational propositions that define and describe the concepts, and the global relational propositions that state the relations between the concepts" (Fawcett, 2023, para. 2). Four foundational metaparadigms that are central to nursing theory development include *person*, *environment*, *health*, and *nursing* (Fawcett, 1984). The metaparadigms have evolved human beings (person), global environment (environment), planetary health (health), and nursing (Fawcett, in press). Later changes acknowledge the global communities and health of all human beings and planetary health and well-being (Fawcett, 2023). These metaparadigms are applicable to *family health* theory because they provide descriptive elements that are essential to the conceptualization of *family health* care across diverse groups and health care systems within different socio-conomic, cultural, and political settings.

Person, Environment, Health, and Nursing

Person

Person(s) refers to the recipient of health care, in this case individual family members, the family subsystems (e.g., dyad, triads), and the family as a unit and community/population. Persons are central to *family health* care. For instance, conceptualizing the person in *family health* care sheds light on how a person's demographic characteristics and involvement as a self-care agent impact *family health* and *family health* care. Self-care active agents are referred to as "individuals, families, and communities that are capable of managing their own health care needs (e.g., health promotion, disease prevention and control; health maintenance and caregiving, coping with illness, disability and death) with or without the support of a health care worker" (WHO, 2024, para. 1).

Health

Health is referred to as a holistic multidimensional aspect that integrates the biological, psychological, social, and spiritual needs of the person during health and illness (Selanders, 2010). Descriptively, health in *family health* care has been conceptualized by understanding the role of *whole health* in person-/patient- and family-centered care. The National Academies of Sciences and Engineering Medicine (2023) defines *whole health* as physical, behavioral, spiritual, and socioeconomic well-being as defined by the person (e.g., individuals, families, and communities). For instance, *family health* theories aim to discover the contexts of whole health that include understanding the biological needs of a person such as the needs for medicine and health care services to prevent, screen, and diagnose as well as treat health conditions. Psychological and social needs such as for social interactions, self-worth, and self-concept as well as spiritual needs should be valued (Selanders, 2010).

Environment

The environment is referred to "the recipients' significant others and surroundings, as well as the settings in which nursing actions occur" (Fawcett, 1989, p. 6). In nursing, Florence Nightingale (1992) was first to theorize the relationship between the person and the environment in promoting health and recovery from illness. Her conceptualization of the environment shed light to the importance of promoting environmental health (clean air, water, ventilation, sunlight, and noise free) to improve *individual health* at the point of inpatient care. Today, the environment entails a much broader view beyond the hospital bedroom/unit and includes the conceptualization of the contextual environment factors that describe the places where families live, play, learn, work, worship, access care, and age and how they impact *family health*. The environment has been central to the role of the social determinants of health in *population health*.

Nursing

The *nursing* metaparadigm refers to "the actions taken by nurses on behalf of or conjunction with the recipient" (Fawcett, 1989, p. 6) and is an important element of *family health* care practice. Nursing actions include activities in assessment, diagnosis, planning, intervention, and evaluation (Fawcett, in press). According to Orem (2001), nursing actions during health alterations include activities such as doing for others (e.g., helping with activities of daily living), providing guidance and supportive care, and providing a healthy environment for professional development through mutual processes. This metaparadigm is useful in delineating heath care professionals' attributes, behaviors, characteristics, and actions/competencies needed to provide quality, safe, and efficient health care to the person during health and illness encounters. Understanding how one's profession roles, actions, and attributes are conceptualized in family relational practice is important in *family health* care. Relational care practice values how health care providers intervene with patients and families at the interpersonal level to influence health outcomes (Doane, 2002). For example, *family health* theories are vital in theorizing patient–clinician communications and relationship (PCR) processes, such as how to assess and assist families in setting mutual goals (self-efficacy) and making family decisions such as using professional services, engaging in self-care, and making lifestyle changes. Other interpersonal factors of interest include family relationships such as marital, intergenerational, and sibling ties (Thomas et al., 2017) that facilitate coping behaviors (Berkman & Glass, 2000; Landstedt et al., 2015, Uchino, 2006).

Philosophical Assumptions

The term *philosophy* refers to "the set of beliefs about the nature of how the world works" (Black, 2014, p. 268). Each discipline has as a set of beliefs on how family is defined and how family works in the world of health, illness, and health care. These beliefs are the building blocks of key concepts or constructs of a theory, conceptual framework, or model development. By definition, a *concept* is "a building block or a primary element of a theory and a *construct* is a concept developed or adopted for use in a particular theory" (National Cancer Institute (NCI), 2005, p. 4). Constructs are considered key concepts within a given theory (NCI et al., 2005). Later in the chapter, different concepts/constructs used in *family health* theories are presented. Assumptions are central to theorizing health and illness in the context of *family health* care and public health. The following are examples of philosophical assumptions of interest to *family health* theorists and scholars:

- Family constitutes perhaps the most important social context within which illness occurs and is resolved. It consequently serves as a primary unit in health and medical care (Litman, 1974).
- The process of "becoming a patient" and availing oneself of the use of various health services encompasses a series of decisions and events involving the interaction of a number of persons, including their families, friends, and professional providers of care (Shwed, 1982).
- Families are an inherent and inevitable participant in the prevention and treatment of diseases and health problems (Doherty, 1991).
- Individuals in all cultures are born into families, and most spend their lives interacting with their family members (Doherty, 1991).
- *Family health* process include *family health* beliefs, the health status of family members, health responses and practices, lifestyle practices, and health care provisions during illness and wellness (Anderson, 2000).
- Family experiences are embedded in the culture, which has an impact on family processes (Kerry, 2003).
- The assessment of the family context includes data about the individuals, family subsystems, and the embedded household contexts (Denham, 2003).
- Family is a hereditary link (Facio et al., 2010).
- Family developmental stages and roles influence the reaction of the family system to illness and illness management (Alderfer & Stanley, 2012).
- Family is central to health and illness by contributing to a positive or negative course and outcome (Alderfer & Stanley, 2012).
- The experiences of health and illness are family affairs (Wright & Leahey, 2013).
- Families can be in all public health issues because they are uniquely important to health of individuals and families in providing immediate context, care and caring, continuity in people's lives, and connections (Weiss et al., 2020).
- The family unit is the community's most essential and fundamental building block of life for generations to come (Adabanya et al., 2023).

Conceptual/Theoretical Frameworks or Models

In the literature, conceptual/theoretical frameworks or models and theories have been used interchangeably. These terms and their development structures are different. By definition, a model/conceptual framework is "a network of interlinked concepts that together provide a comprehensive understanding of a phenomenon or phenomena" (Jabareen, 2009, p. 51). Conceptual/theoretical frameworks or models provide a more broad structure organization of concepts of interests in theories than philosophies (Black, 2004). They also may be based on information from existing theories to help understand a phenomenon of interest (NCI et al., 2005). In terms of applicability, conceptual/theoretical frameworks or models are normally complex but not highly developed or rigorous tested (NCI et al., 2005). They usually present a summary of concepts based on research findings that represent the status of the phenomenon of interest (Kivunja, 2018).

Theory

According to Black (2014), a theory is referred to as an idea, a supposition, a belief system, and a reason for something, an explanation for what we believe to be true about the world we see. Theories are socially constructed descriptions, explanations, or predictions of a given phenomenon (Chinn et al., 2021; Fine & Fincham, 2013). They describe and explain phenomena of interest by specifying a set of defined and interrelated concepts and constructs and are predictive of relationships between constructs and variables (Kivunja, 2018; NCI et al., 2005). By definition, a variable is the "operational form of constructs"; in other words, it "define[s] how a construct is to be measured in a specific situation" (NCI et al., 2005, p. 4). Phenomena of interest such as *family health* events and situations, family knowledge, attitudes, behaviors, and competencies are examples of useful practical areas that make *family health* theories useful in health care. In terms of applicability, theories have been empirically tested to facilitate the understanding of a phenomenon of interest.

There are two major types of theories, namely *grand theories* and *midrange theories* (Fawcett, 2000). Both theories are important in *family health*. In nursing, Higgins and Moore (2000) explain levels of theory from the highest to the lowest as meta-theory, grand theory, middle-range theory, and micro-range theory. A *meta theory* is the most abstract and usually used to inquire theory based on analytical reasoning and logic. A *grand theory* is a broad conceptualization of explanatory constructs that summarize knowledge about phenomena of interest in an interactional way that is empirically untestable (Bonell et al., 2023). A *middle-range theory* is narrow in focus (Black, 2014) and more verifiable through testing across different contexts, interventions, or outcomes (Bonell et al., 2023). The validity of a middle-range theory is usually improved through testing and refinement using empirical evidence from experimental and quasi-experimental research methods. Proof of principle studies are studies that intend to assess a proof of a principle, such as a relationship between constructs, rather than determine the scalability of interventions and usually draw on one middle-range theory (Bonell et al., 2023). For example, in public health evaluation intervention studies, middle-range theories are used to inform intervention theories of change (Bonell et al., 2023). A micro-range theory is the least form of theory that represent a set of hypotheses that are used to categorize a phenomenon (Higgins & Moore, 2000). A middle-range theory can originate from a grand theory or its components or further development of concepts from the micro theory (Higgins & Moore, 2000).

Borrowed and Shared Theories

Different theories have been used in *family health* because no single theory can address the complexities of family-related phenomena alone (Fine & Fincham, 2013). Hence, the majority of *family health* theories or concepts/constructs have been adapted among disciplines such as psychology, family ecology, home economics, educational psychology, nursing, sociology, anthropology, and preventative medicine (Bomar, 1989). The terms *borrowed* or *shared* theories have been used in this regard. *Borrowed* family theories or concepts are described as ideas developed from a topic(s) or from other disciplines and used to address an issue or explain a phenomenon of interest in another topic or discipline (Bengston et al., 2005). If borrowed knowledge is adequately applied/combined within the adopting discipline's theoretical underpinnings (Fawcett, 2005), the new theory developed is described as a *shared* theory (Barnum, 1998).

Theoretical Paradigms

In the language of family theory development, it is important to understand how knowledge about phenomena of interest is constructed to be practical or useful. In this section, empiricism and interpretive and critical paradigms (Khan, 2003) are described as the major family theoretical paradigms in theory development and evidence-based practice in *family health* research and intervention. By definition, a *paradigm* refers to a pattern of shared understanding and assumptions about reality and the world, worldview, or widely accepted value system (Khan, 2003). Scholars who employ an empirical paradigm take into account the deductive and theory-testing approach to generate hard and value-free evidence based on single realities (Monti & Tingen, 1999). Scholars using an interpretive paradigm develop evidence inductively, taking into account multiple socially constructed perceptions of reality (Weaver & Olson, 2006), including one's values, aesthetics, and ethics (Carper, 2012; Monti & Tingen, 1999). Lastly, the critical paradigm is a paradigm that contextualizes evidence from a sociocultural context with intentions to improve equity and reduce disparities in populations and *population health* (Bowleg, 2012). Understanding the sociocultural context is important in *family health* (Barton & Bischop, 2014; Evans et al., 2021).

Conceptual/Theoretical Frameworks and Theories of Family Health

In this section of the chapter, major interdisciplinary theoretical perspectives applied in *family health* science are presented. The most common schools of thoughts include the biomedical, biopsychosocial, trajectory and life course/developmental, systems thinking, and stress and coping perspectives (Doherty, 1991). This list is not exhaustive. Since *family health* is a complex phenomenon, *family health* scholars also incorporate constructs from other schools of thought such as behavioral change and interactional and communication perspectives.

Biomedical Perspective

Description and Application

The traditional biomedical model of illness has been the dominant model in health care when it comes to medical discoveries and treatments in modern medicine (Engel, 1977). Within this model, health and illness are centered around understanding the body (physical or biological aspects) and how the body functions, the impact of the physical world from the natural sciences lens in explaining the causes of disease (e.g., microbiology, biochemistry, etc.), and how medical intervention can be applied to cure and control biological systems (Adibi, 2014). Psychology and social science hold the lower end of the hierarchy of science. The *body* in relation to illness is the focal entity in the biomedical model and not necessarily the individual person (Rocca & Anjum, 2020). The body is best explained by understanding the body structures (human anatomy) and the chemistry and physics of the body structures (human physiology). The *body structure* described entails the least to most complex structure, namely the chemical (atoms/molecules), cellular, tissue, organs and organ systems, and organismal levels. The *organismal level* includes the interactions between the nervous system (signaling), integumentary system, respiratory system (gas exchange), digestive system (energy processing), excretory system (waste), skeletal system (supportive structure), muscular system (movement), circulatory or cardiovascular system, endocrine system (hormones), reproductive system (sexual reproduction), and lymphatic (immune) system. Cognitions and social relations are usually approached from a biomedical perspective (Rocca & Anjum, 2020). This means the "psychosocial system" is also medicalized. For example, disorders, such as attention-deficit hyperactivity disorder (ADHD) is considered a neurobiology disorder that can be addressed through pharmacotherapies (Rocca & Anjum, 2020).

The benefits of the model include understanding the systems of the physical body, their functions, and the related measurable clinical (i.e., biological or somatic) variables. Most importantly, the model is useful in understanding biomarkers in symptom and self-management science (Page et al., 2018). The model conceptualizes the symptom experience (Lenz et al., 1997) and how it is characterized by a person's observable characteristics and traits (also known as a phenotype) and is determined by individuals' behavioral, biological, and clinical data (Cashion et al., 2016). Understanding symptom management strategies from a broader context beyond the individual is crucial (Dodd et al., 2001). *Family health* care professionals benefiting from the biomedical models demonstrate an understanding of role of epidemiology, human anatomy, and pathophysiology in articulating disease burdens and related interventions in the context of relational care.

Limitations

The model has faced criticism for its limited powers in conceptualizing whole health, specifically understanding the role of the psychosocial, behavioral, and political processes influencing health (Engel, 1977). As a result, a more inclusive biopsychosocial framework has been proposed for mental health issues (e.g., somatic disorders; Çetin, & Varma, 2021; Henningsen, 2018). Somatic disorders are medical issues that have been of interest to the medical and *family health* community. As defined by the American Psychiatric Association's *Diagnostic and Statistical Manual of Mental Disorders*, fifth edition (DSM-5), individuals presenting with somatic disorders have physical symptoms that may or may not be associated with a diagnosed medical condition such as pain, weakness, or shortness of breath but result in poor quality of life because of major distress and/or problems functioning (American Psychiatric Association, 2013). The medicalization of disorders such as medically unexplained conditions or syndromes such as chronic pain/fatigue, irritable bowel syndrome, low back pain, general anxiety disorder, posttraumatic stress disorder (PTSD), and burnout has been criticized. Critics believe that intervening at the medical (physical) without examining the social and psychological issue is limiting to the model's explanatory powers of meeting patients as "whole persons" (Rocca, & Anjum, 2020).

Biopsychosocial and Systems Thinking Perspective

Description and Application

The major phenomena of interest in the study and practice of *family health* and *family health* care is understanding health and illness beyond the context of the biomedical model. Biopsychosocial perspectives align well with the Maslow's hierarchy of needs model (Naveen, 2010). Maslow's model brings to light the important universal dynamic biopsychosocial human needs that demonstrate that human health and psychological well-being depend equally on interrelating biological, psychological, social, and environmental domains (Taylor & Seager, 2021). Chapter 3 provides a detailed description of the Maslow's hierarchy of needs.

Theorizing assessment and intervention plans, progress, and priorities about health and illness across the life spans and context of the broader changing socioecological environment is important to advance *family health* science. It requires a good grasp of biological and socio-epidemiology aspects of *family health*, which is well described by the socioecological framework (Fiese & Hammons, 2013) pioneered by the work of Engel (1977) and Bronfenbrenner (1979) and, recently, the application of the biopsychosocial perspective in conceptualization factors relevant to understanding *population health* and health disparities (King et al., 2009). The biopsychosocial perspective acknowledges the multiple influences on health and quality of life, also described as a syndemic: a "set of linked problems involving two or more afflictions, interacting synergistically, and contributing to an excess burden of disease" (King et al., p. 5). Understanding the integration of the multiple levels of influence (i.e., individual, interpersonal, community, societal) within the ecological domains (i.e., biological, behavioral, physical/built environment, sociocultural environment, and healthcare system) is essential in addressing health disparities (National Institute on Minority Health and Health Disparities [NIMHD], 2017).

Family health theories based on a the socioecological framework consider the following relevant contexts in theorizing health and illness: (a) the developmental context; (b) environmental stress, including family-level stressors; (c) maintenance and prevention with particular attention to adherence to medical regimens and the promotion of healthy lifestyles; (d) the intersection of the family with health care institutions and communication with health care providers; and (e) the broader socioeconomic context (Fiese & Hammons, 2013). Thus, the theories intend to explain, describe, or predict factors that address *family health* normative and non-normative challenges within the family's multiple contexts (i.e., the individual, family, and organization level and social environment) over time.

The ecological perspective is useful in *family health* theory development to help theorize intervention points for behavioral changes within the family's multiple contexts as well as changes pertaining to the environment (NCI, 2005). For instance, family-focused health interventions that target behavior change at the family level integrate theoretical perspectives that can be theorized at the interpersonal level. Likewise, reciprocal causations can be conceptualized, for example understanding how a *family health* change strategy can indirectly lead to changes in individual behaviors, and vice versa. A summary of the key ecological constructs and key domains of influence are presented in Table 2.1 and Table 2.2, respectively.

TABLE 2.1 **Common Key Ecological Constructs in Relation to 4HEALTH**

Construct	**Definition**	**Related 4HEALTH Context**
Ecological environment	Conceived topologically as a nested arrangement of structures, each contained within the next structure.	*Individual health, Family health, Population health* and public health
Levels of Influence		
Microsystem (individual/ intrapersonal)	A microsystem is the smallest complex relational system between the developing person and their environment in an immediate setting (e.g., home, school, workplace, etc.). Individual characteristics that influence behavior, such as knowledge, attitudes, beliefs and personality traits.	*Individual health*
Mesosystem (interpersonal)	A mesosystem comprises the interrelations among major settings containing the developing person at a particular point in life. Includes interpersonal processes and primary groups such as families, friends, and peers. These groups provide social identity, support, and role definition.	*Family health*
Exosystem (institutional)	An exosystem is an extension of the mesosystem and embraces other specific social structures, both formal and informal, that do not themselves contain the developing person but impinge on or encompass the immediate settings in which that person is found, and thereby influence, delimit, or even determine what goes on there. Rules, regulations, policies, and informal structures are present that may constrain or promote recommended behaviors within the micro- and mesosystem.	Organizational health (*population health*)
	Social networks and social norms, or standards, which exist as formal or informal among individuals, groups, and organizations.	Community health (*population health*)

Macrosystem (public policy/ societal)	A macrosystem refers to the overarching institutional patterns of the culture or subculture, such as the economic, social, educational, legal, and political systems, of which micro-, meso-, and exosystems are the concrete manifestations. Local, state, and federal policies and laws that regulate or support healthy actions and practices for disease prevention, early detection, control, and management.	Public health

TABLE 2.2 **Key Domains of Influence**

Domain/Level	Description
Biological	Biological processes that help explain mechanisms of observed differences in disease incidence and outcomes that are most relevant for populations (e.g., stress)
Behavioral	Individual behaviors and psychological processes that represent major pathways by which environmental and social exposures affect health
Physical/Built Environment	An environment that encompasses a broad spectrum of factors that threaten *population health*
Sociocultural Environment	Group norms, beliefs, values and social mobility, collective responses within the environment
Health Care Systems	Organizations, institutions, people, and resources whose primary purpose is to promote, restore or maintain health (WHO's definition)
Life Course	An approach or perspective that acknowledges health status is a reflection of cumulative life conditions. Thus, health interventions should be tailored to specific developmental stages and take into account the impact of cumulative social and environmental exposures, both positive and negative (Jones et al., 2019)
Reciprocal Causation	Bidirectional processes/influences between ecological factors/ variables. Individual behavior both influences and is influenced by the environment.

Moreover, traditional family systems based on a systems thinking perspective have origins in general systems theory (vob Bertalanffy, 1972). Within the family systems perspective, a family system is referred to as a "group of individuals and the pattern of relationship between them" (Patterson & Garwick, 1994, p. 131). Historical contributions in family systems theories include the theorizing process of the concept of family as a system by Murray Bowen, a medical family therapy scholar and scientists (Johnson & Ray, 2016). Through his work developing Bowen family systems theory, Bowen conceptualized families as evolving emotional systems that have implications for practitioners' family assessment skills based on the "systems thinking" approach of the interrelations of concepts and variables (Kerr & Bowen, 1988; Whitchurch & Constantine, 1993). The family systems approach follows biopsychosocioecological perspectives, which offer a means of configuring and representing the complex, multifaceted relationships that occur within and between systems and the larger sociocultural environment across time and space. In other words, the theorizing process sheds light on the interrelations and interconnectedness between the biological systems (disease processes), psychological systems (affective function), and the social systems (socialization function; Fiese & Hammons, 2013). These systems reciprocally influence one another, affecting the development and maintenance of wellness and disorder, including traumatic stress within families. Moreover, in nursing, Betty Neuman developed the Neuman systems model (Neuman & Fawcell, 2011). The theory has been applicable to *family health* nursing care (Neuman, 1983). The theory postulates key interrelated variables that are important in theorizing family system. The variables include (a) the psychosocial-cultural relationships of the family (e.g., traditions, behaviors, and practices), (b) the physical health of the family, (c) the development of the family (i.e., family developmental stage and tasks) and, (d) the spiritual influences on the family (family role and ability to support a sense of love, belonging, safety purpose, meaning, hope, forgiveness, creativity, interconnectedness, and transcendence; Neuman & Fawcett, 2011). The theory of prevention as intervention is one of the theories derived from Neuman's (2011) systems model.

Understanding the concept of family as a whole is essential in family systems theory. This means that the health of the family as a whole is affected by *individual health*, and vice versa (Neuman & Fawcett, 2011). In addition, the concept of *family health* being greater than the sum of the health of individual family members is also crucial (Neuman & Fawcett, 2011). The magnitude of influence between the socioecological variables depends on how well the family is functioning and adapting to normative and non-normative family life and health stressors (Neuman & Fawcett, 2011). A family member's illness can influence how other family members respond to how they manage and adjust to the situation.

Application

Overall, the biopsychosocial model and ecological and family systems theoretical perspectives are instrumental in understanding *family health* dimensions of health promotion and risk reduction as well as the process of adaptation to chronic illness or recovery within the *family health* and illness cycle (Patterson & Garwick, 1994). The focus of family systems theories/models is to challenge the status quo of *family health* to move beyond individual and dyadic influences to include the broader environmental contextual influences and examine their direct and indirect pathways of interactions (Bornstein & Sawyer, 2006). A systems theory perspective sheds light on one's understanding of how families stabilize around new interaction patterns after an illness or after the acute phase of treatment and of how they interact with health professionals. Thus, from a systems perspective, family communication and interpersonal processes are important in understanding how families operate in a nonsummative nature (Gavazzi & Lim, 2023) and how they maintain family boundaries (open or closed). For example, some family systems may not be receptive to share or disclose family secrets with others for fear of creating stressful demands on personal and relational health (Afifi et al., 2014). Family systems theory goes beyond simplistic notions of modeling *individual health* behaviors to demonstrating how practices, such as diet, exercise, and smoking, are incorporated into stable family patterns that are difficult to change with simple education and advice.

The fabric of family systems is contained within two critical aspects described from structural and functional perspectives: family structure(s) (the family compositions—who is in and who is out) and the family function(s) (i.e., different dimensions of functioning that define connections between the family members and broader social systems) overtime (Patterson & Garwick, 1994). As mentioned in Chapter 1, the family structure is conceptualized in different ways based on the family form (e.g., nuclear versus extended), type of power structure (e.g., matriarchal versus patriarchal), marital patterns (e.g., exogamy versus endogamy), and subsystems (e.g., parent–child systems, sibling subsystem; Friedman et al., 2003). The changing dynamics of family structures provides a lens of conceptualizing family role structures (Friedman et al., 2003) and family protective and risk factors influencing health and illness over time and across varied spaces (Sharma, 2013). Family roles are crucial for family functioning. For instance, it is important to understand how roles in family systems are conceptualized during heath alterations in *family health* and *family health* care over time.

On the other hand, family functions are important in conceptualizing assessment and intervention strategies at the point of care (Smilkstein, 1984). The five functions most of interest to family systems health care providers and scholars are the affective function, the socialization and social placement functions, the reproductive function, the economic function, and the health care function (Friedman et al., 2003). A healthy family system is conceptualized as a system that is or is attempting to "maintain balanced functioning or homeostasis by using its capabilities (resources and coping behaviors) to meet its demands (stressors and strains)" (Patterson & Garwick, 1994, p. 132). In meeting the health care function, the family system provides health promotion, preventative care, and disease management care for the sick members. Self-care (e.g., education and counseling) is the primary goal of *family health* practice (Friedman et al., 2003). Thus, the concept of self-care is instrumental in facilitating the understanding of how families can be empowered to manage their health and well-being. Pioneered by the work of Dorothea Orem (2001), a nurse theorist, self-care was defined as "the practice of activities that individuals initiate and perform on their own behalf in maintaining life, health, and well-being" (p. 43). The self-care concept continues to evolve beyond *individual health* to include family, community, and *population health* (Hartweg & Metcalfe, 2022). These dimensions have been captured in the WHO's definition, as stated earlier in this chapter. When self-care interventions are promoted, individuals, families, communities, and populations are activated to participate in their own health care to achieve greater self-determination, self-efficacy, autonomy, and engagement in health (WHO, 2020). Table 2.3 provides key constructs important in family systems theories.

TABLE 2.3 **Key Constructs in Family Systems Theories**

Constructs	Definition
Family System	A family system that is at risk, healthy or living with a disease/illness and has self-defined family members or family subsystem(s)
Family Structure	How a family is organized, the manner in which units are arranged and how the units relate to each other (Friedman et al., 2003)
Family Power	The potential or actual ability of individual members to change or influence the behaviors of other family members (Friedman et al., 2003)
Family Function	Are consequences or outcomes of the family structure that represent what the family does to meet the basic need of individual family members, the whole family, and wider society (Friedman et al., 2003)
Family Nonsummativity (Wholeness/Holism)	The view of the family as a whole and not merely the sum of its part (Friedman et al., 2013)
Reciprocal Determinism or Ripple Effect	The reverberating results from changes in a system that happens when any one part of the system either through transitional and situational stressors affects another part of the system (Friedman et al., 2013)
Family as a Hierarchical System	A family comprised of smaller subsystems (e.g., spouse, parent, and siblings) embedded within other larger systems or suprasystems (Friedman et al., 2013)
Family Self-Reflexivity And Goal Setting	Families' ability and tendency to make themselves and their own behaviors the focus of examination and target of explanation (Friedman et al., 2013)
Family Boundaries (Open/Closed/Random Family Systems)	The space or interface rings that actively expands (or open) and retract (or close) according to outside demands and internal needs depending on whether it is an open, closed, or random system (Friedman et al., 2013) Open family system: An open family system actively welcomes the exchange of information, techniques, opportunities, and resources to solve their problems Closed family system: A closed family system has limited permeability, view change as threatening, and are resistant to it and are usually untrusting to strangers Random family system: A random family system values spontaneity, free choice, very fluid norms, and challenges through a loosely regulated process of exchange of information (Friedman et al., 2013)
Family Adaptation	The capacity of the family and its members to modify their behaviors to each other and to their outer world (reject or accept information, energy, or services) in response to external or internal inputs (Friedman et al., 2013)
Family Secret	A common human defense mechanism is to "distance" the self from an event experienced or perceived as shameful such as a loss, abuse, shameful or embarrassing events, and economic events with highly stressful and/or traumatic potential (Termini, 2018)
Family-Related Physiological Variables	Biomedical factors that contribute to the development of health or illness and/or influence health care (Eustace, 2022)
Family-Related Psychological Variables	Mental process and relationships that contribute to the development of health risks and/or influence health care (Eustace, 2022)
Family-Related Sociocultural Variables	Sociocultural variables (socioeconomic, cultural, and political) that contribute to the development of health risks or influence health care (Eustace, 2022)

Family-Related Developmental Variables	Time-sensitive variable developmental processes (age-related or environmental processes) that contribute to the development of health risks and/or influence health care (Eustace, 2022)
Family-Related Spiritual Variables	Family-related spiritual or religious beliefs that contribute to the development of health risks and/or influence health care (Eustace, 2022)
Family Stressors	Tension-producing stimuli (internal or external to the environment) that have the potential to cause system instability (Neuman & Fawcett, 2011)
Environmental Stressors	Modifiable or nonmodifiable family-related environmental stressors derived within (internal) and outside (external) the family system that have the potential to disrupt family stability and sustainability
Protective Lines	Flexible line of defense: A protective buffer system for the family's normal and stable state that prevents stressors' invasions, keeping the system free from stressor reactions or symptomatology Normal line of defense: A dynamic line of defense that represents what the family has become and the state to which the client has evolved over time or the usual wellness level (family cohesion). It is protected by the flexible line of defense Lines of resistance: The lines activated following invasion of the normal line of defense by environmental stressors. Examples include family commitment to each other degree of trust and internal support
Prevention as Intervention	Family interventions that promote family wellness by preventing stressors and reducing risk factors. They can be primary, secondary, or tertiary prevention interventions

Limitations

Family health theories based the biopsychosocial, ecological, and systems theories have been criticized for their complexities and difficulties in operationalizing all the concepts and variables across the broader environment. For example, the need for inclusion of conceptual underpinnings of sophisticated interventions and research methods that capture ecological influences (Wendel et al., 2015), as well as dyads as the unit of analyses is still warranted (Thompson & Walker, 1982). Practically, practitioners using these perspectives may have a harder time meeting the whole person as they tend to care for families from different levels (e.g., biological [physician], psychological [psychologist], and social [social worker]), which if not planned well the whole persons perspective may be fragmented (Rocca & Anjum, 2020; Xiao et al., 2021). Likewise, the models are limiting in their power of explaining how big data on health and biopsychosocial information (Rocca & Anjum, 2020) is linked to understanding health disparities among vulnerable populations (King et al., 2009). Multilevel approaches based on systems thinking and biopsychosocial perspectives are still needed to facilitate desirable patient- and family-centered outcomes (Tramonti et al., 2021). Likewise, the need to engage patient, families, and communities to help the greater understanding of the disease, illness experiences, and decision within the biopsychosocial framework requires attention (Tramonti et al., 2021).

Trajectory Models

Description and Application

The first *family health* theories developed in the family literature came out of the trajectory models that examined the psychosomatic illness beyond the individual to include the family contexts. The models are best studied from different borrowed and shared family theoretical perspectives that are family focused and have adequate empirical support (Doherty, 1991). For example, the *family health* and illness cycle models were derived from biopsychosocial systems and developmental theoretical perspectives. The models recognize that family is central to health and illness and that *family health* problems are biological, psychological, and social in nature. The historical contributions involve the development of the explanatory conceptual model that describe the three factors necessary for development of psychosomatic illness in children: (a) physiological vulnerability; (b) the child's family transactional characteristics of enmeshment, overprotectiveness, rigidity, and lack of conflict resolution; and (c) the sick child's role in the family's patterns of conflict avoidance as a source of reinforcement for the child's symptoms (Minuchin et al., 1975). Later, the development of the chronic illness framework, also known as the family systems and chronic illness framework, helped foster an understanding of how the worlds of illness (types and time phases) and individual and family development (functioning; Rolland, 1984, 1987) can be theorized. In an attempt to organize the literature on *family health* and illness experiences, the *family health* and illness cycle model was pioneered by Doherty and McCubbin (1985). The model continued to evolve through the work of Doherty (1991) and later Danielson Hamel-Bissell and Winstead-Fry (1993). The health and illness perspective illustrates how health care can be enhanced by taking families and *family health* into account. The model depicts a cycle process that includes phases of a family's experience, namely (a) health promotion and risk reduction, then (b) family vulnerability and disease onset or relapse, (c) family illness appraisal, (d) family acute response, (e) family adaptation to illness and recovery, and finally (f) death/end of life. In the model, the family system is considered an interactional system whereby the family affects individual's health, and vice versa, across all stages of the *family health*-illness life cycle. The phases help *family health* care professionals identify intervention points for health promotion, health protection, disease prevention, management of health and illness/diseases, as well as end-of-life care. Tables 2.4 and 2.5 provide a summary of the key constructs in models using the trajectory and developmental perspective, respectively.

TABLE 2.4 **Common Key Trajectory Constructs Based on the *Family Health*-Illness Life Cycle Models**

Constructs	Definition
Family Health Promotion and Risk Reduction	Family beliefs and behavior patterns that either help family members stay healthy or put them at a long-term risk of developing disease
Vulnerability and Disease Onset/Relapse	Life events and experiences of the family that make family members more susceptible to becoming ill or to having a relapse of a chronic illness

Illness Appraisal	Family beliefs about a family member's illness and family decisions about how to deal with the illness within a context of the availability and accessibility of health care
Acute Response	The aftermath of the illness for the family
Family Adaptation to Illness and Recovery	How a family reorganizes itself around a chronic illness or disability of a family member and the ways that a family adapts to the recovery of an ill member
Time Phases of Illness Approach/Way	A way for the clinician to think longitudinally and to reach a fuller understanding of chronic illness as an ongoing process with landmarks, transitions, and changing demands
The Crisis Phase	Includes any symptomatic period before actual diagnosis and the initial period of readjustment and coping after the problem has been clarified through a diagnosis and initial treatment plan
The Chronic Phase	Whether long or short, the time span between the initial diagnosis and readjustment period and the third phase when issues of death and terminal illness predominate. It is an era that can be marked by constancy, progression, or episodic change. In this sense, its meaning cannot be grasped by simply knowing the biological behavior of an illness. Rather, it is more a psychosocial construct that has been referred to as "the long haul," or a phase of day-to-day living with chronic illness
The Last or Terminal Phase	Includes the preterminal stage of an illness wherein the inevitability of death becomes apparent and dominates family life. This phase is distinguished by issues surrounding separation, death, grief, resolution of mourning, and resumption of "normal" family life beyond the loss
Care Continuum	A series of initiating, continuing, and concluding care events that result when the patient seeks providers in one or more environments within the healthcare system (McBryde-Foster & Allen, 2005)

TABLE 2.5 **Key Constructs in Family Developmental Theories**

Constructs	**Definition**
Trajectory	Change in roles and statuses that represents a distinct departure from prior roles and statuses (Hutchison, 2018)
Family Trajectories	The whole sequence of family events during the life course in shaping health outcomes
Transitions	Long-term pattern of stability and change, which usually involves multiple transitions (Hutchison, 2018).
Life Events	Significant occurrence involving a relatively abrupt change that may produce serious and long-lasting effects (Hutchison, 2018)
Cohort	A group of persons who were born during the same time/period and who experience particular social changes within a given culture in the same sequence and at the same age (Hutchison, 2018)
Life Expectancy	A health indicator that tells the average number of years of life a person who has attained a given age can expect to live (Centers for Disease Control, 2023)
Lifestyle	A system of meanings, attitudes, and values within which the subject acts that define individual and collective models of health practices within social, historical, and cultural contexts (Brivio et al., 2023)

Life Stage	A phase in a sequence of age statues and/ roles Stage 1: Beginning families (married couple without children) Stage 2: Childbearing families (oldest child, birth to 30 months) Stage 3: Families with preschool children (oldest child 2.5–6 years) Stage 4: Families with school children (oldest child 6–13 years) Stage 5: Families with teenagers (oldest child 13–20 years) Stage 6: Families as launching centers (first child gone to last child's leaving home) Stage 7: Families in the middle years (empty nest to retirement) Aging families (retirement to death of one or both spouses)

Application

Trajectory models are useful in providing an understanding in how family systems engage and make decisions in care provisions throughout the continuum of care (Evashwick, 1989). In this case, the concept of a care continuum is defined as a "series of initiating, continuing and concluding care events that result when the patient seeks providers in one or more environments within the healthcare system" (McBryde-Foster & Allen, 2005. p. 630). For example, theorizing about *family health* and *family health* care can take place along the cancer care continuum (pretreatment, in-treatment, post-treatment, recurrence), HIV care continuum (diagnosis, linked to care, received or were retained in care and viral suppression), or stroke care continuum (acute treatment, secondary prevention, rehabilitation and community care). Trajectory models based on a family life course / developmental perspective have played a major role in theorizing family lived experiences, normative and non-normative transitions, developmental tasks across life stages, span (Duvall, 1988), settings, and cultures (Dilworth-Anderson & Burton, 1996). The "time thinking" approach in relation to human growth, experiences, and learning overtime is a fundamental basic assumption of family developmental theories. These theories have been instrumental in studying the *family health* dimension of health promotion and risk reduction as well as the process of adaptation to illness or recovery within the *family health* and illness cycle across time. Table 2.6 summarizes key constructs of family life stages in family developmental theories.

TABLE 2.6 **Key Family Life Stage Constructs in Family Developmental Theories**

Major Stages and Description	**Developmental Tasks**	***Population Health***	**Examples of Health Concerns/Needs**
Stage 1: Single family, dating/nondating but living alone or sharing residence with others (without children)	Dating/nondating but living alone or sharing residence with others (without children)	Adolescent, adult, or older adult	Family planning education and counseling

Stage 2: Beginning families, married/cohabiting couple without children)	Navigating how to live together Adjusting relationships with families of origin and social networks to include a partner	Adolescents or adult or older adult couples	Family planning education and counseling, Prenatal education and counseling
Stage 3: Childbearing families (oldest child, birth to 30 months)	Preparing and adjusting the family system to accommodate children Developing roles as parents Redefining roles with extended families	Infant, children with adolescents, adults, or older adult parents	Preparation for birth experiences, transition to parenthood, infant care, well-baby checks, immunizations, normal growth and development, safety measures, family planning, family interaction, good health practices (e.g., sleep, nutrition and exercise)
Stage 4: Families with preschool children (oldest child 2.5–6 years)	Socializing, educating, and guiding children Assessing and adjusting parenting roles as children age and more children join the family	Children with adolescents, adult, or older adult parents	Communicable disease of children, accident prevention and home safety (e.g., falls, burns, poisoning), marital relationship, sibling relations, family planning, growth and development needs, parenting issues, child abuse and neglect and good health practices
Stage 5: Families with school children (oldest child 6–13 years)	Providing guidance to children while collaborating with outside resources (e.g., school, extracurricular activities)	Children with adolescents, adult, or older adult parents	Health challenges to children (e.g., vision, hearing, speech), dental health, child abuse and neglect, substance abuse, communicable diseases, chronic conditions, behavior problems and good health
Stage 6: Families with teenagers (oldest child 13–20 years)	Adjusting parent–child relationships with adolescents to provide more independence with safe limits Tending to parents' midlife relationship and career issues	Adolescents with adult or older adult parents	Accidents (e.g., driving), sport injuries, drug and alcohol misuse, birth control, teenage pregnancy, sex education, marital relationships, adolescent–parent relations, good health practices

Stage 7: Families as launching centers (first child gone to last child's leaving home)	Navigating adult-to-adult relationships with children Resolving midlife issues Caring for aging family members	Children or adolescents with adult or older adult parents	Communication issues between parents and young adults, role transitional problems for husband and wife, emergence of chronic health problems, family planning for young adults, menopause concerns, effects associated with prolonged drinking, smoking, poor dietary practices, and wellness lifestyle
Stage 8: Families in the middle years (empty nest to retirement)	Adjusting to being a couple without children living at home Caring for aging family members	Adult or older adult parents	Good health practices, marital relationship, communication with and relating to children, in-laws, grandchildren and aging parents, caregiver concerns, adjustment to physiological changes of aging
Stage 9: Aging families (retirement to death of one or both spouses)	Learning new roles related to retirement, becoming grandparents, losing a partner, and health-related changes	Older adult (grandparents)	Increasing functional disabilities, mobility impairment, chronic illness, diminished physical rigor and function, long-term care services, caregiving, social isolation, grief/depression, cognitive impairment

Limitations

Both the *family health* and illness and developmental perspectives have limitations in interpretation and explanatory powers. For example, the family cycle of health and illness model (Doherty, 1991) presents with the following basic limitations:

- Cycle deals with the family's experience of a particular member's illness, not the complex dynamics created by multiple illnesses.
- Cycle is more elaborative in the illness area than disease prevention and health promotion.
- Cycles focus mostly on family's interactions with other important social groups aside from the health care professionals.
- Cycle separates processes that can overlap or occur simultaneously in certain situations.

Stress and Coping Perspective

Description and Applications

Family stress and coping theories are middle-range theories. They have been instrumental in studying the *family health* dimension of vulnerability and disease onset and acute response, as well as the process of adaptation to illness or recovery within the *family health* and illness cycle, discussed earlier. Family stress perspectives have evolved from the pioneering work and conceptualization of diverse scholars (i.e., Boss, 1999; Burr, 1973; Hansen & Johnson, 1979; Hill, 1949, 1958; McCubbin & Patterson, 1982). The family stress and coping perspectives emphasize how families experience, respond, and adapt to stressful life events, including health and illness. Four key factors theorized to explain family response to stressful events, include (a) the stressful event (e.g., acute illness: A); (b) the family's resources for dealing with the event (e.g., financial, social, psychological: B); (c) the family's definition or perception or meaning of the event (e.g., catastrophic, manageable, potentially helpful: C); and (d) the degree of crisis (X; i.e., the ABC-X model pioneered by Hill, 1958). Family stressful events have been described as a change within the family or a family demand that can be normative and non-normative, ongoing family strains such as unresolved issues, insidious tensions, and daily hassles (Daneshpour, 2017). Normative demands are defined as "typical life cycle and societal changes affecting everyone" (Patterson, 2002, p. 238). Non-normative demands are demands that happen unexpectedly such as disasters, birth of an unexpected child, diagnosis of an illness, and so on. Family demands are also conceptualized as either "actual" demands or familial risk factors. For example, a family demand could be family risks for adverse childhood experiences such as low income and high conflict and negative communication styles.

McCubbin and Patterson's (1982) extended Hill's work to include an adaptation phase (i.e., postcrisis stage) that emphasizes variability in family's ability to recover when there is a pile of stressors, the need of new resources, redefinition of the stressful event, and outcomes on family's coping strategies (the double ABCX model). The degree of crisis is dependent on how vulnerable the family is and the family's regenerative/recovery power(s) (Daneshpour, 2017). In other words, families may change or resist change depending on their capabilities or resources (i.e., "tangible and psychosocial resources (what the family has) and coping behaviors (what the family does)") and their perceptions or definitions of the stressors (Daneshpour, 2017, p. 4). Capabilities have also been referred to as protective factors or family strengths (Patterson, 2002). Examples of family protective processes include family cohesiveness and degree of flexibility, family communication, and family meanings (Patterson, 2002). Family demands and capabilities can emerge from the individual, family, community, and sociocultural contexts (Patterson, 2002).

Family vulnerability and regenerative power vary across families that withstand stress and recover from crisis and those that do not (McCubbin & Patterson, 1983). A crisis state is usually inevitable when families are unable to adapt positively to the stressors that caused the change and hence need further help within or outside the family system. Family adaptation to stressful events can also be influenced by family ambiguous loss in boundaries and roles (Boss, 2016).

Family resilience is key concept in conceptualizing family stress and coping. It has been embedded within the family adjustment and adaptation response (FAAR) model (Patterson, 1988, 2002). The term *resilience* is referred to as the ability to withstand and rebound from crisis and adversity (Walsh, 1996, 2006, 2011). This is an important concept that goes beyond the articulation of families' immediate responses to demands in the original theorization of family crisis and adjustment to the inclusion of how families deal with the long-term aftermath of chronic illnesses (Walsh, 1996). The key assumption in this perspective is that families have potential to rebound in the midst of adversities if they demonstrate healthier models of dealing with the demand of a challenge at hand (Walsh, 1996).

Theorists, using a resilience perspective, assume that every family is unique on how it deals with family demands; thus, there is no one size fits all pathway (Walsh, 1996). Family relational resilience is important when it comes to family-level assessment and intervention (Patterson, 2002; Walsh, 1996). Patterson (2002) conceptualized family-level ecological outcomes using the family core family functions as key outcomes for assessing family competence in being resilient (i.e., whether the family meets or does not meet the membership and family formation, economic support, nurturance, education, socialization, and protection of vulnerable members functions or individual family members and society). Furthermore, healthy family functions that incorporate routines, rituals, and beliefs that guide behavior and meaning making are important for promoting family resilience and positive health outcomes (Fiese & Hammons, 2013).

How families perceive, appraise, or construct meanings to the life demands and capabilities matters to family stress, coping, and adaptation theorists (Lazarus, 1966; Lazarus & Folkman, 1984; Patterson & Garwick, 1994). Thus, a family's definition, perception, or meaning of a family stressful event is essential in understanding family adaptation because it influences how families cope (Patterson, 2002), adopt self-care behaviors, and ultimately be resilient (Baker & Stern, 1993). Compared to resources, perceptions have been identified as good predictors of which families manage high stress and which ones fall into crisis (Boss, 1992). Family scholars have studied ways families develop meaning of a stressful event, such as diagnosis of a chronic illness and their capability of managing a chronic illness by utilizing symbolic interactionist and constructive lenses (Knyahnytska, 2014). The symbolic interaction perspective pioneered by George Herbert Mead (1934) has been instrumental in facilitating the theorizing family processes and actions of family perceptions in family communication, family decision-making, family role enactment, and socialization. Of recent interest in *family health* and the health care is the application of the symbolic interaction perspective to understand trust through patient–clinician interactions and communication in health care encounters to build trusting relationships (Elwood, 2023; Knyahnytska, 2014;

Shattell, 2004). Likewise, stressful events can be conceptualized in many ways: (a) situational meanings, (b) family identity, and (c) family worldview. Situational meaning refers to the "individual's and family's subjective definitions of their demands, their capabilities, and of these two factors relative to each other" (Patterson & Garwick, 1994, p. 5). Family identity meaning refers to how families view themselves (family structure and functioning) in relation to demands and capabilities. Lastly, the family worldview is conceptualized as the family's orientation toward the outside world, "how they interpret reality, what their core assumptions are about their environment, as well as their existential beliefs, such as the family's purpose in life" (Patterson & Garwick, 1994, p. 5). Family shared meanings are constructed through interactions between family members and within a family–health care provider interaction (Meiers & Brauer, 2008).

The evidence in relation to family coping in family stress and coping theory is derived from a continuous cyclical transactional process. The theory of stress and coping by Lazarus and Folkman (1984) conceptualizes coping as a cognitive appraisal process of psychological stress, which includes primary appraisal (meaning making) and secondary appraisal (what can be done). Problem-focused (directly aimed to manage the stressor) and emotion-focused (aimed to regulate arising emotions) coping actions are enacted when a situation is primarily appraised as a stressful. Lazarus and Folkman's work has evolved, and new ways of categorizing coping behaviors have emerged. For example, Skinner et al. (2003) conceptualized family adaptive functions, which entail developing competence (ability), relatedness (reliance onto others), and autonomy (preference within available options) as coping behaviors and strategies for problem solving or information seeking across different contexts. Anticipatory, preventative, and proactive coping strategies have been emphasized in improving health targets and strategies to minimize stressors (Cooper & Quick, 2017).

Most important is the emphasis of a strengths-based perspective that it is patient, family, and resource centered as opposed to a deficit-based thinking approach. Strength-based approaches posit that family systems have valuable skills and experiences to manage demands or difficulties in family nursing and *family health* care. The key values that inform strengths-based practice are summarized as "health and healing, uniqueness, holism/embodiment, subjective reality/created meaning, person-environment integral, self-determination, learning-readiness-timing, and collaborative partnership" (Gottlieb & Gottlieb, 2017, p. 323). A strength-based perspective has the potential to increase positive involvement, confidence in roles, stability, relationship, resilience, and well-being at individual/family and community/population levels. At the organizational level, a strength-based approach may increase value, reduce cost, and increase positive adaptability, patient and staff satisfactions, and provider well-being. Key constructs are family stress and coping theories and are summarized in Table 2.7.

TABLE 2.7 **Key Constructs in Family Stress and Coping Theories**

Constructs	Definition
Family System	The whole family unit of analysis
Family Resilience	The capacity of a family to successfully manage challenging life circumstances (Walsh, 1996) Characteristics, dimensions, and properties of families that help families be resistant to disruption in the face of change and adaptive in the face of crises (McCubbin & McCubbin, 1988)
Family Demands	Comprise (a) normative and nonnormative stressors (discrete events of change); (b) ongoing family strains (unresolved, insidious tensions); and (c) daily hassles (minor disruptions of daily life)
Family Capabilities	Include (a) tangible and psychosocial resources (what the family has) and (b) coping behaviors (what the family does)
Family (Shared) Meanings	The interpretations, images, and views that have been collectively constructed by family members as they interact with each other; as they share time, space, and life experiences; and as they talk with each other and dialogue about these experiences
Family Adjustment/Adaptation	A process of restoring balance between capabilities and demands at two levels of transaction: (a) between family members and the family unit and (b) between a family unit and the community
Family Stressor Event	Life events or occurrences of sufficient magnitude to bring about change in the family systems
Family Crisis	A period of significant disequilibrium, disorganization, and disruptiveness in the family (Patterson, 2002)
Family Boundary Ambiguity	Family not knowing who is in and who is out of the system; a state in which family members are uncertain in their perception about who is in or out of the family and who is performing what roles and tasks within the family system
Interaction	A social behavior between the two or more people in which certain types of communication (verbal and nonverbal) occur so that each person responds to the situation and changes their behavior as a result (Burr et al., 1979)

Limitations

Family stress and theories are without limitations despite their capability as middle-range theories. Generalizations of the theoretical approaches have limitations due to conceptual diversities on how stress, stressors, and coping strategies are perceived and how constructs are measured across settings and time (Folkman, 2011).

Conclusion

Understanding the foundation of *family health* theories is vital in the 21st-century public health efforts. This chapter provided knowledge on how different *family health* theoretical perspectives contribute unique insights regarding conceptual underpinnings of health and illness at the family level. Although an integrated *family health* theoretical model is lacking (Fiese & Hammon, 2014), the theories discussed, shed light on key general concepts and constructs that are important to family and *family health* care. The theories provide valuable theoretical compliments that offer great insights into practice (i.e., assessment and intervention), research, and policy targets for health and illness within in the immediate family environment (e.g., family subsystems, family relational resilience, family risks and protective factors, family roles and decision-making, beliefs, routines, health-promotion behaviors, etc.), the healthcare system, and the broader environment. The information shared in this chapter provided the foundational aspects of understanding the importance of the role of social determinants of health, patient and family engagement, interprofessional education and practice, and more.

Suggested Websites

Family health model: https://internationalfamilynursing.org/2015/01/30/family-health-model/
Neuman's systems model: https://nursology.net/nurse-theories/neumans-systems-model/
The National Institute on Minority Health and Health Disparities' (NIMHD) minority health and health disparities research framework: https://www.nimhd.nih.gov/about/overview/research-framework/
The Bowen Center for the Study of the Family: https://www.thebowencenter.org/

Suggested Readings

General Theoretical Perspectives

Barton, A. W., & Bishop, R. C. (2014). Paradigms, processes, and values in family research. *Journal of Family Theory & Review, 6*(3), 241–256.

Burr, X. V. R., Hill, R., Nyc, F. L., & Reiss, I. L. (1979). *Contemporary theories about the family* (Vol. 2). The Free Press.

Doherty, W. J. (1991). Family theory and *family health* research: Understanding the *family health* and illness cycle. *Canadian Family Physician, 37*, 2423–2428.

Fawcett, J. (1984). The metaparadigm of nursing: Present status and future refinements. *The Journal of Nursing Scholarship, 16*(3), 84–87.

Kerry. D. (2003). Family theory versus the theories families live by. *Journal of Marriage and Family, 65*(4), 771–784.

Ecological Perspectives

Bronfenbrenner, U. (1977). Toward an experimental ecology of human development. *American Psychologist, 32*(7), 513–531.

Bronfenbrenner, U. (1979). *The ecology of human development: Experiments by nature and design.* Harvard University Press.

National Institute on Minority Health and Health Disparities. (2017). *NIMHD research framework.* https://nimhd.nih.gov/researchFramework

System Perspectives

Anderson, K. H. (2000). The *family health* system approach to family systems nursing. *Journal of Family Nursing, 6*(2), 103–119.

Bornstein, M. H., & Sawyer, J. (2006). Family systems. In K. McCartney & D. Phillips (Eds.), *Blackwell handbook of early childhood development* (pp. 381–398). Blackwell. https://doi.org/10.1002/9780470757703.ch19

Johnson, B. E., & Ray, W. A. (2016). Family systems theory. In *Encyclopedia of Family Studies*, 1–5 John Wiley & Sons, Inc. DOI: 10.1002/9781119085621

Whitchurch, G. and Constantine, L. (1993) Systems Theory. In: Boss, P., Doherty, W., LaRossa, R., Schumm, W. and Tenmetz, S. (Eds.), *Sourcebook of Family Theories and Methods* (pp. 325–355). Plenum, New York, http://dx.doi.org/10.1007/978-0-387-85764-0_14

Developmental Perspectives

Dilworth-Anderson, P., & Burton, L. M. (1996). Rethinking family development: Critical conceptual issues in the study of diverse groups. *Journal of Social and Personal Relationships* , *13*(3), 325–334.

Duvall, E. M. (1988). Family development's first forty years. *Family Relations*, *37*, 127–134.

Scott. C, J., & Bradford, K. (2021). Multidimensional family development theory: A reconceptualization of family development. *Journal of Family Theory & Review*, *13*(2), 202–223.

Family Stress and Coping Perspectives

Boss, P. G. (1988). *Family stress management*. SAGE.

Boss, P., & Greenberg, J. (1984). Family boundary ambiguity: A new variable in family stress theory. *Family Process*, *23*(4), 535–546.

Hill, R. (1958). Generic features of families under stress. *Social Casework*, *39*,139–159.

Patterson, J. M., & Garwick, A. W. (1994). Levels of meaning in family stress theory. *Family Process*, *33*(3), 287–304.

Patterson, J. M. (2002). Integrating family resilience and family stress theory. *Journal of Marriage and Family*, *64*(2), 349–360.

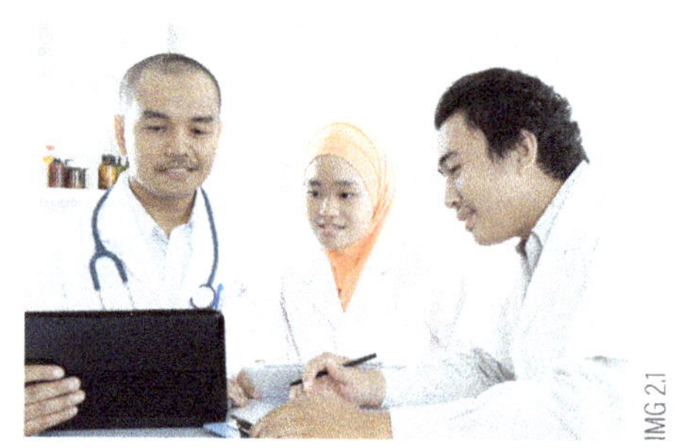

IMG 2.1

Reflection Questions

Think about a *family health* stressor (life health event) that you are interested in and reflect on these questions:

1. What is your philosophical perspective about this *family health* stressor (life health event)?
2. What question(s) would you ask to learn more about the *family health* stressor (life health event) if you were using a developmental perspective?
3. Why should care about interpersonal relationships when studying this *family health* (live health event) stressor?

References

Adabanya, U., Awosika, A., Moon, J. H., Reddy, Y. U., & Ugwuja, F. (2023). Changing a Community: A Holistic View of the Fundamental Human Needs and Their Public Health Impacts. *Cureus*, *15*(8), e44023. https://doi.org/10.7759/cureus.44023

Adibi, H. (2014). Health: Its Implications within the Biomedical and Social Models of Health—A Critical Review. *Cyber Journals: Multidisciplinary Journals of Science and Technology*, *4*(2), 16–23.

Afifi, T. D., Merrill, A. F., & Davis, S. M. (2014). Examining family secrets from a communication perspective. In L.Turner, & R. West (Eds.), *The Sage handbook of family communication* (pp. 169–183). Sage Publications.

Alderfer, M. A., & Stanley, C. M. (2012). Health and illness in the context of the family. In A. Baum, T. A. Revenson, & J. Singer (Eds.), *Handbook of health psychology* (pp. 493–516). Psychology Press.

Anderson, K. H. (2000). The *family health* system approach to family systems nursing. *Journal of family nursing, 6*(2), 103–119.

Baker, C., & Stern, P. N. (1993). Finding meaning in chronic illness as the key to self-care. *The Canadian journal of nursing research = Revue canadienne de recherche en sciences infirmieres, 25*(2), 23–36.

Barton, A. W., & Bishop, R. C. (2014). Paradigms, processes, and values in family research. *Journal of Family Theory & Review, 6*(3), 241–256.

Berkman, L. F., & Glass, T. (2000). Social integration, social networks, social support, and health. *Social epidemiology, 1*(6), 137–173.

Bengtson, V. L., Acock, A. C., Allen, K. R., Dilworth-Anderson, P., & Klein, D. M. (2005). Theory and Theorizing in Family Research: Puzzle Building and Puzzle Solving. In V. L. Bengtson, A. C. Acock, K. R. Allen, P. Dilworth-Anderson, & D. M. Klein (Eds.), *Sourcebook of family theory & research* (pp. 3–33). Sage Publications, Inc.

Black, P. B. (2014). *Professional Nursing: Concepts and Challenges* (7th ed.). Elsevier.

Bomar, P. J. (1989). *Nurses and family health promotion: Concepts, assessment, and interventions* (2nd ed.). Saunders.

Bonell, C., Ponsford, R., Meiksin, R., & Melendez-Torres, G. J. (2023). Testing and refining middle-range theory in evaluations of public-health interventions: Evidence from recent systematic reviews and trials. *J Epidemiol Community Health, 77*(3), 147–151.

Bornstein, M. H., & Sawyer, J. (2006). Family Systems. In K. McCartney & D. Phillips (Eds.), *Blackwell handbook of early childhood development* (pp. 381–398). Blackwell. https://doi.org/10.1002/9780470757703.ch19

Boss, P. (1992). Primacy of perception in family stress theory and measurement. *Journal of Family Psychology, 6*(2), 113–119. https://doi.org/10.1037/0893-3200.6.2.113

Boss, P. (1999). *Ambiguous loss: learning to live with unresolved grief.* Harvard University Press.

Boss, P. (2016). The context and process of theory development: The story of ambiguous loss. *Journal of Family Theory & Review, 8*(3), 269–286.

Boss, P., & Greenberg, J. (1984). Family boundary ambiguity: A new variable in family stress theory. *Family process, 23*(4), 535–546.

Bowleg, L. (2012). The problem with the phrase women and minorities: intersectionality—An important theoretical framework for public health. *American journal of public health, 102*(7), 1267–1273.

Brivio, F., Viganò, A., Paterna, A., Palena, N., & Greco, A. (2023). Narrative Review and Analysis of the Use of "Lifestyle" in Health Psychology. *International journal of environmental research and public health, 20*(5), 4427. https://doi.org/10.3390/ijerph20054427

Burr, W. R. (1973). Theory construction and the sociology of the family. Wiley.

Burr, X. V. R., Hill, R., Nyc, F. l., & Reiss, I. L (1979). *Contemporary theories about the family* (Vol. 2). The Free Press.

Carper, B. A. (2012). Fundamental patterns of knowing. In P. G. Reed & N. C. Shearer (Eds.), *Perspectives on nursing theory* (6th ed., pp. 139–148). Wolters Kluwer Health / Lippincott Williams & Wilkins

Cashion, A. K., Gill, J., Hawes, R., Henderson, W. A., & Saligan, L. (2016). National Institutes of Health symptom science model sheds light on patient symptoms. *Nursing Outlook, 64*(5), 499–506. https://doi.org/10.1016/j.outlook.2016.05.008

Çetin, Ş., & Varma, G. S. (2021). Somatic symptom disorder: Historical process and biopsychosocial approach. *Psikiyatride Guncel Yaklasimlar, 13*(4), 790–804.

Chinn, P. L., Kramer, M. K., & Sitzman, K. (2021). *Knowledge development in nursing e-book: Theory and process.* Elsevier Health Sciences.

Cooper, C., & Quick, J. C. (Eds.). (2017). *The handbook of stress and health: A guide to research and practice*. Wiley.

Daneshpour, M. (2017). Examining family stress: Theory and research. *Quarterly of Clinical Psychology Studies, 28*, 1–7.

Danielson, C. B., Hamel-Bissell, B., & Winstead-Fry, P. (1993). *Families, health & illness: Perspectives on coping and intervention*. Mosby.

Denham, S. A. (2003). Relationships between family rituals, family routines, and health. *Journal of Family Nursing, 9*(3), 305–330.

Dodd, M., Janson, S., Facione, N., Faucett, J., Froelicher, E. S., Humphreys, J., ... & Taylor, D. (2001). Advancing the science of symptom management. *Journal of advanced nursing, 33*(5), 668–676.

Doherty W. J. (1991). Family Theory and *Family Health* Research: Understanding the *family health* and illness cycle. *Canadian family physician, 37*, 2423–2428.

Doherty, W. J., & McCubbin, H. I. (1985). Families and health care: An emerging arena of theory, research, and clinical intervention. *Family Relations: An Interdisciplinary Journal of Applied Family Studies, 34*(1), 5–11. https://doi.org/10.2307/583751

Doane, G. H. (2002). In the spirit of creativity: The learning and teaching of ethics in nursing. *Journal of Advanced Nursing, 39*(6), 521–528.

Dilworth-Anderson, P., & Burton, L. M. (1996). Rethinking family development: Critical conceptual issues in the study of diverse groups. *Journal of Social and Personal, 13*(3), 325–334.

Duvall, E. M. (1988). Family development's first forty years. *Family Relations, 37*, 127–134.

Elwood W. N. (2023). Trust as a dyadic mechanism of action: a call to explore patient-provider relationships in the twenty-first century. *Journal of communication in healthcare, 16*(4), 370–374. https://doi.org/10.1080/17538068.2023.2267830

Engel, G. L. (1977). The need for a new medical model: A challenge for biomedicine. *Science, 196*(4286), 129–136.

Eustace, R. W. (2022). A Theory of *Family Health*: A Neuman's Systems Perspective. *Nursing Science Quarterly, 35*(1), 101–110.

Evans, R. G., Barer, M. L., & Marmor, T. R. (Eds.). (2021). *Why are some people healthy and others not? The determinants of health of populations*. Walter de Gruyter.

Evashwick C. (1989). Creating the continuum of care. *Health Matrix, 7*(1), 30–39.

Facio, F. M., Feero, W. G., Linn, A., Oden, N., Manickam, K., & Biesecker, L. G. (2010). Validation of My *Family Health* Portrait for six common heritable conditions. *Genetics in Medicine, 12*(6), 370–375.

Fine, M. A., & Fincham, F. D. (Eds.). (2013). *Handbook of family theories: A content-based approach*. Routledge.

Fiese, B. H., & Hammons, A. (2013). Theories of *family health*: An integrative perspective and look towards the future. In M. A. Fine & F. D. Fincham (Eds.), *Handbook of family theories: A content-based approach* (pp. 398–416). Routledge/Taylor & Francis Group.

Fawcett, J. (1984). The metaparadigm of nursing: Present status and future refinements. *The journal of nursing scholarship, 16*(3), 84–87.

Fawcett, J. T. (1989). Networks, linkages, and migration systems. *International migration review, 23*(3), 671–680.

Fawcett, J. (2000). *Analysis and evaluation of contemporary nursing knowledge: Nursing models and theories*. F. A. Davis.

Fawcett, J. (2005). Contemporary nursing knowledge: Analysis and evaluation of nursing models and theories (2nd ed.). F. A. Davis.

Fawcett, J. (2023, January 14). Evolution of One Version of Our Disciplinary Metaparadigm. *Nursology*. https://nursology.net/2023/01/17/evolution-of-one-version-of-our-disciplinary-metaparadigm/

Gavazzi, S. M., & Lim, J. Y. (2023). Family systems theory. In R. J. R. Levesque Editor, *Families with Adolescents: Bridging the Gaps Between Theory, Research, and Practice* (pp. 35–45). Springer.

Gottlieb, L. N., & Gottlieb, B. (2017). Strengths-based nursing: A process for implementing a philosophy into practice. *Journal of family nursing, 23*(3), 319–340.

Hansen, D, A., & Johnson, V. A. (1979). Rethinking family stress theory: Definitional aspects. In W. Burr, R. Hill, F. Nye, & I. Reiss (Eds.), *Contemporary Theories About the Family* (Vol. 1, pp. 582–603). The Free Press.

Hartweg, D. L., & Metcalfe, S. A. (2022). Orem's self-care deficit nursing theory: Relevance and need for refinement. *Nursing science quarterly, 35*(1), 70–76.

Henningsen, P. (2018). Management of somatic symptom disorder. *Dialogues in clinical neuroscience, 20*(1), 23–31.

Higgins, P. A., & Moore, S. M. (2000), Levels of theoretical thinking in nursing. *Nursing Outlook, 48*(4), 179–183.

Hill, R. (1949). *Families Under Stress.* Harper and Row.

Hill, R. (1958). Generic features of families under stress. *Soc Casework, 39*, 139–159.

Hutchison, E. D. (2018). *Dimensions of human behavior: The changing life course* (6th ed.). SAGE.

Jabareen, Y. (2009). Building a conceptual framework: Philosophy, definitions, and procedure. *International journal of qualitative methods, 8*(4), 49–62.

Jones, N. L., Gilman, S. E., Cheng, T. L., Drury, S. S., Hill, C. V., & Geronimus, A. T. (2019). Life course approaches to the causes of health disparities. *American journal of public health, 109*(S1), S48–S55.

Johnson, B. E., & Ray, W. A. (2016). Family systems theory. In *Encyclopedia of Family Studies*, 1–5 John Wiley & Sons, Inc. DOI: 10.1002/9781119085621

Kerr, M. E., & Bowen, M. (1988). *Family evaluation.* Norton.

Kerry, D. (2003). Family theory versus the theories families live by. *Journal of Marriage and Family, 65*(4), 771–784.

Khan, H. A. (2003). On paradigms, theories and models. *Problemas del Desarrollo, 34*(134), 149–155.

Kivunja, C. (2018). Distinguishing between theory, theoretical framework, and conceptual framework: A systematic review of lessons from the field. *International journal of higher education, 7*(6), 44–53.

King, D. W., Hurd, T. C., Hajek, R. A., & Jones, L. A. (2009). Using a biopsychosocial approach to address health disparities—One person's vision. *J Cancer Educ.*, 24(2), S26–S32. https://doi.org/10.1080/08858190903412091

Knyahnytska, Y. (2014). Looking through a different window: Chronic disease management in public health. Application of symbolic interactionism and institutional ethnography. *The Qualitative Report, 19*(21), 1–9.

Landstedt, E., Hammarström, A., & Winefield, H. (2015). How well do parental and peer relationships in adolescence predict health in adulthood? *Scandinavian journal of public health, 43*(5), 460–468.

Lazarus, R. S. (1996). The role of coping in the emotions and how coping changes over the life course. In C. Magai & S. H. McFadden (Eds). *Handbook of emotion, adult development, and aging* (pp. 289-306). Academic Press.

Lazarus, R. S., & Folkman, S. (1984). *Stress, appraisal, and coping.* Springer.

Lenz, E. R., Pugh, L. C., Milligan, R. A., Gift, A., & & Suppe, F. (1997). The middle-range theory of unpleasant symptoms: An update. *Advances in Nursing Science, 19*, 14–27.

Litman T. J. (1974). The family as a basic unit in health and medical care: A social-behavioral overview. *Social science & medicine, 8*(9–10), 495–519. https://doi.org/10.1016/0037-7856(74)90072-9

McBryde-Foster, M., & Allen, T. (2005). The continuum of care: A concept development study. *Journal of Advanced Nursing, 50*(6), 624–632.

McCubbin, H. I., & McCubbin, M. A. (1988). Typologies of resilient families: Emerging roles of social class and ethnicity. *Family relations, 37* (3), 247–254.

McCubbin, H. I., & Patterson, J. M. (1982). The family stress process: The Double ABCX Model of adjustment and adaptation. In H. I. McCubbin, A. E., Cauble, & J. M. Patterson (Eds.), *Family stress, coping, and social support* (pp. 169–188). Haworth Press.

McCubbin, H. I., & Patterson, J. M. (1983). Family transitions: Adaptation to stress. In H. I. McCubbin & C. R. Figley (Eds.), *Stress and the family: Vol. 1. Coping with normative transitions* (pp. 5–25). Brunner/Mazel.

Mead, G. H. (1934). *Mind, self, and society* (Vol. 111). The University of Chicago Press.

Meiers, S. J., & Brauer, D. J. (2008). Existential caring in the *family health* experience: A proposed conceptualization. *Scandinavian Journal of Caring Sciences, 22*(1), 110–117.

Minuchin, S., Baker, L., Rosman, B. L., Liebman, R., Milman, L., & Todd, T. C. (1975). A conceptual model of psychosomatic illness in children: Family organization and family therapy. *Archives of general psychiatry, 32*(8), 1031–1038.

Monti, E. J., & Tingen, M. S. (1999). Multiple paradigms of nursing science. *Advanced Nursing Science,* 21(4), 64–80. http://journals.lww.com/advancesinnursingscience/

Muskin, P. R. (2021, August). *What is Somatic Symptom Disorder?* American Psychiatric Association. https://www.psychiatry.org/patients-families/somatic-symptom-disorder/what-is-somatic-symptom-disorder

National Cancer Institute. (2017). *Theory at a glance: A guide for health promotion practice* (2nd ed). U.S. Department of Health and Human Services, National Institute on Minority Health and Health Disparities.

Naveen, K. (2010). Abraham Maslow (1908–1970). *Archives of Mental Health, 11*(1), 31–32.

Neuman, B. (1983). *Family intervention using the Betty Neuman health care systems model.* In I. W. Clements & F. B. Roberts (Eds.), *Family health: A theoretical approach to nursing care* (pp. 239–254). Wiley.

Neuman, B. (2011). The Neuman systems model. In B. Neuman & J. Fawcett (Eds.), *The Neuman systems model* (5th ed., pp. 3–33). Pearson.

Neuman, B., & Fawcett, J. (Eds.). (2011). *The Neuman systems model* (5th ed.). Pearson.

Nightingale, F. (1992). *Notes on nursing: What it is, and what it is not.* Lippincott Williams & Wilkins.

Orem, D. (2001). Nursing: Concepts of practice. Mosby Year Book.

Page, G. G., Corwin, E. J., Dorsey, S. G., Redeker, N. S., McCloskey, D. J., Austin, J. K., ... & Grady, P. (2018). Biomarkers as common data elements for symptom and self-management science. *Journal of Nursing Scholarship, 50*(3), 276–286.

Patterson, J. M. (1988). Families experiencing stress: I. The Family Adjustment and Adaptation Response Model: II. Applying the FAAR Model to health-related issues for intervention and research. *Family systems medicine, 6*(2), 202–237.

Patterson, J. M. (2002). Integrating family resilience and family stress theory. *Journal of marriage and family, 64*(2), 349–360.

Patterson, J. M., & Garwick, A. W. (1994). Levels of meaning in family stress theory. *Family process, 33*(3), 287–304.

Pauline, B., & Boss, P. (2009). *Ambiguous loss: Learning to live with unresolved grief.* Harvard University Press.

Rocca, E., & Anjum, R. L. (2020). Complexity, Reductionism and the Biomedical Model. In R. L. Anjum, S. Copeland, & E. Rocca (Eds.), *Rethinking Causality, Complexity and Evidence for the Unique Patient.* Springer. https://doi.org/10.1007/978-3-030-41239-5_5

Rolland, J. S. (1984). Toward a psychosocial typology of chronic and life-threatening illness. *Family Systems Medicine, 2*(3), 245–262. https://doi.org/10.1037/h0091663

Rolland, J. S. (1987). Chronic illness and the life cycle: A conceptual framework. *Family Process, 26*(2), 203–221.

Selanders, L. C. (1998). The power of environmental adaptation: Florence Nightingale's original theory for nursing practice. *Journal of Holistic Nursing, 16*(2), 247–263.

Sharma, R. (2013). The family and family structure classification redefined for the current times. *Journal of family medicine and primary care, 2*(4), 306–310.

Shattell, M. (2004). Nurse–patient interaction: A review of the literature. *Journal of clinical nursing, 13*(6), 714–722.

Shwed, J. A. (1982). *An empirical investigation of the micro dimensions of a social ecological model for health status, health behavior, and illness behavior.* The Ohio State University Press.

Skinner, E. A., Edge, K., Altman, J., & Sherwood, H. (2003). Searching for the structure of coping: A review and critique of category systems for classifying ways of coping.*Psychological Bulletin, 129*(2), 216–269. https://doi.org/10.1037/0033-2909.129.2.216

Smilkstein, G. (1984). The physician and family function assessment. *Family Systems Medicine, 2*(3), 263–278. https://doi.org/10.1037/h0091661

Taylor, L., & Seager, M. (2021). Maslow revised: How COVID-19 highlights a circle of needs, not a hierarchy. *Psychreg Journal of Psychology, 5*, 115–127.

Thomas, P. A., Liu, H., & Umberson, D. (2017). Family Relationships and Well-Being. *Innovation in aging, 1*(3), igx025. https://doi.org/10.1093/geroni/igx025

Thompson, L., & Walker, A. J. (1982). The dyad as the unit of analysis: Conceptual and methodological issues. *Journal of Marriage and the Family, 44*(4), 889–900.

Tramonti, F., Giorgi, F., & Fanali, A. (2021). Systems thinking and the biopsychosocial approach: A multilevel framework for patient-centred care. *Systems Research and Behavioral Science, 38*(2), 215–230.

Von Bertalanffy, L. (1972). The history and status of general systems theory. *Academy of management journal, 15*(4), 407–426.

Uchino, B. N. (2006). Social support and health: A review of physiological processes potentially underlying links to disease outcomes. *Journal of behavioral medicine, 29*, 377–387.

Walsh, F. (1996). The concept of family resilience: Crisis and challenge. *Family Process, 35*(3), 261–281.

Walsh, F. (2006). Strengthening family resilience (2nd ed.). Guilford.

Walsh, F. (2011). Family resilience: A collaborative approach in response to stressful life challenges. *Resilience and mental health: Challenges across the lifespan, 12*, 149–161.

Weaver, K., & Olson, J. K. (2006). Understanding paradigms used for nursing research. *Journal of Advanced Nursing, 53*(4), 459–469. https://doi.org/10.1111/j.1365-2648.2006.03740.x

Weiss-Laxer, N. S., Crandall, A., Hughes, M. E., & Riley, A. W. (2020). Families as a cornerstone in 21st century public health: Recommendations for research, education, policy, and practice. *Frontiers in Public Health, 8*, 503.

Wendel, M. L., Garney, W. R., & McLeroy, K. R. (2015). Ecological approaches. *American Journal of Public Health, 86*, 674–677.

Whitchurch, G. G., & Constantine, L. L. (1993). Systems theory. In P.Boss, W.J. Doherty, R. LaRossa, W. R. Schumm & S. K, Steinmetz. (Eds.) *Sourcebook of family theories and methods: A contextual approach* (pp. 325–355). Springer.

World Health Organization. (2020). *What do we mean by self-care? Sexual and reproductive health.* https://www.who.int/reproductivehealth/self-care-interventions/definitions/en/

World Health Organization. (2024, February 1). *Self-care interventions for health.* https://www.who.int/health-topics/self-care#tab=tab_1

Wright, L. M., & Leahey, M. (2013). *Nurses and families: A guide to family assessment and intervention* (6th ed.). F.A. Davis.

Xiao, X., Song, H., Sang, T., Wu, Z., Xie, Y., & Yang, Q. (2021). Analysis of Real-World Implementation of the Biopsychosocial Approach to Healthcare: Evidence from a Combination of Qualitative and Quantitative Methods. *Frontiers in Psychiatry, 12*, 725596.

Figure credit

CHAPTER 3

Social Determinants of Family Health

Realize that everything connects to everything else.

—Leonardo da Vinci

Learning Objectives

By the end of this chapter, learners will do the following:

- Describe the meaning of social determinants of health (SDoH).
- Describe the characteristics of a healthy family and healthy community.
- Describe *family health* as an upstream social determinant of health.
- Compare and contrast *population health* data across local, regional, national, and global levels to determine patterns of disease burden and health disparities.
- Demonstrate an understanding of ways to integrate the Maslow's hierarchy of needs model and social determinants of *family health* within the 4HEALTH context, namely *individual health*, *family health*, *population health*, and public health.

Before you read on, consider the following questions:

- What are the characteristics of a healthy family?
- What life challenges/stressors/disturbances within and outside the family systems influence a health family?
- Is family a determinant of health and illness?
- Is health and Illness a determinant of *family health*?
- Which factors protect *family health*, and which factors harm *family health*?
- How are *family health* measures as a *population health* indicator?

Biologically, human body cells progress through a normal wear-and-tear process due to natural aging (Prake & Yeo, 2013). Subsequently, in the natural form, the aging body reaches the final stage of growth of "timely" or "natural" death. Unfortunately, for many individuals, timely deaths due to aging are not always achievable due to other genetic and contextual factors influencing the pace of wear-and-tear processes resulting in premature deaths, living with chronic diseases and disabilities, or being at risk for health problems. Human-related illnesses/diseases (i.e., acute or chronic illness/disease, communicable or noncommunicable [see definitions in Table 3.4]) triggered by genetics or environmental factors can cause abnormal progressive damage to human bodies, resulting in premature deaths or disabilities. In addition, family genetics can cause diseases such cancers, diabetes, and cardiovascular diseases (IOM, 2006). Similarly, environmental factors such as COVID-19, war, unsafe drinking water, or family life stressors can cause health insufficiencies, resulting in premature death or sickening from acute and chronic illness and/or living with a disability. These factors affect how individuals, families, and communities/populations thrive and survive within and outside health systems. Consequently, there has been much interest in the scientific communities uncovering the causes of health and illness/disability and death at the local, national, and international levels. The purpose of this chapter is to provide a basic understanding of social determinants of health (SDoH) and how the determinants can be translated in *family health* care within the broader perspective of the 4HEALTH framework.

Determinants of Health and SDoH Defined

Population health is influenced by many factors, collectively known as the *determinants of health*, that contribute to the development of chronic illnesses and global mortality. These determinants are categorized as medical (genetics), behavior, environmental and physical influences, medical care, and social factors (Centers for Disease Control and Prevention [CDC], 2019). For example, genetics determine one's life span, healthiness, and the likelihood of developing certain disorders caused by either gene mutation, a combination of gene mutations and environmental factors, or damaged chromosomes (National Human Genome Research Institute [NHGRI], 2018). Sickle cell disease, an inherited disease from parents, is a prime example of a genetic disease. Environmental determinants that account for population deaths include exposure to air pollution (including indoor smoke and occupational exposure; 14%), tobacco smoking and second-hand smoke (13%), high plasma levels of sodium (6%), and high consumption of alcohol (5%; Lim, 2012).

With the culture shifting from a biomedical approach of health care to a biopsychosocial model (discussed in the previous chapter), there has been a growing interest on studying the nonmedical determinants, referred to as the *social determinants of health* (SDoH). By definition, SDoH are defined as conditions in which people are born, grow, work, live, worship and age and the wider set of forces and systems shaping the conditions of daily life (Office of Disease Prevention and Health Promotion, n.d.; WHO, 2024). The SDoH account for between 30%–55% of health outcomes (WHO, 2023). In the United States, traditional medical care accounts for about 10%–20% of modifiable contributors compared to 80%–90% accounted for SDoH (Hood et al., 2016). In the United States, SDoH are categorized in five major domains: economic stability, education access and quality, health care access and quality, neighborhood and built environment, and social and community contexts. The goal of health systems and related systems around the world is to address

SDoH is to achieve health equity, eliminate health disparities, and improve health for all, especially the most vulnerable (Office of Disease Prevention and Health Promotion, n.d.; WHO, 2024). *Health equity* is "the attainment of the highest level of health for all people. Achieving health equity requires valuing everyone equally with focused and ongoing societal efforts to address avoidable inequalities, historical and contemporary injustices, and the elimination of health and health care disparities" (Healthy People 2030, 2022 para. 1). *Health disparity* is defined as "a particular type of health difference that is closely linked with social, economic, and/or environmental disadvantage. The health disparity adversely affected groups include racial or ethnic groups; religion; socioeconomic status; gender; age; mental health; cognitive, sensory, or physical disability; sexual orientation or gender identity; geographic location; or other characteristics historically linked to discrimination or exclusion" (Healthy People 2030, 2022, para. 1).

Other terminologies used to conceptualize SDoH include *upstream*, *midstream*, and *downstream* determinants. Upstream determinants are SDoH that affect community health in a broader way across race and locations (Ray et al., 2023). Examples include socioeconomic, cultural, and political factors such as education and income disparities, discrimination, and social marginalization (Castrucci & Auerbach, 2019). Midstream determinants are SDoH that represent individual and family social needs that affect one's health. These include homelessness, food insecurities, poor access to education and health, and trauma (Castrucci & Auerbach, 2019). Downstream determinants are related

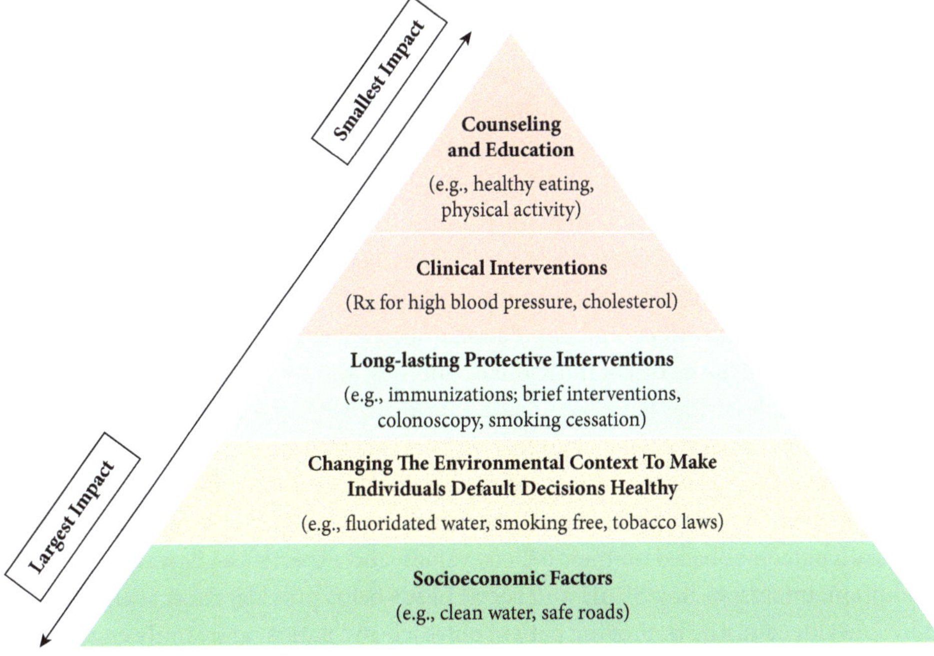

FIGURE 3.1 CDC public health interventions health impact pyramid (Frieden, 2010).

to the provision of clinical care at the individual level, such as providing medical and health interventions, screening, and disease management (Castrucci & Auerbach, 2019).

According to the SDoH and social needs model (Castrucci & Auerbach, 2019), strategies used to address upstream determinants include improving community conditions through law, policies, and regulation tactics. Midstream strategies address individual and family social needs by using tactics that involve patient screening about social needs like housing and food access. The data generated is used to inform care and provide referrals. Downstream strategies include providing clinical needs, such as providing medical and health care interventions. Unfortunately, most of the evidence translated today on SDoH is focused on downstream strategies (Brownson et al., 2010). More effort is needed to design strategies to intervene with SDoH at the population and systems levels beyond individual and family point of care (Braveman et al., 2011). The CDC health impact pyramid (Frieden, 2010) has been proposed to facilitate a better understanding of the need to consider upstream strategies (see Figure 3.1).

Family Health as an Upstream Social Determinant of Health

Family health is considered an upstream context for health (Weiss-Laxer et al., 2020). In other words, the family is an essential setting for improving *population health* through activities that promote health, prevent diseases, facilitates early detection and treatment, and promotes coping with illness, injury, disability, and death. As discussed in Chapter 1, families provide a context for health, care and caring, intergenerational continuity, and connections (Weiss-Laxer et al., 2020). In addition, families are impacted by SDoH, and vice versa. For example, a family living with HIV and without health insurance maybe at increased risk for poor health due to lack of medication and lack of access to follow-up care. Likewise, a family with uncontrolled HIV status due to the mentioned SDoH is likely to live with poor health outcomes (e.g., quality of life or death). Hence, it is unrealistic to conceptualize *individual health* and *population health* determinants and outcomes without including the family unit as a contextual determinant of health. There has been substantial improvement in assessing SDoH through the lived experiences of individuals, families, and populations. Social needs and SDoH data are vital to assess and improve the health of individuals, families, and communities (Gottlieb et al., 2016). For example, strides have been made to prioritize SDoH for individual patients at the point of care as part of health systems investments (Magnan, 2017). The term *social needs* instead of SDoH is common at the point of care (Wilkinson & Marmot, 2003). Subjective indicators used include patients/clients' needs, health care decision-making, and health outcomes based on their beliefs, values, and experiences (Street et al., 2012). In addition, understanding SDoH and social needs helps providers and health systems address health equity by improving patient outreach and patient and family engagement efforts (Simon et al., 2020).

Of interest today is assessing the common family-level social determinant of health known as *adverse childhood experiences* (ACEs) that reduce health and increase health disparities across race, place, and class (McEwen & Gregerson, 2019). For instance, studies that examine the unique impact of home and community environments have demonstrated higher risk homes with increased ACEs (Giovanelli & Reynolds, 2021; Maguire-Jack et al., 2021). By definition, ACEs are "intense and frequent occurring traumatic events that occur in childhood (0–17 years) such as abuse, or neglect; violence between parents or caregivers; other kinds of serious household dysfunction such as alcohol and substance abuse; having a family member/peer attempt or die by suicide, incarceration, separation/divorce in families, and collective violence" (CDC, 2023; para 1). Every family is vulnerable for ACEs; however, some families are at increased risk depending on their life experiences within the broader socioecological contexts where people eat, live, pay, worship, learn, and age. If not prevented, cumulative stress from ACEs affects one's health and well-being in childhood and later in adult life as well as across generations.

According to the CDC (2023), effects from ACEs include increased "risks of injury, sexually transmitted infections, maternal and child health problems (including teen pregnancy, pregnancy complications, and fetal death), involvement in sex trafficking, and a wide range of chronic diseases that lead to death, such as cancer, diabetes, heart disease, and suicide" (para. 1). Likewise, among children, prolonged stress can affect brain development, immune systems and stress-response systems, making them vulnerable for poor attention span, decision-making and learning, and relationships; unstable work histories as adults; and depression throughout the life span, as well as further exposure to toxic stress related to discrimination and poverty (CDC, 2023). Figure 3.2 demonstrates how ACEs influence health and well-being throughout the life span.

Overall, measures of aggregated data at the point of care help determine prevention and intervention strategies to address SDoH, particularly among high-risk groups. For example, the measurement of ACEs has been in place at the point of care through an ACE index score. Unfortunately, a key barrier to the ACEs index score is that it does not

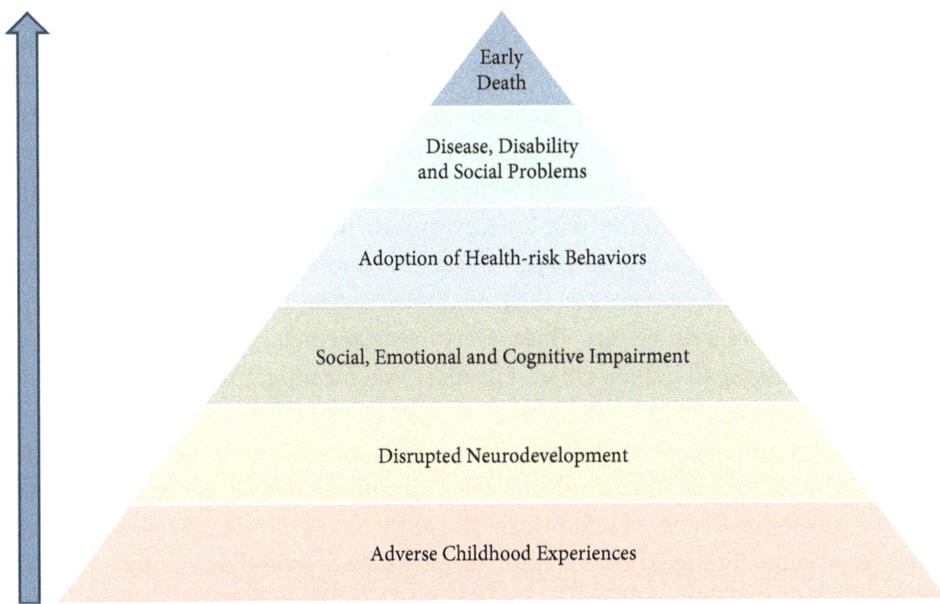

FIGURE 3.2 Mechanism by which ACEs influence health and well-being throughout the life span (CDC, 202a; Felitti et al., 1998).

capture the broader impacts to the populations affected (McEwen & Gregerson, 2019). For instance, studies that examine unique impact of home and community environments have demonstrated higher sociodemographic risk homes with increased ACEs (Giovanelli & Reynolds, 2021; Maguire-Jack et al., 2021).

Furthermore, SDoH mainly focus on individual and *population health* outcomes (National Academies of Sciences, Engineering, and Medicine, 2019). The lack of "family" in SDoH evidence (Deatrick, 2017) and lack of or minimal inclusion of the family and *family health* in the nation's *population health* goals and metrics is a public health concern (Weiss-Laxer et al., 2020).

It is unrealistic to conceptualize *individual health* and *population health* determinants and outcomes without including the family unit as a contextual determinant of health. Thus, it is important for *family health* professionals to have a basic understanding of how the available data on *population health* is of interest to *family health* within the boarder concepts of individual, population and public health contexts. *Population health* data facilitates the determination of *population health* trends and hence guiding prioritization of care and prevention efforts (Gottlieb et al., 2016). The next section discusses strategies that are useful in prioritizing *family health*-related SDoH targets and *population health* indicators within the 4HEALTH context.

Prioritizing SDoH and Social Needs in Family Health

Social and SDoH Needs

The traditional Maslow's hierarchy of needs (Naveen, 2010) is considered a promising basic foundational model that has the potential to identify and prioritize social needs and SDoH within individual/family, community, and systems-level determinants (Beran, 2014; Donaldson, 2018; Howell et al., 2023). The model postulates that individuals are motivated to achieve basic holistic needs cumulatively to reach their highest potential of health well-being or wellness. To do so, the individuals have to meet their physiological needs, safety needs, love, and belonging needs and esteem needs and finally achieve self-actualization. At the basic level, every individual needs to meet *physiological* needs (appropriate food, water, air as part of survival and well-being). Thereafter, *safety* needs that protect one from violence, theft, emotional instability, health insecurities, and financial insecurities must be met. Once safety needs are met, individuals feel the need for *love and belonging* to build a sense of purpose and meaning through positive social interactions and connections with intimate partners, family, friends, significant others, and professionals. In addition, once this need is met, *sense of esteem* needs that involve feeling respected, valued, and dignified as a person with confidence for personal growth and accomplishments need to be fulfilled to feel self-worth (*self-esteem*). Lastly are needs of self-improvement to maximize fulfillment (*self-actualization*), when the individual achieves a sense of awareness of being "healthy" and adopting a growth mind-set (Perry, 2024; see Figure 3.3).

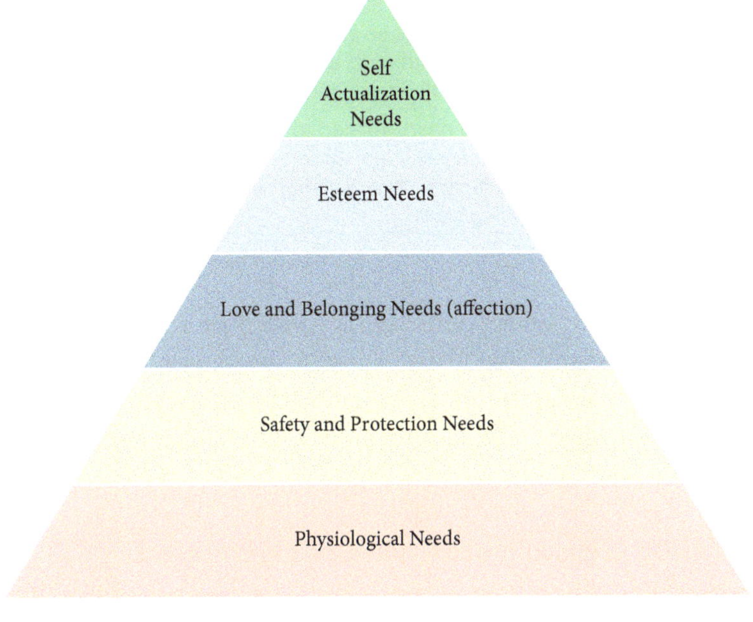

FIGURE 3.3 Maslow's hierarchy of needs.

Characteristics of a Health Family and Healthy Community

Maslow's hierarchy of needs can also be applied to *family health*. Although what constitutes a normal family varies, there is some consistency between basic Maslow needs and some evidence-based characteristics of a "healthy" functioning family (see Table 3.1).

TABLE 3.1 **Examples of Characteristics of a Healthy Family**

Family Function	Evidence-Based Characteristics
Affection	Has well-developed capacity for empathy and expression of affection; parents are devoted to each other, appreciate each other, have quality time together, are committed to family members For married couples, they have a strong marriage (shared power, intimacy, and cooperation), family closeness, and support; are open to share feelings (warmth, humor, and mutual concern), and promote intimacy and autonomy; develop a sense of trust; have a sense of play and humor, develop and maintain mutual nurturance, maintain an atmosphere of mutual respect, bond, develop a rounded sense of separateness and connectedness, show compassion, attend to other's needs
Socialization	Family presents with characteristics such as positive parental discipline encouragement and growth of all family members, positive spiritual well-being and good communication, strong problem-solving skills; meaningful participation of family members in activities outside the home, with a clear open systems view of the world, demonstrates clear boundaries (distinct roles with assertiveness), affirm and support one another, admits and seeks help with problems (ego strength), shares leisure time and prevents social loneliness

Economic	Families view hard work as a success , provides and allocates sufficient resources (financial, space and material) to meet basic needs of food, clothing, shelter, health care, and protections against danger. Also, family provides healthy financial literacy to its members.
Health Care Function	Family attends to needs related to *family health* promotion and disease prevention and disease management, coping with health issues needs in a balanced manner through effective self-care management and problem-solving skills

Sources: Gladding (1998); Friedman et al. (2003); Kaakinen et al. (2015)

Where families live, play, worship, learn, and age matters for health. Thus, understanding what a "healthy" community looks like is important for *family health*. Similar to healthy families, examples of characteristics and processes defining a healthy community mirror the basic needs in Maslow's model that are needed for self-improvement and self-actualization (see Table 3.2).

TABLE 3.2 **Healthy Community Characteristics and Processes**

Characteristics	Processes
Equity (lack of disparities)	Engage multisector participation
A strong economy and employment opportunities (lack of poverty)	Strong economy and employment opportunities
Access to health care and preventive health services	Employ environmental strategies
Housing/shelter	Use data to guide and measure efforts
Opportunities for active living	Inclusive, equitable, and broad community participation
Transportation	Collaboration between partners
Access to healthy food	The capacity to access and address its own health concerns
A stable, sustainable ecosystem and environment	Civic engagement
Safety	
Education	
An empowered population	
Healthy child development	
Healthy public policy	
Inclusive, equitable, and broad community participation	
Collaboration between partners	
The capacity to access and address its own health concerns	
Civic engagement	

The Role of Epidemiology in Family Health

Epidemiology is the "study of distribution and determinants of health-related states among specified populations and the application of that study to the control of health problems" (CDC, n.d). Knowledge in epidemiology of things such as key terms facilitates a better understanding of SDoH and intervention targets for relational care. Table 3.3 outlines some basic epidemiological terms used to describe the disease/illness burdens.

TABLE 3.3 **Definitions of Basic Epidemiological Terms**

Key Term	Definition
Health Indicator	A measure that reflects, or indicates, the state of health of persons in a defined population (e.g., the infant mortality rate).
Population	The total number of inhabitants of a given area or country. In sampling, the population may refer to the units from which the sample is drawn, not necessarily the total population of people.
High-Risk Group	A group in the community with an elevated risk of disease.
Mortality Rate	A measure of the frequency of occurrence of death in a defined population during a specified interval of time.
Infant Mortality Rate	A ratio expressing the number of deaths among children under 1 year of age reported during a given time period divided by the number of births reported during the same period. The infant mortality rate is usually expressed per 1,000 live births.
Morbidity	Any departure, subjective or objective, from a state of physiological or psychological well-being.
Prevalence	The number or proportion of cases or events or conditions in a given population.
Prevalence Rate	The proportion of persons in a population who have a particular disease or attribute at a specified point in time or over a specified period of time.
Incidence	The measurement of people who newly develop a disease within the subset of a given population
Incidence Rate	A measure of the frequency with which an event, such as a new case of illness, occurs in a population over a period of time. The denominator is the population at risk; the numerator is the number of new cases occurring during a given time.
Public Health Surveillance	The systematic collection, analysis, interpretation, and dissemination of health data on an ongoing basis to gain knowledge of the pattern of disease occurrence and potential in a community in order to control and prevent disease in the community.
Age-Adjusted Mortality Rate	A mortality rate statistically modified to eliminate the effect of different age distributions in the different populations.
Risk Factor	An aspect of personal behavior or lifestyle, an environmental exposure, or an inborn or inherited characteristic that is associated with an increased occurrence of disease or other health-related event or condition.
Years of Potential Life Lost	A measure of the impact of premature mortality on a population, calculated as the sum of the differences between some predetermined minimum or desired life span and the age of death for individuals who died earlier than that predetermined age.
Chronic diseases	Chronic diseases are defined broadly as conditions that last 1 year or more and require ongoing medical attention or limit activities of daily living or both (e.g., heart disease, cancer, diabetes, asthma)
Communicable Disease	An illness caused by an infectious agent or its toxins that occurs through the direct or indirect transmission of the infectious agent or its products from an infected individual or an animal, vector, or the inanimate environment to a susceptible animal or human host
Noncommunicable Diseases (NCDs)	Also known as chronic diseases; not passed from person to person. They are of long duration and generally slow progression.

Centers for Disease Control and Prevention, *Epidemiology Glossary*, Centers for Disease Control and Prevention, 2024.

Moreover, Maslow's needs model sheds light on the relationship among individual and *family health* needs, community/population needs, and public health needs (Warner et al., 2023), also known as the 4HEALTH context. Population-level data is needed to facilitate a better understanding of disease/illness/condition epidemiology and burdens that affect and are affected by *family health*. The population demographic, general health, and *population health* indicators are tracked and reported either locally at the county/state/district/regional/national/international levels. For example, Healthy People 2030 in the United States and the Canadian Institute for Health Information (CIHI) in Canada are examples of country-level data sources. The WHO has developed the Global Health Observatory as a global data resource. Other sources include vital statistic sources such as Census tracks and birth, death, disease registries. (See examples of data sources at the end of the chapter.) The Census tracks and population data have been useful in tracking family-related factors such as family size and family structure.

Tables 3.4 and 3.5 provide snapshots of how *population health* data facilitates the identification and understanding of family-level intervention targets to meet SDoH and social needs. Specifically, in Table 3.4 global data from the WHO website is used to present a snapshot of disease burdens and potential family intervention targets across diverse population groups of interest to *family health*. The intervention targets in Table 3.4 reflect the relational uniqueness of the role of family to health (i.e., contexts, care and caring, connections and continuity; Weiss et al., 2020).

TABLE 3.4 **Example of *Population Health* Indicators Across the Life Span**

Population Health	**Example of Health Indicator**	**Examples of Facts on a Global Burden for the World Health Organization Website**	**Examples of Family-Level Intervention Targets**
Preconception Health	Infertility	Infertility is a global health issue affecting millions of people of reproductive age worldwide. Available data as of 2023 suggests that globally one in six people experience infertility in their lifetime.	Family engagement Family therapy Family communication Family empowerment Pregnancy prevention Family shared decision-making Family self-care management
Neonate/Infant Health	Newborns survival and well-being	Globally, 2.4 million children died in the first month of life in 2019.	Family psychosocial Family-level educational and support Sibling Support Family engagement Family disease management Parent education *Family health* promotion and disease prevention Family therapy Parent education

<table>
<tr><td rowspan="5">Child Health</td><td>Childhood cancer</td><td>In 2020, almost 280,000 children and adolescents (aged 0–19 years) were diagnosed with cancer worldwide and almost 110,000 children died from cancer</td><td rowspan="6">Family Life Education
Family caregiver support
Family engagement
Family communication
Family empowerment
Family bereavement support
Family shared decision-making
Family self-care management</td></tr>
<tr><td>Child maltreatment</td><td>Nearly three in four children, or 300 million children, aged 2–4 years regularly suffer physical punishment and/or psychological violence at the hands of parents and caregivers.</td></tr>
<tr><td>Children survival and well-being</td><td>In 2019 an estimated 5.2 million children under 5 years died from preventable and treatable causes such as preterm birth complications, birth asphyxia/trauma, pneumonia, congenital anomalies, diarrhea and malaria.</td></tr>
<tr><td>Infant and young child feeding</td><td>Undernutrition is associated with 45% of child deaths.</td></tr>
<tr><td>Mortality among children aged 5–14 years</td><td>Almost 10 million children aged 5–14 years will die between 2019 and 2030.</td></tr>
<tr><td>Adolescence Health</td><td>Traffic injuries</td><td>Injuries (including road traffic injuries and drowning), interpersonal violence, self-harm, and maternal conditions are the leading causes of death among adolescents and young adults.</td></tr>
<tr><td>Women Health</td><td>Maternal mortality rates</td><td>Every day in 2020, almost 800 women died from preventable causes related to pregnancy and childbirth.</td><td rowspan="2">Family health promotion and disease prevention
Family support (spousal support)
Family engagement
Family life education
Family resource management
Family communication
Family bereavement support
Family shared decision-making
Family self-care management</td></tr>
<tr><td>Men Health</td><td>Cancer screenings</td><td>Overall, global health data is scarce for this population.
In Europe the data shows that cancer screening is limited for men. Many men are unsure of their prostate health, despite the growing prevalence of prostate cancer and other prostate diseases.</td></tr>
</table>

Elderly Health	Elderly maltreatment	Around one in six people 60 years and older experienced some form of abuse in community settings during the past year.	Family caregiving support *Family health* promotion and disease prevention Family disease management Family resource management Family engagement Family communication Family bereavement support Family shared decision-making Family self-care management
	Falls	Falls are the second leading cause of unintentional injury deaths among the elderly worldwide.	
	Mental health	Over 20% of adults aged 60 and over suffer from a mental or neurological disorder (excluding headache disorders), and mental health accounts for 6.6% of all disability.	

Table 3.5 provides a snapshot of the integration of the Maslow's hierarchy of need's in identifying and prioritizing SDoH/social needs and structural/policy targets that go beyond individual and family targets. The table provides a summary of understanding the complexities of SDoH/social needs and implications for multilevel intervention targets to facilitate optimal health at the individual, family, community, population, and public health levels.

TABLE 3.5 **Prioritizing ACEs SDoH / Social Needs Within 4HEALTH**

Maslow's Hierarchy of Needs	**4HEALTH Context**			
	Individual Health	***Family Health***	***Population Health***	**Public Health**
Self-Actualization	High-risk individuals suffering from ACEs and its consequences because of lack of individual-level interventions	High-risk families suffering from ACEs and its consequences because of lack of family-level interventions	High-risk communities and populations suffering with ACEs and health inequities due to lack of policy changes because of poor public health performance at the local level (demonstrated by a lack of implementing the recommended policy or plans or laws changes to adopt and support family-friendly policies, such as paid family leave and flexible work schedules). Improve access to high-quality childcare by expanding eligibility, activities offered, and family involvement. Support community programs and policies that provide safe and healthy conditions for all children and families.	High-risk public health system in managing ACEs due to lack of policy changes. As a result, public health fails to protect and promote the health of individual, families, and communities or populations and systems affected with ACEs (demonstrated by the lack of implementing the recommended policy/plans/laws to adopt and support family-friendly policies, such as paid family leave and flexible work schedules). Improve access to high-quality childcare by expanding eligibility, activities offered, and family involvement. Support community programs and policies that provide safe and healthy conditions for all children and families.

Esteem	Perceived discrimination, racism, trauma due to toxic stress related to ineffective individual-level prevention strategies	Perceived experience of discrimination, racism, trauma due to toxic stress related to ineffective family-level prevention strategies	Perceived ineffectiveness in creating, championing, and/or implementing local policies, plans, and laws that impact the allocating of resources that empower and value communities and populations affected by discrimination, racism, and trauma due to ACEs' toxic stress	Perceived ineffectiveness in creating, championing, and/or implementing policies, plans, and laws that impact the allocating of resources that empower and value the public affected by discrimination, racism, and trauma due to ACEs' toxic stress
Belonging and Love	Children and youth who do not feel close to their parents/caregivers and feel like they can't talk to them Children and youth with few or no friends or with friends who engage in aggressive or delinquent behavior Families that are isolated from and not connected to other people (extended family, friends, neighbors)	Children and youth who do not feel close to their parents/caregivers and feel like they can't talk to them Children and youth with few or no friends or with friends who engage in aggressive or delinquent behavior Families that are isolated from and not connected to other people (extended family, friends, neighbors)	Neighbors who don't know or look out for each other low community involvement among residents Lack of local policies and programs that promote healthy living and reduce social isolation for families with ACEs or are at risk for ACEs Lack of local policies and programs that support school connectedness and engage parents	Lack of policies that promote healthy living and reduce social isolation for families with ACEs or are at risk for ACEs Lack of policies that promote school connectedness and engage parents
Safety and Security	Individuals experiencing caregiving challenges related to	Experiencing caregiving challenges related to children with special needs Dating early or engaging in sexual activity early Caregivers having a limited understanding of children's needs or development Caregivers who were abused or neglected as children Families with young caregivers or single parents Families with low SES status High parenting stress or economic stress High conflict and negative communication styles	Communities with high rates of violence and crime Communities with high rates of poverty and limited educational and economic opportunities Communities with high unemployment rates Communities with easy access to drugs and alcohol Communities with few community activities for young people Communities where families frequently experience food insecurity Communities with high levels of social and environmental disorder Lack of policies that support assessment for ACEs and referral services in health care systems and communities Lack of policies that ensure public safety and economic opportunities for vulnerable families	Lack of policies that support assessment for ACEs and referral services in health care systems and communities Lack of policies that ensure public safety and economic opportunities for vulnerable families

Physiological	Unstable housing Frequent food insecurities	Unstable housing Frequent food insecurities	Unstable housing Frequent food insecurities Lack of local housing and food policies and program to support victims and families in need	Lack of policies that support safety net housing for at-risk, low-income families and emergency housing for victims of violence Lack of food security policies to support food programs for ACEs' victims and low-income families (e.g., nutrition assistance program for families at different setting such as schools, community, etc.)

Conclusion

This chapter shed light on the importance of understanding *population health* determinants from a biopsychosocial perspective. Specifically, the chapter shed light on how *family health* is a health determinant and how *family health* care professionals can apply priority-setting strategies to identify trends related to SDoH to inform policy targets for health and social care. Articulating the global burden of disease/health conditions and potential targets for family engagement strategies is a great example of demonstrating the importance of *family health* in individual and family as well as population and public health. In the next chapter, you will be introduced to the topic on patient and family engagement in health care.

Suggested Websites

CDC: https://www.cdc.gov/nchs/
CDC ACES: https://www.cdc.gov/violenceprevention/aces/index.html
Eurostat: https://ec.europa.eu/eurostat/web/main/about-us/who-we-are
Office of Disease Prevention and Health Promotion, Healthy People 2030: https://health.gov/healthypeople/priority-areas/social-determinants-health
Organization for Economic Co-operation and Development (OECD): https://data.oecd.org/pop/population.htm
The U.S. Census Bureau: https://www.census.gov/
WHO Global Health Observatory: https://www.who.int/data/gho/data/themes/mortality-and-global-health-estimates

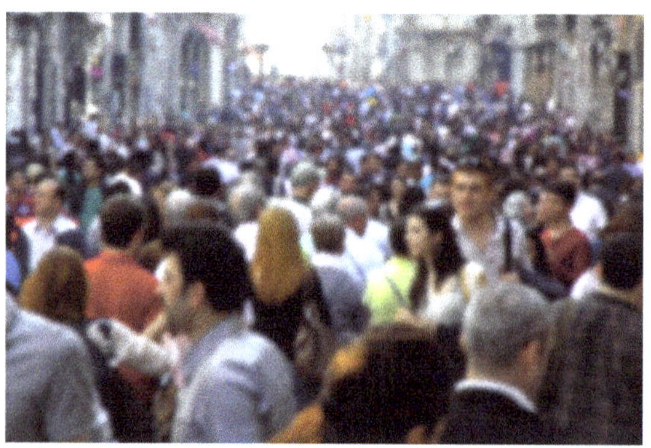

IMG 3.1

Reflection Questions

Think about your general family life and what you learned in this chapter and reflect on these questions:

1. What are your possible family social needs?
2. What potential SDoH can you identify in your neighborhood?
3. Why should care about ACEs?

References

Beran D. (2014). Developing a hierarchy of needs for Type 1 diabetes. *Diabetic Medicine: A Journal of the British Diabetic Association*, *31*(1), 61–67. https://doi.org/10.1111/dme.12284

Braveman, P., Egerter, S., & Williams, D. R. (2011). The social determinants of health: Coming of age. *Annual Review of Public Health*, *32*, 381–398.

Brownson, R. C., Seiler, R., & Eyler, A. A. (2010). Measuring the impact of public health policy. *Prev Chronic Dis*, 7(4), A77. http://www.cdc.gov/pcd/issues/2010/jul/09_0249.htm

Centers for Disease Control and Prevention (CDC). (2014). Epidemiology Glossary, from https://www.cdc.gov/reproductivehealth/data_stats/glossary.html

Castrucci B., & Auerbach J. (2019, January 16). *Meeting individual social needs falls short of addressing social determinants of health.* Health Affairs. https://www.healthaffairs.org/do/10.1377/forefront.20190115.234942/

Centers for Disease Control and Prevention. (2019, December 19). *What are Social Determinants of Health?* https://www.cdc.gov/nchhstp/socialdeterminants/faq.html# :~:text=Health%20is%20influenced%20by%20many,These%20five%20categories%20are%20interconnected

Centers for Disease Control and Prevention (2021, April 6). About the CDC—Kaiser ACE Study. https://www.cdc.gov/violenceprevention/aces/about.html

Centers for Disease Control and Prevention. (2023, June 29). *Adverse childhood experiences, or ACEs.* https://www.cdc.gov/violenceprevention/aces/index.html

Centers for Disease Control and Prevention (CDC) (n.d). Introduction to Public Health. In: Public Health 101 Series. Atlanta, GA: U.S. Department of Health and Human Services, CDC; 2014. Available at: https://www.cdc.gov/publichealth101/epidemiology.html.

Deatrick, J. A. (2017). Where is "family" in the social determinants of health? Implications for family nursing practice, research, education, and policy. *Journal of Family Nursing*, *23*(4), 423–433.

Donaldson, S. (2018, May 24). Community-Centered Health Home: Life on the Other Side of the Wall. *Prev Chronic Dis*, *15*, 170510. http://doi.org/10.5888/pcd15.170510external icon

Foley, J. (2013, July, 25). Defining Healthy Communities. *Health Resource in Action*, https://hria.org/wp-content/uploads/2016/10/defininghealthycommunities.original.pdf

Frieden, T. R. (2010). A framework for public health action: The health impact pyramid. *American journal of public health*, *100*(4), 590–595. https://doi.org/10.2105/AJPH.2009.185652

Friedman, B., Bowden, V. R., & Elaine, G. Jones. (2003). Family nursing: Research, theory and practice (5th ed.). Prentice Hall.

Giovanelli, A., & Reynolds, A. J. (2021). Adverse childhood experiences in a low-income Black cohort: The importance of context. *Preventive medicine*, *148*, 106557.

Gladding, S. T. (1998). Family therapy. History, theory and practice (2nd ed.). Prentice Hall.

Gottlieb, L., Tobey, R., Cantor, J., Hessler, D., & Adler, N. E. (2016). Integrating social and medical data to improve *population health*: opportunities and barriers. *Health Affairs*, *35*(11), 2116–2123.

Howell, C. R., Harada, C. N., Fontaine, K. R., Mugavero, M. J., & Cherrington, A. L. (2023). Perspective: Acknowledging a Hierarchy of Social Needs in Diabetes Clinical Care and Prevention. Diabetes, metabolic syndrome and obesity : targets and therapy, 16, 161–166. https://doi.org/10.2147/DMSO.S389182

Institute of Medicine. (2006). Committee on Assessing Interactions Among Social, Behavioral, and Genetic Factors in Health. In L. M. Hernandez, D. G. Blazer (Eds)*Genes, Behavior, and the Social Environment: Moving Beyond the Nature/Nurture Debate.* Washington (DC): *National Academies Press* (US), 3, *Genetics and Health.* https://www.ncbi.nlm.nih.gov/books/NBK19932/

Kaakinen, J. R., Coehlo, D. P., Steele, R., Tabacco, A., & Hanson, S. M. H. (Eds.). (2015). *Family health* care nursing: Theory, practice, and research. F.A Davis.

Magnan, S. (2017, October, 9). Social Determinants of Health 101 for Health Care: Five Plus Five. [Discussion Paper]. *NAM Perspectives.* National Academy of Medicine, Washington, DC. https://doi.org/10.31478/201710c

Maguire-Jack, K., Font, S., Dillard, R., Dvalishvili, D., & Barnhart, S. (2021). Neighborhood poverty and adverse childhood experiences over the first 15 years of life. *International journal on child maltreatment: Research, policy and practice, 4,* 93–114.

McEwen, C. A., & Gregerson, S. F. (2019). A critical assessment of the adverse childhood experiences study at 20 years. *American journal of preventive medicine, 56*(6), 790–794.

National Academies of Sciences, Engineering, and Medicine. (2019). *Integrating social care into the delivery of health care: moving upstream to improve the nation's health.* Washington, DC: The National Academies Press, https://doi.org/10.17226/25467

Naveen, K. (2010). Abraham Maslow (1908–1970). *Archives of Mental Health, 11*(1), 31–32.

Office of Disease Prevention and Health Promotion. (n.d.). *Social Determinants of Health.* Healthy People 2030. https://health.gov/healthypeople/priority-areas/social-determinants-health

Park, D., C. & Yeo, S., G. (2013). Aging. *Korean J Audiol, 17,* 39–44.

Perry, E. (2024, January 25). How to make a self-care checklist (and 7 examples). *Wellbeing.* Better Up. https://www.betterup.com/blog/self-care-checklist

Ray, R., Lantz, P. M., & Williams, D. (2023). Upstream Policy Changes to Improve *Population Health* and Health Equity: A Priority Agenda. *The Milbank Quarterly, 101*(S1), 20–35.

Simon, M., Baur, C., Guastello, S., Ramiah, K., Tufte, J., Wisdom, K., Johnston-Fleece, M., Cupito, A., & Anise, A. (2020). Patient and Family Engaged Care: An Essential Element of Health Equity. NAM perspectives, 2020, 10.31478/202007a. https://doi.org/10.31478/202007a

Street, R. L., Elwyn, G., & Epstein, R. M. (2012). Patient preferences and healthcare outcomes: An ecological perspective. *Expert review of pharmacoeconomics & outcomes research, 12*(2), 167–180.

Warner, T. D., Leban, L., Pester, D. A., & Walker, J. T. (2023). Contextualizing adverse childhood experiences: the intersections of individual and community adversity. *Journal of youth and adolescence, 52*(3), 570–584.

Weiss-Laxer, N. S., Crandall, A., Hughes, M. E., & Riley, A. W. (2020). Families as a cornerstone in 21st century public health: Recommendations for research, education, policy, and practice. *Frontiers in Public Health, 8,* 503.

Wilkinson, R. G., & Marmot, M. (Eds.). (2003). Social determinants of health: The solid facts (2nd ed.). World Health Organization.

World Health Organization. (2018). *Adverse Childhood Experiences International Questionnaire.* https://www.who.int/publications/m/item/adverse-childhood-experiences-international-questionnaire-(ace-iq)

World Health Organization. (2024, February 2). *Social determinants of health.* https://www.who.int/health-topics/social-determinants-of-health#tab=tab_1

Figure credit

IMG 3.1: Copyright © 2012 Depositphotos/katatonia82.

CHAPTER 4

Patient and Family Engagement, and Levels of Professional Involvement in Family Health Care

Families are the tie that reminds us of yesterday, provide strength and support today, and give us hope for tomorrow.

—Bill Owens

Learning Objectives

By the end of this chapter, learners will do the following:

- Describe the foundational concepts of patient and family engagement in health and health care.
- Examine the importance of patient and family engagement science in improving quality and safe health care.
- Describe the multidimensional framework for patient and family engagement in health and and its use in patient engagement.
- Describe a range of major determinants of patient and family engagement within the 4HEALTH context (*individual health*, *family health*, *population health* and public health).
- Demonstrate motivation to support and adjust patient and family engagement strategies at various levels of the 4HEALTH contexts.

Before you read on, consider the following questions:

- Why are unengaged patients and their families in health care a public health problem?
- What are the levels of patient engagement in health care?
- Where can you engage patients and families in health care?
- When should you engage patients and families in health care?
- How can you effectively engage with patients and families in health care?
- Whom should you include during patient and family engagement in health care?

The Importance of Patient and Family Engagement in Health and Health Care

It is difficult to imagine how you can involve and engage patients and families in diverse health care settings if you do not know why and you do not have the knowledge, attitude, and skills to do so (what, where, when, how, and whom). The questions that begin the chapter are impetuses for you to start thinking about practicing patient and family engagement in health care. This chapter introduces the concept of engagement science in the context of patient and family engagement. Thus, why should you care about patient and family engagement in the context of health care and health outcomes?

Sample Facts on the Importance of Patient Engagement

Quality Care and Patient Safety and Patient Engagement

According to the WHO (2023), the following are true:

- Around one in every 10 patients is harmed in health care due to unsafe care.
- More than 3 million deaths occur annually due to unsafe care, with death occurring at a rate of four in 100 people in low- to middle-income countries.
- Almost more that 50% of the harm is preventable.

The indirect cost of harm amounts to trillions of dollars each year, potentially reducing global economic growth by 0.7% a year. If done well, patient engagement is a good return on investment: It can reduce the burden of harm by 15%.

Self-Care Management and Patient Engagement

According to the WHO (2023), the following are true:

- One in five of the world's population are now living in humanitarian crises, and health systems are challenged to deliver essential services.
- By 2030, the estimated global shortage of health workers to achieve and sustain universal health care (UHC) is expected to grow to 15 million health workers.
- On average, individuals spend less than 1 hour in a year with a health care worker versus over 8,700 hours a year in self-care.
- Self-care recognizes individuals as active agents in managing their own health care in areas including health promotion; disease prevention and control; self-medication; providing care to dependent persons; and rehabilitation, including palliative care. It does not replace the healthcare system, but instead provides additional choices and options for health care.
- Evidence-based self-care interventions promote individuals' active participation in their own health care and are a push toward greater self-determination, self-efficacy, autonomy, and engagement in health with or without the support of a health care provider.

Population Health Indicators and Outcomes

According to the Healthy People 2023 health behavior and communication indicators, there are existing gaps and points for intervention for improving patient engagement (U.S. Department of Health and Human Services, 2023). This is reflected in the status of key national *population health* metrics on some of patient engagement goals as follows:

- In 2017, 8.9% of the people over 18 years old still had trouble talking with their health care providers
- In 2020, most people over 18 years of age (52%) wanted to participate in making decisions about their health.
- In 2020, 72% of adults aged 18 and over were offered online access to their medical record to better track and manage their care
- In 2020–2021, 39.8% of the adolescents aged 12 to 17 years spoke privately with a health care provider without another adult in the room during preventive medical visits in the past month (.
- In 2020, 86.9% of adults aged 18 years and over reported having social support (e.g., having friends or family members whom they talk to about their health)

Various national and international organizations, as well as individuals, have made calls to action on patient engagement as a global priority (see examples at the end of the chapter). Of interest to family professionals and scholars is the advancement of engagement science and practical application of patient engagement to improve engagement and health outcomes. The focused targeted outcomes include better care, better culture, better health, lower costs (Frampton et al., 2017), better productivity, and workforce engagement (WHO, 2023).

The patient engagement outcomes indicators represent a multifaceted concept spanning measurable behavioral markers of patients' compliance and symptom management and cognitive and relational factors to markers related to building partnerships (Barello et al., 2012). Subsequent empirical evidence has also demonstrated better outcomes in coordination of care, patient satisfaction (Gao et al., 2022), health outcomes, and health care costs (Carman et al., 2013). Other outcomes include improvement in family presence, family support, and family contributions to care (Olding et al., 2016), better outcomes in communication, and empowered shared decision-making processes (Galle et al., 2021). Such attributes of patient engagement are essential to the implementation of patient- and family-centered care (PFCC; Carman et al., 2013; Smith et al., 2021). As mentioned earlier, most important is the impact of patient engagement for patient safety and quality outcomes (Angood et al., 2010).

Conceptual Background of Patient and Family Engagement in Health Care

Engagement science, defined as a science of meaningful participation, involvement, collaboration, and partnership among health care stakeholders, is vital to patient- and family-centered health service research outcomes (Cope et al., 2019; Patient-Centered Outcomes Research Institute [PCORI], 2024). The science refocuses the health care field from a disease-focused care model that is based on the idea that health care providers "know better" (Rolland, 2015) to value a whole person–centered care model whereby persons (including patients) and families are collaborators or partners (Vick & Wolff, 2021) as well as health experts or educators (Rowland et al., 2019). Including the diverse patient and family perspectives and choices is important in improving health care service delivery and outcomes (Lehmann & Liao, 2021).

The concept of patient engagement has been referenced in the literature since the 1960 from multidisciplinary perspectives, including scholars from fields of medicine, nursing, public health, and psychology (Higgins et al., 2017). Over the years, conceptual clarity has been lacking resulting into different conceptual definitions and terminologies in the health care literature (Barello et al., 2014; Hickmann et al., 2022). These terms include *adherence*, *compliance*, *patient* and/or *family involvement*, *activation*, *empowerment*, *engagement*, *self-care and self-management*, *co-production of health* (Vick & Wolff, 2021), and *participation* (Wyskiel et al., 2015). The concept of patient engagement has been systematically explored in both clinical (CORI) and in nonclinical settings (Rooke & Oudshoorn, 2020, July). The term has received much more attention in contexts of chronic disease management (Bennett et al., 2020; Vick & Wolff, 2021), family presence in the intensive care unit (ICU; Burns et al., 2017), and family caregiving burden (CDC, 2019; WHO, 2022). Patient engagement is patient-level characteristics that provides a better understanding of the quality of health care through patient experiences beyond medical treatment (OECD, 2019).

For the purpose of this chapter, the term *patient and family engagement* (PFE) is used interchangeably to patient engagement. The evolving engaged model known as the multidimensional framework for patient and family engagement in health and health care (Carman et al., 2013) is presented as an example of valuable conceptual approach to understand PFE in health care service research and practice. Within the framework, PFE is referred to as "patients, families, their representatives (non-family members), and health professionals working in active partnership at various levels across the healthcare system—direct care, organizational design and governance, and policy making—to improve health and health care" (Carman, Dardess, Maurer et al., 2013, p. 224). The term broadly reflects the inclusion of key stakeholders within health care organizations and communities (Bennett et al., 2020). The multidimensional framework for PFE helps health care providers, health systems administrators, and policy makers conceptualize priority areas in PFE strategies across the continuum of engagement (i.e., from consultation and involvement to partnership and shared leadership) and across three levels of PFE engagement (i.e., direct patient care, health system or organizational, and community/policy levels; Carman et al., 2013). The framework has been useful in delineating priority areas in policymaking, research, and practice to ensure effective implementation of PFE strategies in patient safety (Park & Giap, 2020). Likewise, it has been useful in evidence mapping of PFE strategies and potential PFE measures and outcomes (Bennett et al., 2020).

Levels of Engagement

According to Carman et al. (2013), at the *consultation/information* (minimum) level of engagement, the power of engagement lies within the health care provider. During the *involvement* level, patients are active agents in the patient–health professional/service provider/system relationship. However, the power in the relationship lies with health care professional/service provider/system. Lastly, at the level of *partnership/shared leadership* (highest), patients are active agents and share power with the health care professional/ service provider/system.

Level of the Healthcare System Engagement

Direct Patient Care

Direct patient care refers to the strategies that "directly inform patients' own treatment decisions, health behaviors, or outcomes (e.g. self-management support, shared decision making, and communication strategies)" (Bennett et al., p. 14). Examples of direct patient care engagement strategies at the individual and family level include family assessment techniques such as conducting a functioning assessment and drawing family genograms. Other strategies include conducting family conferences (Botelho et al., 1996) and task sharing whereby nurses delegates tasks to the patient's family and conduct patient and family education strategies (i.e., self-management programs; Wyskiel, et al., 2015). Task sharing increases nurses' availability for other tasks. Providing online patient portal communication (Vicki & Wolff, 2021) as well as helping the patient and family in seeking online health information and resources is also a direct patient care strategy (Carman, Dardess, Maurer et al., 2013). Recently, the COVID-19 pandemic accelerated the adoption of digital patient and family engagement strategies in health care settings (Gaugler & Mitchell, 2022; Shin et al., 2023). A positive impact on PFE strategies with health information technology initiatives have been reported in the engagement literature (Leung et al., 2019). PFE strategies in health IT other than online portals include virtual reality / games, videoconferencing, emails, mobile phone messaging (Cené et al., 2016), and mobile health apps (Leung et al., 2019).

Systems/Organizational

A health system strategy is defined as "a strategy that engages patients and families in organizational activities and/or decision-making and informs the delivery of care within a health care system, beyond the individual patient's care (e.g., participation in an advisory committee or board membership)" (Bennett et al., 2020, p. 37). PFE strategies at the systems level include family participation or engagement in advisory and decision-making councils or engagement in development and revision of health care policies (Dworetzky et al., 2023); using a multidisciplinary, team-based approach; and training/educating patients and health care providers as strategies to engage patients and families in the use of health IT (Leung et al., 2019). Other systems-level strategies include structural designs such as a family-friendly physical environment (Vick & Wolff, 2021) and including surveillance to assess patients' experiences and satisfaction (Bennett et al., 2020).

Community or Policy

A community- or policy-level strategy can be defined as "as a strategy that engages patients, consumers, or citizens in policymaking or that engages communities in health care policies" (Bennett et al., 2020, p. 39). Examples include hospital–neighborhood partnerships and disease-specific patient lobbyist and community advocate groups. Very few evidence is available for PFE strategies and outcomes at the systems and community or policy levels.

The activities with patients and families may take place with or without the interactions with minimal levels of engagement to the shared or collaborative active engagement (Carman, Dardess, Maurer et al., 2013). For instance, at the consultation/involvement level, patients and families can receive information about their specific health issues through one-way communication from their health care provider/other service provider at the practice organization level. At the involvement level, patients and families actively participate in provider-led discussions or other service providers/organizational discussions/activities. At the shared or partnership level, the patient and immediate provider/systems service provider/system engage as equals. Table 4.1 provides examples of levels of engagement.

TABLE 4.1 **Examples of Levels of Engagement**

Level of Engagement	Continuum of Engagement		
	Consultation/ Information	**Involvement**	**Partnership/Shared Leadership**
Direct Patient Care	Provider shares a patient and family education brochure with patient	Patient completes a satisfaction or experience survey as part of the health organization policy	Patient and provider collaborate in designing, implementing, and evaluating the survey or video result
Systems/Organization	Provider completes the admission checklist and shares the aggregate published data with patient	Patient and family codesign the admission checklist and provider collects the data. Providers use the data for staff quality improvement	Patient and family colead education sessions on the codesigned admission checklist with new hires during orientation
Community or Policy	Hospital accreditation body visits the patient and family and queries about the checklist usage. Patient unaware of why the visit occurred	Hospital accreditation committee and patient champion prepare for the visit, including for the use of the implementation checklist	Accreditation body, hospital accreditation committee, and patient champions work together to prepare for the visit, including for use of the implementation checklist and outcomes

Although not mentioned within the framework, it is important to articulate the PFE aviator who will be the target of the PFE strategies. Research in PFE demonstrates varied compositions or memberships that range from individual patients and their families to family subsystems, for instance the parent subsystems (Uding et al., 2007), such as the child–father subsystem (Ali, & Dean, 2015; Boman et al., 2014; Katz & Krulik, 1999), child–grandparent subsystem (Pulgaron et al., 2016), couple subsystem (Meis et al., 2013; Sayers et al., 2006), and the sibling subsystem (Hilario, 2022). Other PFE compositions include peer-to-peer subsystems that are tailored toward building meaningful relationships and support through shared lived expertise among specific family-to-family groups within an organization and community (Greer et al., 2017).

Determinants of PFE in Health Care

People-centered health care is a key characteristic of service delivery in health system(s) (WHO, 2007). In theory, services are expected to be responsive and acceptable to targeted patients and families. The consumers of the services are also expected to participate and engage in the design and assessment of the services. In reality, these expectations have not been met across health systems despite the mounting evidence on barriers and facilitators of PFCC. There has been a call to integrate patient and family engagement into the healthcare system building blocks of service delivery, health workforce, health information, access to essential medicine, financing, and leadership/governance as part of health systems' performance monitoring (Lazarus, 2014).

The PFE approach continues to present multilevel determinants that influence effective implementation in health system(s) for better health outcomes. Following is an outline of some of the key determinants of PFE examined through the lens of the *4HEALTH* context to shed light on gaps and opportunities for advancing *family health* care that is equitable, efficient, and responsive and that provides social and risk protection. The 4HEALTH context assumes that PFE strategies and outcomes are not only individual and family focused but are also population and public health focused. As you will notice, the PFE determinants discussed herein build on the discussion of barriers to implementation of *family health* care at different levels of influence (see Chapter 1).

Individual Health

One of the key determinants of PFE is the ongoing culture of care focusing on the individual. Health systems rooted in the individual-focused traditional models consider PFE a philosophy of inclusion, but in reality some patients and families are indirectly excluded (Gao et al., 2022). Specific vulnerable communities that include families from racial and ethnic minorities, rural and urban areas, those who identify as LBGTQ, families with disabilities, individuals from low-income families, individuals without insurance, and individuals dealing with comorbidities are at increased risk of being excluded (Simon et al., 2020). Some of the facilitating exclusion factors include lack of patient/family motivation, lack of knowledge, attitudes and beliefs, lack of experience with health care, poor self-efficacy, poor health literary, and poor health status (Carman, Dardess, Maurer et al., 2013). Other barriers include family distress and ethical conflicts (McAndrew et al., 2020). The exclusions in PFE can be at the levels of consultation or involvement or at the stakeholder partnership phases.

Family Health

One of the key family-level determinants of patient and family engagement is the lack of routine monitoring of *family health* indicators in national health surveys and performance measures (Weiss-Laxer et al., 2020a). This is partly attributed to the lack of conceptual clarity on the definitions of family and *family health* (Weiss-Laxer et al., 2020a) and the ongoing focus on diseases and individual risk behaviors without acknowledging the contexts of unhealthy and healthy behaviors (Weiss-Laxer et al., 2020b). Health systems continue to demonstrate their commitment to support the role of family in PFCC but underutilize families, especially in the areas of health promotion and disease prevention (Barnes et al., 2020; Ho et al., 2022). The majority of family involvement strategies continue to focus on advancing the family's role in disease management through the lens of family caregiving, which is described as "informal caregiving that involves unpaid assistance to family members who are unable to function independently" (Hopps et al., 2017, p. 437). Despite the benefits of caregiving for the growing aging population and individuals with disabilities, family caregiving is a public health issue (CDC, 2019). Family burden as an outcome of family involvement in caregiving has had negative impacts on people's ability to work, relate with others, and maintain good physical and mental health (Talley & Crews, 2007). Likewise, gender disparities associated with family caregiving ire concerning, with female caregivers suffering the most (Stall et al., 2023).

A conceptual framework of the multilevel determinants of family nurses' engagement with families has been proposed. The theory of nurse-promoted engagement with families' framework delineates determinants of family nurses' supportive care in the ICU setting, an evolving area in family nursing engagement research (McAndrew et al., 2020). Barriers to engagement include family distress, ethical conflicts, nurses' workload demands and resources, and family exclusion policies and practices (McAndrew et al., 2020). The facilitators to engagement in ICU settings include family adaptation factors such as preexisting family strengths and strong patient and family connections. Other factors are related to organization, such as the ICU nursing culture (e.g., skills and comfort with family care, nurse moral resilience), unit support factors (e.g., health ICU work environment, leadership involvement in family care), and factors related to organizational responsiveness (e.g., nurse–family resources, recognitions of the unique contributions of nurses, active mitigation of moral distress/burnout).

Overall, these observations suggest the need for health systems to improve family involvement and participation to ensure a safe and satisfying experience for patients, families, and the health care team (Dehghan et al., 2015; Gilliss et al., 2019; Jazieh et al., 2018).

For effective implementation of family involvement to take place, a cultural and organizational shift toward working with families is warranted. There must be shared goals among all members of the clinical team, including the leaders of the organization (Eassom et al., 2014). The shared goals should include implementing strategies that adequately prepare staff to work with families and family-friendly policies that favor a balanced workload to ensure success of PFE (Bélanger et al., 2017). In addition, there is a need to integrate the role of family, family interventions, and *family health* outcomes into *population health* initiatives and outcomes (Weiss-Laxer et al., 2020a).

Some possible risks among individuals and families that are related to lack of poor PFE at the direct service delivery in acute care settings include inadequate support, poor health assessment, embarrassment, time being wasted, disappointment, and potential threat to the patient, family, and provider relationship (Haines et al., 2017). Provider-level risk can include professional pride, feeling threatened by patients and family, lack of value of PFE, and limited knowledge or lack of new insights from lessons learned (Haines et al., 2017). The ultimate risks include poor individual and *family health* outcomes, especially for those who are the most vulnerable.

Population Health

As mentioned earlier, it is important to address organizational cultural factors that hinder engagement, such as organizational goals and policies and practices to promote patient and family engagement for better *population health* outcomes (Carman, Dardess, Maurer et al., 2013). For example, lack of family presence policies or electronic medical records, lack of opportunities to serve on boards/councils, and lack of physical comfort such as access to a family room and privacy are health systems challenges that need to be addressed at the organization/system level of influence (Bélanger et al., 2018). Involving patients and families as champion stakeholders throughout PFE policy development and program design, implementation, and evaluation while ensuring mutual needs are met is beneficial to the health systems and the communities served (Petts, 2008). Patients and families must be willing to engage in the shared decision-making processes (Rowe & Calnan, 2006). Just having informed patients and families is not enough.

One of the notable determinants that cuts across the levels of engagement and continuum of engagement is the lack of trust (Gilson, 2006). Patients and families with self-trust issues have limited opportunities to engage with health systems as patient experts and health educators. Trust is a relational process that is essential for effective patient- and family–provider relationships (Dinç & Gastmans, 2013). The essential attributes of the relationships include empathy, presence, contact, authenticity, trust, and reciprocity (Allande-Cussó et al., 2022). Trusting relationships build healthy positive encounters and family support and promote family involvement in health care (Lynn-McHale & Deatrick, 2000; Thorne & Robinson, 1988b). Patients report more beneficial health behaviors, less symptoms, higher quality of life, and more satisfaction with treatment when they have higher levels of trust in their health care professional (Birkhäuer et al., 2017). Additionally, trust in patient and family engagement promotes teamwork, job satisfaction, and efficient care (Dinç & Gastmans, 2013; Gilson, 2006). Unfortunately, it is difficult to build meaningful, engaging, and trustworthy relationships if you do not have enough time to know someone (Pratt et al., 2021). Thus, addressing "time," a barrier for PFCC, is an essential determinant of PFE at the provider and organizational level.

Likewise, overall public trust in health systems has been an ongoing public health issue (Gille et al., 2015). In some settings, it is also alarming to realize that despite advancement in technology, integrated health information–sharing systems are still not favorable by the public due to trust issues (Platt et al., 2018). Public lack of trust deters positive relational coproduction care that facilitates meaningful consensus dialogues and exchange of information for health communication actions among the stakeholders involved (Batalden et al., 2016)—for example, lack of public trust and knowledge regarding the use of real-world data (RWE), referred to as "information derived from studies analyzing real-world data derived from sources other than randomized controlled trials (e.g. patient registries, patient cohorts, administrative claims, or electronic health records)" (Oehrlein, Graff, Perfetto, Mullins, et al., 2018, p. 111). Privacy issues in RWE usage is a key trust barrier to patient engagement (Han et al., 2020; Oehrlein et al., 2019) despite its benefits in the implementation of precision medicine (study of genes, diseases, and treatments; Fendrick & Shope, 2018). Lack of RWE usage denies health systems and organizations the ability to clarify the best use of regulatory agency-approved treatments and added precisions to value assessment and clinical decision-making. Likewise, privacy concerns are central to RWE usage in relation to precision *population health* management (Han et al., 2020), an evolving approach (Steenkamer et al., 2017) that is "people-centered, data-driven and proactive in managing the health and well-being of a defined population, considering the differences within that population and their social determinants of health" (WHO, 2023, p. 2). Organization/health systems that do not have the capability or infrastructure and capacity to adopt a precision public health management approach face the risk of poor PFE outcomes as they cannot meet clients where they are in terms of where they live, play, learn, worship, and age.

The possible risk factors for poor or lack of PFE care at the systems/organizational level include litigation risks as well as increased use of resources and cost (Haines et al., 2017). Organizations/health systems that are unable to recognize PFE targets for intervention are at risk of unnecessary resource and funding waste (Van der Schee et al., 2006). For example, in tracking barriers and facilitators of PFE in the UK health systems, Calnan and Sanford (2004), demonstrated that patient–provider relational and professional competency determinants were the more important targets for PFE interventions than organizational health care service operations and financing. In this case, organization/health systems efforts should be tailored to ensuring a well-trained health care workforce in PFE strategies to support direct patient care as part of routine clinical work (e.g., promoting knowledge, skills, and attitudes in improving self-care to empower individuals, families, and communities to promote health, prevent diseases, and maintain health as well as cope with illness and disability).

Overall, the barriers call for cultural shifts within organizations and health systems in delivery and payment models. For example, a culture shift needs to happen on how time allowance in the delivery of effective PFCC should be conceptualized and reimbursed. The culture shift requires a representative team of all key stakeholders who are equipped to participate at the level of partnership and share leadership engagement across the direct patient care and systems/organizational level of engagement for mutual winning outcomes.

Community Level

Although patient populations in organizations are made up of multiple families within communities, most health care systems continue to underutilize families as an upstream health context in population and public health initiatives (Weiss-Laxer et al., 2020b). Lack of or inadequate *population health* management data sources to measure the state of family-level outcomes in relational care is one of the barriers to public health initiatives that are family focused (Weiss-Laxer et al., 2020b). Moreover, despite the positive benefits of community engagement (O'Mara-Eves et al., 2015), if not done properly using promising evidence approaches such as the use of community participatory methods (Rhodes, 2014), it can be a barrier to PFE among disadvantaged populations. To facilitate effective patient and family activation for at-risk populations, health systems should strive to promote *population health* management champions, both frontline clinical and nonclinical public health professionals and leaders, who can assess, assemble community resources, and engage all key stakeholders (government and nongovernment entities) that represent the community they serve (WHO, 2023). Thus, preparing diverse groups of stakeholders to work together to build consensus on issues of interest is beneficial in building public trust in public health (SteelFisher, et al., 2023). Likewise, the role of civic engagement should not be underestimated in building public trust for population and community health. Engaging community stakeholders and leaders to work together in assessing their communities through platforms like community health advisory boards and setting PFE visions, missions, and designs as well as implementing and evaluating programs is crucial. Poor engagement or lack of community member and organization or institution engagement propels public mistrust, and, similar to organizations/health systems, communities may endure the same risk for litigation, poor resource allocations, and ultimately poor *population health* outcomes.

Public Health

The majority of the PFE determinants require organizational- / health system-level changes, which can take years because of lack of capacity, infrastructure, and capability. For example, the lack of individual/family or organizational level evidence-based PFE policies is a barrier for effective engagement outcomes. Public health efforts should create, champion, and implement policies, plans, and laws that impact and support PFE within health systems.

In addition, although many health systems worldwide have embraced whole health care approaches, the gap is still wide for many as they continue to struggle to put patients, families, and communities at the center of PFCC, one of the pillars of quality care (National Academics of Science, Engineering and Medicine, 2023). For instance, there is still lack of effective means that assess and address psychosocial patient and family needs (Bergman et al.,1993). Integrating social care into health care delivery systems can have drawbacks if not planned well. PFE strategies that engage patients and families in screening for social needs, such as activating patients to engage in shared decisions, are needed (National Academics of Science, Engineering and Medicine, 2019). Thus, public health efforts should include building a diverse and skilled workforce to be able to screen and offer information, mobilize communities, develop appropriate partnerships, and build and maintain a strong *population health* management infrastructure to achieve *whole health care* and *whole health systems* (see Table 4.2). Unfortunately, the lack of standardized *population health* data sets across health systems and organizations is still a challenge (Han et al., 2020). Thus, there is a need to develop public health strategies that engage key stakeholders to ensure the public is aware of inconsistencies on country-specific national, state, and local plans on key PFE outcomes; how the plans are translated at the local policies; and what is/should be done to modernize the data. This should include establishing safe public health IT infrastructure.

TABLE 4.2 **Definitions of Whole Health, Whole Health Care, and Whole Heath System**

Term	Definitions
Whole Health	Physical, behavioral, spiritual, and socioeconomic well-being as defined by individuals, families, and communities
Whole Health Care	An interprofessional, team-based approach anchored in trusted longitudinal relationship to promote resilience, prevent disease, and restore health. It aligns with as person's life mission, aspiration, and purpose.
Whole Health System	A collaborative health system that encompasses conventional programs, social services, and public health. It addresses the five foundational elements of whole health: people-centered-holistic and comprehensive, upstream-focused, equitable, accountable, and team well-being

Source: National Academics of Science, Engineering and Medicine (2023)

Innovations such as patients' health portals with patients' engagement IT functionalities are essential for public health policy decisions to improve patient safety (Upadhyay et al., 2022). However, their use is impacted by lack of trust with existing health information systems. For instance, in the United States, the majority of the public has issues with integrated health information–sharing system modalities because of privacy concerns (Platt et al., 2018). Ensuring that health systems are accountable by utilizing legal and regulatory actions that promote safe IT to protect the public is essential.

Moreover, there have been concerns about which PFE models are best to promote relational care and health systems/organizational rewards for effective PFCC and the uptake and spread of evidence-based decision-making strategies. To promote relational care, public health efforts should include measures to assure a competent work force by monitoring educational and training preparation through regulatory bodies—for example, reassuring a skilled workforce in communication training that promotes patient engagement (e.g., the Johns Hopkins patient engagement program; Schechter & Wegener, 2022) and ensuring a public health force that is equipped with indispensable high-performance skills that include community engagement, systems thinking, and strategic thinking; change management; effective communication; data-driven decision-making; justice, equity, diversity, and inclusion; resources management and finances; policy engagement; and cross-sectoral partnership (Yu, 2022).

In addition, policies that support and reward health systems grounded on value-based health care (VBHC) need to be developed or adapted to ensure effective access and delivery of equitable services and care. VBHC encompass "a range of considerations beyond only considering value for money in selection processes, by making sure that this estimated value of care/services is passed on to patients and corresponds to their interpretation of value. It includes ensuring health improvement at the patient level, responsiveness of the health system to patient needs, financial protection, efficiency and equity" (WHO, 2021, p. 1).

Public health efforts to support ongoing research in patient and family engagement science are needed. For example, more research is needed to understand how to effectively engage patients in advisory roles and collaborative teams at the level of direct care service in a VBHC context (van der Voorden et al., 2023). Equally, models that capture the complex role of patients in the uptake of evidence beyond clinician and health systems targets are needed (Moore et al., 2015). Another example is the need for supporting and funding further research to test proposed practice model that address specific national PFE-related targets (e.g., the health literate model—an engagement model that facilitates understanding of patients' heath literacy challenges and options for engagement) to improve interests such as health literacy (Koh et al., 2013).

Conclusion

This chapter focused on the evolving concept of PFE and the related determinants. PFE determinants are multilevel in nature and thus require multilevel solutions. One of the important determinants at the individual level is the ability of health care provider to provide relational care through interdisciplinary and multisectoral approaches. In the next chapter, levels of involvement with families and interprofessional practice in *family health* care are introduced.

Suggested Websites

World Health Organization, Patient Safety: https://www.who.int/teams/integrated-health-services/patient-safety

CDC, Family Caregiving: https://www.cdc.gov/aging/caregiving/caregiver-brief.html

Suggested Readings

Carman, K. L., Dardess, P., Maurer, M., Sofaer, S., Adams, K., Bechtel, C., & Sweeney, J. (2013). Patient and family engagement: A framework for understanding the elements and developing interventions and policies. *Health Affairs*, *32*(2), 223–231.

Frampton, S. B., Guastello, S., Hoy, L., Naylor, M., Sheridan, S., & Johnston-Fleece, M. (2017). Harnessing evidence and experience to change culture: A guiding framework for patient and family engaged care. *NAM perspectives*. Discussion Paper, National Academy of Medicine, Washington, DC. https://doi.org/10.31478/201701f

McAndrew, N. S., Schiffman, R., & Leske, J. (2020). A theoretical lens through which to view the facilitators and disruptors of nurse-promoted engagement with families in the ICU. *Journal of Family Nursing*, *26*(3), 190–212.

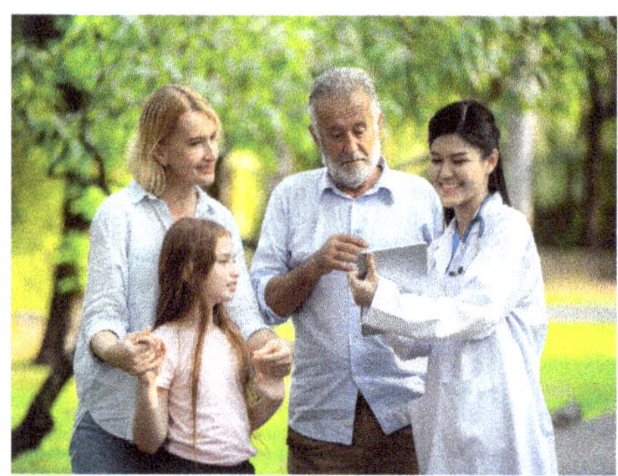

IMG 4.1

National Academies of Sciences, Engineering, and Medicine. (2019). Integrating social care into the delivery of health care: Moving upstream to improve the nation's health. National Academies Press. https://doi.org/10.17226/25467

National Academies of Sciences, Engineering, and Medicine. (2023). *Achieving whole health: A new approach for veterans and the nation*. National Academies Press. https://doi.org/10.17226/26854.

Yu, E. (Ed.). (2022). *Strategic skills: Community engagement*. American Public Health Association.

Reflection Questions

Think about how your community, and reflect on these questions:

1. What is your philosophical perspective about patient and family engagement in your community?
2. Mention, three people in your community who you think would be your advocate for matters related to patients, family, and community engagement with your local health systems.
3. Why did you select the three people in question 2?

References

Ali, M. M., & Dean, D., Jr. (2015). The influence of nonresident fathers on adolescent and young adult cigarette smoking. *Families, Systems, & Health*, *33*(3), 314–323. https://doi.org/10.1037/fsh0000137.

Allande-Cussó, R., Fernández-García, E., & Porcel-Gálvez, A. M. (2022). Defining and characterising the nurse-patient relationship: A concept analysis. *Nursing ethics*, *29*(2), 462–484.

Angood, P., Dingman, J., Foley, M. E., Ford, D., Martins, B., O'Regan, P., ... & Denham, C. R. (2010). Patient and family involvement in contemporary health care. *Journal of Patient Safety*, *6*(1), 38–42.

Barello, S., Graffigna, G., & Vegni, E. (2012). Patient engagement as an emerging challenge for healthcare services: Mapping the literature. *Nursing research and practice*. https://doi.org/10.1155/2012/905934

Barello, S., Graffigna, G., Vegni, E., & Bosio, A. C. (2014). The challenges of conceptualizing patient engagement in health care: a lexicographic literature review. *Journal of Participatory Medicine*, *6*(11), 259–267.

Barnes, M. D., Hanson, C. L., Novilla, L. B., Magnusson, B. M., Crandall, A. C., & Bradford, G. (2020). Family-centered health promotion: Perspectives for engaging families and achieving better health outcomes. *INQUIRY: The Journal of Health Care Organization, Provision, and Financing, 57.*

Batalden, M., Batalden, P., Margolis, P., Seid, M., Armstrong, G., Opipari-Arigan, L., & Hartung, H. (2016). Coproduction of healthcare service. *BMJ Qual* Saf, *25*(7), 509–517. https://doi.org/10.1136/bmjqs-2015-004315

Bélanger, L., Bussières, S., Rainville, F., Coulombe, M., & Desmartis, M. (2017). Hospital visiting policies-impacts on patients, families and staff: A review of the literature to inform decision making. *J Hosp Adm*, *6*(6), 51–62.

Bélanger, L., Desmartis, M., & Coulombe, M. (2018). Barriers and facilitators to family participation in the care of their hospitalized loved ones. *Patient Experience Journal*, *5*(1), 56–65.

Bennett, W. L., Pitts, S., Aboumatar, H. M., Sharma, R., Smith, B. M., Das, A., Day, J., Holzhauer, K. & Bass, B. E. (2020). *Strategies for Patient, Family, and Caregiver Engagement* (Report No. 20-EHC017). Agency for Healthcare Research and Quality.

Bergman, A., Wells, L., Bogo, M., Abbey, S., Chandler, V., Embleton, L., ... & Urman, S. (1993). High-risk indicators for family involvement in social work in health care: A review of the literature. *Social Work*, *38*(3), 281–288.

Birkhäuer, J., Gaab, J., Kossowsky, J., Hasler, S., Krummenacher, P., Werner, C., & Gerger, H. (2017). Trust in the health care professional and health outcome: A meta-analysis. *PloS one*, *12*(2), e0170988.

Boman, Å., Povlsen, L., Dahlborg-Lyckhage, E., Hanas, R., & Borup, I. K. (2014). Fathers of children with type 1 diabetes: Perceptions of a father's involvement from a health promotion perspective. *Journal of family nursing*, *20*(3), 337–354.

Botelho, R. J., Lue, B. H., & Fiscella, K. (1996). Family involvement in routine health care: A survey of patients' behaviors and preferences. *Journal of Family Practice*, *42*(6), 572–577.

Burns, K. E., Misak, C., Herridge, M., Meade, M. O., & Oczkowski, S. (2018). Patient and family engagement in the ICU. Untapped opportunities and underrecognized challenges. *American journal of respiratory and critical care medicine*, *198*(3), 310–319.

Calnan, M. W., & Sanford, E. (2004). Public trust in health care: the system or the doctor? *BMJ Quality & Safety*, *13*(2), 92–97.

Carman, K. L., Dardess, P., Maurer, M., Sofaer, S., Adams, K., Bechtel, C., & Sweeney, J. (2013). Patient and family engagement: A framework for understanding the elements and developing interventions and policies. *Health affairs*, *32*(2), 223–231.

Cené, C, W., Johnson, B. H., Wells, N., Baker, B., Davis. R., & Turchi, R. (2016). A Narrative Review of Patient and Family Engagement: The "Foundation" of the Medical "Home." *Med Care*, *54*(7), 697–705. https://doi.org/10.1097/MLR.0000000000000548

Centers for Disease Prevention and Control. (2019). *Caregiving for Family and Friends—A Public Health Issue*. https://www.cdc.gov/aging/caregiving/caregiver-brief.html

Cope, E., Angove, R., Dungan, R., & Peay, H. (2019). Engagement science: An overview of the landscape of engaged research. *Post Academy Health*. www.academyhealth. org/blog/2019-01/engagementscience-overview-landscape-engaged-research

Dehghan Nayeri, N., Gholizadeh, L., Mohammadi, E., & Yazdi, K. (2015). Family involvement in the care of hospitalized elderly patients. *Journal of Applied Gerontology*, *34*(6), 779–796.

Dinç, L, & Gastmans, C. (2013). Trust in nurse–patient relationships: A literature review. *Nursing Ethics*, *20*(5), 501–516. https://doi.org/10.1177/0969733012468463

Dworetzky, B., Hoover, C. G., & Walker, D. K. (2023). Family Engagement at the Systems Level: A Framework for Action. *Maternal and child health journal*, *27*(6), 969–977. https://doi.org/10.1007/s10995-023-03619-2

Eassom, E., Giacco, D., Dirik, A., & Priebe, S. (2014). Implementing family involvement in the treatment of patients with psychosis: A systematic review of facilitating and hindering factors. *BMJ open*, *4*(10), e006108.

Fendrick, M., & Shope, M. (2018). Precision benefit design: Using clinical benefit to guide how health care dollars are spent. *J Clin Pathw*, *4*(7), 39 –40. https://doi.org/10.25270/JCP.2018.09.00032

Frampton, S. B., Guastello, S., Hoy, L., Naylor, M., Sheridan, S., & Johnston-Fleece, M. (2017). Harnessing evidence and experience to change culture: A guiding framework for patient and family engaged care. *NAM perspectives*. Discussion Paper, National Academy of Medicine, Washington, DC. https://doi.org/10.31478/201701f

Galle, A., Plaieser, G., Van Steenstraeten, T., Griffin, S., Osman, N. B., Roelens, K., & Degomme, O. (2021). Systematic review of the concept "male involvement in maternal health" by natural language processing and descriptive analysis. *BMJ global health*, *6*(4), e004909.

Gao, Y., Abonyi, S., Downe, P., Baerg, K., & Ward, H. A. (2022). Patient and family engagement: Bridging together interprofessional practice and patient- and family-centred care. *Patient Experience Journal*, *9*(1), 54–61. https://doi.org/10.35680/2372-0247.1580

Gaugler, J. E., & Mitchell, L. L. (2022). Reimagining family involvement in residential long-term care. *Journal of the American Medical Directors Association*, *23*(2), 235–240.

Greer, A. M., Amlani, A. A., Buxton, J. A., & the PEEP team. (2017). Peer Engagement Principles and Best Practices: A guide for BC Health Authorities and Other Providers (Version 2). BC Centre for Disease Control.

Gille, F., Smith, S., & Mays, N. (2015). Why public trust in health care systems matters and deserves greater research attention. *Journal of health services research & policy*, *20*(1), 62–64.

Gilliss, C. L., Pan, W., & Davis, L. L. (2019). Family involvement in adult chronic disease care: Reviewing the systematic reviews. *Journal of Family Nursing*, *25*(1), 3–27.

Gilson, L. (2006). Trust in health care: theoretical perspectives and research needs. *Journal of health organization and management*, *20*(5), 359–375.

Katz, S., & Krulik, T. (1999). Fathers of children with chronic illness: Do they differ from fathers of healthy children? *Journal of Family Nursing*, *5*(3), 292–315.

Koh, H. K., Brach, C., Harris, L. M., & Parchman, M. L. (2013). A proposed "health literate care model" would constitute a systems approach to improving patients' engagement in care. *Health affairs*, *32*(2), 357–367.

Haines, K. J., Kelly, P., Fitzgerald, P., Skinner, E. H., & Iwashyna, T. J. (2017). The Untapped Potential of Patient and Family Engagement in the Organization of Critical Care. *Critical care medicine*, *45*(5), 899–906. https://doi.org/10.1097/CCM.0000000000002282

Han, A., Isaacson, A., & Muennig, P. (2020). The promise of big data for precision *population health* management in the US. *Public Health*, *185*, 110–116.

Ho, Y. L., Mahirah, D., Ho, C.Z., & Thumboo, J. (2022). The role of the family in health promotion: A scoping review of models and mechanisms. *Health Promot Int*, *37*(6) https://doi.org/10.1093/heapro/daac119

Hopps, M., Iadeluca, L., McDonald, M., & Makinson, G. T. (2017). The burden of family caregiving in the United States: work productivity, health care resource utilization, and mental health among employed adults. *Journal of multidisciplinary healthcare*, *10*, 437–444. https://doi.org/10.2147/JMDH.S135372

Hickmann, E., Richter, P., & Schlieter, H. (2022). All together now–patient engagement, patient empowerment, and associated terms in personal healthcare. *BMC health services research*, *22*(1), 1–11.

Higgins, T., Larson, E., & Schnall, R. (2017). Unraveling the meaning of patient engagement: A concept analysis. *Patient Education and Counseling*, *100*(1), 30–36.

Hilario, A. P. (2022). Sibling caring roles and responsibilities when a child suffers from a chronic illness. *Sociology Compass, 16*(1), e12950.

Jazieh, A. R., Volker, S., & Taher, S. (2018). Involving the family in patient care: A culturally tailored communication model. *Global Journal on Quality and Safety in Healthcare, 1*(2), 33–37.

Lazarus. J. V. (2014, August 22). *A new era for the WHO health systems building blocks?* Health Systems Global. https://healthsystemsglobal.org/news/a-new-era-for-the-who-health-system-building-blocks/

Lehmann, C., & Liao, W. (2021). The patient voice: Participation and engagement in family medicine practice and residency education. *Family Medicine, 53*(7), 578–579.

Leung, K., Lu-McLean, D., Kuziemsky, C., Booth, R. G., Rossetti, S. C., Borycki, E., & Strudwick, G. (2019). Using patient and family engagement strategies to improve outcomes of health information technology initiatives: A scoping review. *Journal of medical Internet research, 21*(10), e14683.

Lynn-McHale, D. J., & Deatrick, J. A. (2000). Trust between family and health care provider. *Journal of family Nursing, 6*(3), 210–230.

McAndrew, N. S., Schiffman, R., & Leske, J. (2020). A Theoretical Lens Through Which to View the Facilitators and Disruptors of Nurse-Promoted Engagement With Families in the ICU. *Journal of family nursing, 26*(3), 190–212. https://doi.org/10.1177/1074840720936736

Meis, L. A., Griffin, J. M., Greer, N., Jensen, A. C., MacDonald, R., Carlyle, M., ... & Wilt, T. J. (2013). Couple and family involvement in adult mental health treatment: A systematic review. *Clinical psychology review, 33*(2), 275–286.

Moore, J. E., Titler, M. G., Low, L. K., Dalton, V. K., & Sampselle, C. M. (2015). Transforming patient-centered care: Development of the evidence informed decision making through engagement model. *Women's Health Issues, 25*(3), 276–282.

National Academies of Sciences, Engineering, and Medicine. (2019). *Integrating social care into the delivery of health care: Moving upstream to improve the nation's health.* National Academies Press. https://doi.org/10.17226/25467

National Academies of Sciences, Engineering, and Medicine. (2023). *Achieving whole health: A new approach for veterans and the nation.* National Academies Press. https://doi.org/10.17226/26854

Oehrlein, E. M., Graff, J.S., Perfetto, E. M., Mullins, C, D., Dubois, R, W., Anyanwu, C., & Onukwugha, E. (2018). Peer-reviewed journal editors' views on real-world evidence. *Int J Technol Assess Health Care, 34*(1), 111–119. https://doi.org/10.1017/S0266462317004408.

Oehrlein, E. M., Graff, J. S., Harris, J., & Perfetto, E. M. (2019). Patient-community perspectives on real-world evidence: Enhancing engagement, understanding, and trust. *The Patient-Patient-Centered Outcomes Research, 12*, 375–381.

Olding, M., McMillan, S. E., Reeves, S., Schmitt, M. H., Puntillo, K., & Kitto, S. (2016). Patient and family involvement in adult critical and intensive care settings: A scoping review. *Health Expectations, 19*(6), 1183–1202.

O'Mara-Eves, A., Brunton, G., Oliver, S., Kavanagh, J., Jamal, F., & Thomas, J. (2015). The effectiveness of community engagement in public health interventions for disadvantaged groups: a meta-analysis. *BMC public health, 15*, 1–23.

Organization for Economic Co-operation and Development. (2019). *Patient-reported indicators for assessing health system performance.* https://www.oecd.org/health/health-systems/Measuring-what-matters-the-Patient-Reported-Indicator-Surveys.pdf

Park, M., & Giap, T. T. T. (2020). Patient and family engagement as a potential approach for improving patient safety: a systematic review. *Journal of advanced nursing, 76*(1), 62–80.

Patient-Centered Outcomes Research Institute. (2024, February 26). *The Value of Engagement in Research.* https://www.pcori.org/engagement/value-engagement

Petts, J. (2008). Public engagement to build trust: false hopes? *Journal of Risk Research, 11*, 821–835.

Platt, J. E., Jacobson, P. D., & Kardia, S. L. (2018). Public trust in health information sharing: A measure of system trust. *Health services research, 53*(2), 824–845.

Pratt, H., Moroney, T., & Middleton, R. (2021). The influence of engaging authentically on nurse–patient relationships: A scoping review. *Nursing Inquiry*, *28*(2), e12388.

Prey, J. E., Woollen, J., Wilcox, L., Sackeim, A. D., Hripcsak, G., Bakken, S., Restaino, S., Feiner, S. & Vawdrey, D. K. (2014). Patient engagement in the inpatient setting: A systematic review. *Journal of the American Medical Informatics Association*, *21*(4), 742–750.

Pulgaron, E. R., Marchante, A. N., Agosto, Y., Lebron, C. N., & Delamater, A. M. (2016). Grandparent involvement and children's health outcomes: The current state of the literature. *Families, Systems, & Health*, *34*(3), 260.

Rhodes, S. D. (2014). Authentic community engagement and community-based participatory research for public health and medicine. In S. Rhode (Ed.), *Innovations in HIV prevention research and practice through community engagement*, (pp 1–10). Springer, New York, NY. https://doi.org/10.1007/978-1-4939-0900-1_1

Rolland, J. S. (2015). Advancing family involvement in collaborative health care: Next steps. *Families, Systems, & Health*, *33*(2), 104–107. https://doi.org/10.1037/fsh0000133

Rooke, T., & Oudshoorn, A. (2020, July). Patient engagement in the nonclinical setting: A concept analysis. *Nursing Forum*, *55*(3), 497–504.

Rowe, R., & Calnan, M. (2006). Trust relations in health care—the new agenda. *The European Journal of Public Health*, *16*(1), 4–6.

Rowland, P., Anderson, M., Kumagai, A. K., McMillan, S., Sandhu, V. K., & Langlois, S. (2019). Patient involvement in health professionals' education: A meta-narrative review. *Advances in Health Sciences Education*, *24*, 595–617.

Sayers, S. L., White, T., Zubritsky, C., & Oslin, D. W. (2006). Family involvement in the care of healthy medical outpatients, *Family Practice*, *33*(3), 317–324. https://doi.org/10.1093/fampra/cmi114

Schechter, N. E., & Wegener, S. T. (2022). The Johns Hopkins Patient Engagement Program: Improving Patient Engagement, Improving Patient Outcomes. *Quality Management in Healthcare*, *31*(2), 105–106.

Shin, J. W., Choi, J., & Tate, J. (2023). Interventions using digital technology to promote family engagement in the adult intensive care unit: An integrative review. *Heart & Lung*, *58*, 166–178.

Simon, M., Baur, C., Guastello, S., Ramiah, K., Tufte, J., Wisdom, K., Johnston-Fleece, M., Cupito, A., & Anise, A. (2020). Patient and Family Engaged Care: An Essential Element of Health Equity. *NAM Perspect*. https://doi.org/10.31478/202007a

Stall, N. M., Shah, N. R., & Bhushan, D. (2023, June). Unpaid Family Caregiving—The Next Frontier of Gender Equity in a Post pandemic Future. *JAMA Health Forum*, *4*(6), e231310.

SteelFisher, G. K., Findling, M. G., Caporello, H. L., Lubell, K. M., Vidoloff Melville, K. G., Lane, L., ... & Ben-Porath, E. N. (2023). Trust In US Federal, State, And Local Public Health Agencies During COVID-19: Responses And Policy Implications: Study reports the results of a survey of public trust in US federal, state, and local public health agencies' performance during the COVID-19 pandemic. *Health Affairs*, *42*(3), 328–337.

Steenkamer, B. M., Drewes, H. W., Heijink, R., Baan, C. A., & Struijs, J. N. (2017). Defining *population health* management: A scoping review of the literature. *Population health management*, *20*(1), 74–85.

Talley, R., & Crews J. (2007). Caring for the Most Vulnerable: Framing the Public Health of Caregiving. *Am J Public Health*, *97*, 224–228.

Thorne, S. E., & Robinson, C. A. (1988b). Reciprocal trust in health care relationships. *Journal of Advanced Nursing*, *13*, 782–789.

Uding, N., Sety, M., & Kieckhefer, G. M. (2007). Family involvement in health care research: The "building on family strengths" case study. *Families, Systems, & Health*, *25*(3), 307.

Upadhyay, S., Opoku-Agyeman, W., Choi, S., & Cochran, R. A. (2022). Do Patient Engagement IT Functionalities Influence Patient Safety Outcomes? A Study of US Hospitals. *Journal of Public Health Management and Practice, 28*(5), 505–512.

U.S. Department of Health and Human Services (2023, February 4). *Heathy People 2023.* https://health.gov/healthypeople

Van der Schee, E., Groenewegen, P. P., & Friele, R. D. (2006). Public trust in health care: A performance indicator? *Journal of Health Organization and Management, 20*(5), 468–476.

Van der Voorden, M., Sipma, W. S., de Jong, M. F., Franx, A., & Ahaus, K. C. (2023). The immaturity of patient engagement in value-based healthcare—A systematic review. *Frontiers in Public Health, 11,* 1144027.

Vick, J. B., & Wolff, J. L. (2021). A scoping review of person and family engagement in the context of multiple chronic conditions. *Health services research, 56,* 990–1005.

Weiss-Laxer, N. S., Crandall, A., Okano, L., & Riley, A. W. (2020a). Building a foundation for *family health* measurement in national surveys: A modified Delphi expert process. *Maternal and Child Health Journal, 24,* 259–266.

Weiss-Laxer, N. S., Crandall, A., Hughes, M. E., & Riley, A. W. (2020b). Families as a cornerstone in 21st century public health: Recommendations for research, education, policy, and practice. *Frontiers in Public Health, 8,* 503.

World Health Organization. (2007). *People-centred health care: A policy framework.* https://iris.who.int/bitstream/handle/10665/206971/9789290613176_eng.pdf?sequence=1

World Health Organization. (2021). *From value for money to value-based health services: A twenty-first century shift.* https://iris.who.int/bitstream/handle/10665/340724/9789240020344-eng.pdf?sequence=1

World Health Organization. (2022, June 28). *Caregiving impacts on unpaid informal carers' health and well-being—A gender perspective.* https://cdn.who.int/media/docs/librariesprovider2/euro-health-topics/child-health/caregiving-impacts-on-unpaid-informal-carers--health-and-well-being---a-gender-perspective.pdf?sfvrsn=cc247fb9_3&download=true

World Health Organization. (2023). *Population health management in primary health care: A proactive approach to improve health and well-being.* https://iris.who.int/bitstream/handle/10665/368805/WHO-EURO-2023-7497-47264-69316-eng.pdf?sequence=1

World Health Organization (September 11, 2023). Patient Safety: Key Facts. https://www.who.int/news-room/fact-sheets/detail/patient-safety

Wyskiel, R. M., Chang, B. H., Alday, A. A., Thompson, D. A., Rosen, M. A., Dietz, A. S., & Marsteller, J. A. (2015). Towards expanding the acute care team: Learning how to involve families in care processes. *Families, Systems, & Health, 33*(3), 242.

Yu, E. (Ed.). (2022). *Strategic Skills: Community Engagement.* American Public Health Association.

Figure credit

PART II

GENERALIST ENTRY-LEVEL FAMILY HEALTH CARE COMPETENCIES ACROSS MULTIPLE DISCIPLINE

CHAPTER 5

Levels of Health Care Workers' Involvement in Family Health Care

Alone we can do so little; together we can do so much.

—Hellen Keller

Learning Objectives

By the end of this chapter, learners will do the following:

- Define the following terms: primary prevention, secondary prevention and tertiary prevention, interprofessional, interdisciplinary, transdisciplinary, multidisciplinary, task sharing, task shifting, integrated health care, whole health care, health care professional burnout.
- Describe the importance of a diverse health care workforce in *family health* and whole health care health systems.
- Describes theoretical foundations of health care professional involvement and collaboration with families in whole health care.
- Discuss major occupational challenges and opportunities in strengthening the *family health* care workforce within the 4HEALTHS.
- Using an interprofessional perspective of care, demonstrate an understanding of how competent *family health* care professionals can support a family living or impacted by a *family health* issue of interest as a team.

Before you read on, consider the following questions:

- Can interventions for *family health* be delivered without the health care provider?
- How would you work/intervene with families in your clinical practice?
- Which part of health will you focus on (i.e., body, mind and spirit)? Why?
- Who is/will be part of your health care team?
- Who are the health care providers within your own disciplines (registered nurses working with advanced practice nurses, nursing assistants, medical doctors, physician assistants, medical specialists, medical assistant, etc.)?

- Is there a difference in how health care workers within one's discipline work with families?
- What barriers and facilitating factors promote health care provider involvement with families?

In addition, think through the following case exemplars of health care workforce indicators.

Global Health Care Workforce Trends as of 2024

- Nursing was the largest health profession occupation (59%).
- Eighteen million more health workers were needed to achieve Universal Health Coverage (UHC) by 2030 in low- and lower middle–income countries.
- Certain occupational risks, such as injuries, noise, carcinogenic agents, airborne particles and ergonomic risks, accounted for a substantial part of the burden of chronic diseases: 37% of all cases of back pain, 16% of hearing loss, 13% of chronic obstructive pulmonary disease, 11% of asthma, 8% of injuries, 9% of lung cancer, 2% of leukemia and 8% of depression. (WHO, 2017)

Health Care Workforce in the United States in 2022

- Over 14.5 million people aged 10 and older were employed in health care occupations (9.3% of total employment).
- The largest occupation was registered nurses (3.4 million, or one out of every five health care workers).
- Personal care aides (1.4 million) and nursing assistants (1.2 million) were the second and third largest occupations, respectively.
- Education attainment varied across health care occupations.
- Sixty percent of home health aids, 49% of personal care aides and 47% of nursing assistants had high school diplomas.
- Worldwide, the 2030 health care worker demand is estimated to be 80.2 million, which almost twice the 2013 estimates (48.3 million).
- Only 17% of all employed people aged 25 and older in the nation held advanced degrees.
- All physician and nearly all nurse practitioners held advanced degrees (master's, professional, and doctoral degrees).
- Ninety-two percent of speech language pathologists had advanced degrees.
- About eight to 10 workers in all health care occupations are women.
- Occupations with a high concentration of women are speech language pathologists (98%), dental hygienists (96%), dental assistants (94%), and nursing assistants (90%).
- Women were slightly underrepresented among physicians (44%).

- Six in 10 workers in all health occupations were White. Whites accounted for veterinary technologists and technicians (83%), occupational therapists (80%), dental hygienists (79%, physical therapists (79%), and physician assistants (78%).
- Although Asian made up 6% of all employed people in the nation, physicians (22%), pharmacists (19%), and clinical laboratory technologists and technicians (15%) had the largest shares of Asian workers.
- Although Black workers accounted for 12% of employment in all occupations, they made up 34% of nursing assistants, 29% of licensed practical and license vocational nurses, and 28% of home health aides. In addition, 25% of personal care aids and other health care support workers (23%), which included orthotic and prosthetic aids, were Black.
- Foreign-born employees made up the largest share of home health aides, personal care aides, and physicians.
- Massage therapists had high shares of self-employment (42%); other therapists such as art, hydro, and music therapists made up 22%.
- Only 12% of physicians were self-employed.
- Self-employed numbers for clinical laboratory technologists and technicians and pharmacist technicians were effectively zero.
- Nearly half (45%) of speech language pathologists were employed in the public sector.
- Twenty-five percent of dietitians and nutritionists and 20% personal aides were more likely to be employed in the public sector than other workers.
- Physicians averaged the most hours at work (47.9 hours per week). Nurse practitioners and physician assistants averaged 40.1 hours per week. Others averaged 38.6 hours per week. Massage therapists and dental hygienist worked fewer hours, 30 and 32.9 hours, respectively. (U.S. Bureau of Labor Statistics, 2024)

Fact Sheet

- Decent work is good for mental health.
- Poor working environments—including discrimination and inequality, excessive workloads, low job control, and job insecurity—pose a risk to mental health.
- Fifteen percent of working-age adults were estimated to have a mental disorder in 2019.
- Globally, an estimated 12 billion working days are lost every year to depression and anxiety at a cost of $1 trillion per year in lost productivity.
- There are effective actions to prevent mental health risks at work, protect and promote mental health at work, and support workers with mental health conditions.

Risks to mental health at work can include the following:

- underuse of skills or being underskilled for work
- excessive workloads or work pace, understaffing
- long, unsocial, or inflexible hours
- lack of control over job design or workload
- unsafe or poor physical working conditions
- organizational culture that enables negative behaviors
- limited support from colleagues or authoritarian supervision
- violence, harassment, or bullying
- discrimination and exclusion
- unclear job role
- under- or overpromotion
- job insecurity, inadequate pay, or poor investment in career development
- conflicting home/work demands (WHO, 2017)

The Importance of a Diverse Health Care Workforce in Family Health and Whole Health Care Health Systems

In this chapter, the essential role of the public health care workforce in improving *family health* and whole health care is discussed from the lens of prevention as an intervention, levels of involvement with families, levels of collaboration, and interprofessional practice. The 4HEALTH context is also presented. The data reports important indicators that are of interest to the welfare of the public health care workforce. The health workforce is a vital building block of any health system (WHO, 2010a). The other building blocks include service delivery, leadership and governance, health information technology, medical products, vaccines and technologies, and health systems financing (WHO, 2010a). By definition, health care workers are all people who engage in actions with a primary intent to enhance the health of individuals, families, populations, and communities (WHO, 2010a). Health care workers are also known for being the helping professionals: "occupations that provide health and education services to individuals and groups, including occupations in the fields of psychology, psychiatry, counseling, medicine, nursing, social work, physical and occupational therapy, teaching, and education" (American Psychological Association, 2018, 1). There are many different compositions of the health care workforce responsible for delivering essential public health services for health to improve health coverage, quality, and safety, as well as health outcomes. Table 5.1 presents the main WHO's (2019) global classification of health care workers and their descriptions, namely health professionals, health associate professionals, personal care workers in health services, health management and support personnel, and other health service providers not elsewhere classified.

TABLE 5.1 **The 2019 WHO Classification of Health Workers by Five Broad Groupings**

Health Care Worker Category	Description and Roles
Health Professionals	Health professionals have the role of studying, advising on, or providing preventive, curative, rehabilitative and promotional health services based on an extensive body of theoretical and factual knowledge in diagnosis and treatment of disease and other health problems. They have different levels of educational background that include a first degree or higher.
Health Associate Professionals	Health associate professionals have the role of performing technical and practical tasks to support the diagnosis and treatment of illness, disease, injuries, and impairments and to support the implementation of health care, treatment, and referral plans, usually established by medical, nursing, and other health professionals. They have different formal qualifications that includes associate degrees, and in some they demonstrate relevant work experience and on-the-job training.
Personal Care Workers in Health Services	Personal care workers provide direct personal care services in health care and residential settings, assist with health care procedures, and perform a variety of other tasks of a simple and routine nature for the provision of health services. They usually have education equivalent to a high school diploma and related certificates.
Health Management and Support Personnel	Health management and support personnel include a wide range of other types of health systems personnel, such as health service managers, health economists, health policy lawyers, biomedical engineers, medical physicists, clinical psychologists, social workers, medical secretaries, ambulance drivers, building maintenance staff, and other general management, professional, technical, administrative, and support staff.
Other Health Service Providers Not Elsewhere Classified	These include the armed forces occupations and interns or trainees who provide clinical services as part of the medical team. Health professionals have the role of studying, advising on, or providing preventive, curative, rehabilitative, and promotional health services based on an extensive body of theoretical and factual knowledge in diagnosis and treatment of disease and other health problems. They have different levels of educational background that include a first degree or higher.

World Health Organization, *Classifying Health Workers: Mapping Occupations to the International Standard Classification*, p. 1, 6, 10, 14.

The Public Health Workforce and Essential Health Services in Family Health Care

As mentioned in previous chapters, patient- and family-centered care or person-centered care is vital for whole health. Hence, there is a growing need for a diverse health care workforce grounded in family science and *family health* for delivering essential health services for whole health care. Table 5.2 provides an overview of how the public health workforce made of multidisciplinary *family health* professionals fits within the concepts of mind, body, and spirit; developmental orientation; definitions of health and whole health; and family science. Later in this chapter, essential health services needs in *family health* care and the engagement and the involvement of multiple disciplines and professionals in meeting the needs in whole health care are introduced.

TABLE 5.2 **The Interrelationship Between Whole Health, the Health Care WORKFORCE, Public Health Care Workforce, and Family Science Professionals Perspectives**

Body-mind-spirit perspectives (Mantri, 2008)	**Developmental oriented perspective (Miller & Bruce, 1991)**	**Health Perspective)**	**Whole Health perspective**	***Health care workforce perspective (Foldspang et al., 2014)**	***Other perspectives: Public health workers (Foldspang et al., 2014) and *population health* care workers (National Academies of Sciences, Engineering, and Medicine, 2023)**
Body	Physiological and pharmacological (biological level)	Physical well-being	Physical well-being	Nurses/midwives Nurse practitioners Physicians Assistants Doctors/physicians Podiatrists Speech pathologists Audiologists Nutritionists/dietitians Occupational therapists Pharmacists Nursing assistants	*Persons*: Public health professionals *Field of work*: Comprehensive public health *Persons*: Politicians, teachers, police officers, architects, and others *Field of work*: Varies (e.g., policy, the classroom, the street, the architect's drawing room, etc.) *Persons*: *Population health* care workers *Field of work*: Aggregates or populations as opposed to individuals
Mind and emotions	Developmental, psychosocial, and emotional (psychologic level)	Mental/psychological well-being	Behavioral well-being	Psychologists	
	Integrated and interactive relationship between individual and family social systems (e.g., child-family-school-peer contexts) (social level)	Social well-being	Socio-economic well-being	Social workers	

Spirit/Soul		Spiritual well-being	Spiritual well-being	Chaplain, clergy, ministers	
Other compositions: community health workers, lay workers, informal caregivers					
*All public health care workers and *population health* care workers can also be identified as *family health* professionals if they have appropriate education/training and/or credentials. Family science professionals: Scholars and professionals in family science, family life education, human development, marriage and family therapy, sociology, psychology, anthropology, social work, theology, child development, health, and more Primary goals are the discovery, verification, and application of knowledge about the family Application of the knowledge: Guided by the levels of public health practice (Minnesota Department of Health, 2019) with a 4HEALTH context: • Individual/family: This practice is directed to individuals and families at risk of health conditions or issues and those who are healthy. The goal is to change knowledge, attitudes, beliefs, practices, and behaviors of individuals and families. • Community: This practice is directed at populations and communities. The goal is to change community norms, attitudes, awareness, practices, and behaviors. • Systems: The practice is directed to systems/organizations that impact public health. The goal is to change systems policies, practices, laws, protocols, and so on to have lasting impact					

Public health has a greater focus on the role of government and does not prioritize the role of the healthcare system or other partners, while *population health* includes partners such as social services, community members (individuals and CBOs), policymakers, and academic research partners.

The Theoretical Foundations of Health Care Professional Involvement and Collaboration With Families in Whole Health Care

A whole health approach is person centered, comprehensive and holistic, upstream-focused, equitable, and accountable (National Academies of Sciences, Engineering, and Medicine, 2023). The approach values quality provider–person partnerships, personal experiences, and longitudinal trusting relationships. In addition, effective, coordinated, and integrated interprofessional teams of *family health* care professionals engage in delivering comprehensive and holistic essential services that address physical health issues as well as upstream conditions within and outside accountable health system(s) to advance health equity.

The direct essential services span three levels of prevention classified as primary (health promotion and disease prevention strategies), secondary (screening and early treatment strategies) and tertiary prevention (strategies to manage health and minimize disability and injury such as chronic disease management, palliation, and rehabilitation to prevent of relapse and complications; Froom & Benbassat, 2000). Although these levels of prevention have been criticized as not being specific enough for various clinical interventions (Froom & Benbassat, 2000), the framework remains useful in understanding and determining goals for PFE and levels of *family health* care professional involvement (Friedman et al., 2023; Myers-Walls et al., 2011). *Family health* care actions or interventions encompass all three levels of prevention across the life course, from birth to death. Apart from assuring service delivery to targeted populations, *family health* professional specialists also engage in assessing, monitoring, and investigating family-related *population health* data. Those with expertise in family policy promote *family health* through family policy development and advocacy (Bogenschneider, 2014; Pratt, 1995). More details about the nature of *family health* interventions (FHI) and family policy will be presented late in the book (see Chapter 9). Table 5.3 provides an overview of the typology of the stage of *family health*, levels of prevention, and examples of key family interventions provided by diverse *family health* care professionals depending on their level of involvement.

TABLE 5.3 **Stages of *Family Health*, Levels of Prevention, and Family Interventions**

Level of Prevention	Stage of *Family Health* and Family Illness/ Health Condition	Examples of Family Interventions	Family Policy Strategies
Primary	Healthy family	Patient and family education Parent and family life education Family education and support	Related to health promotion and disease prevention
Secondary	Family with high risk for health problem(s) or concern(s) Family with a prediagnostic crisis	Family screening Family support Family psychoeducation, Family case management	Related to screening and early treatment
Tertiary	Family with a postdiagnostic health crisis or family dealing with a chronic problem	Family case management Family therapy	Related to disease management, rehabilitation

Levels of Family Health Care Professional Involvement With Families

Over the years, multidisciplinary scholars in the field of family science have conceptualized different levels of *family health* care professional involvement that depict a disciplinary scope of practice, training, and education preparation. Doherty and Baird (1986) pioneered the first *family health* care professional involvement with families' model known as the level of physician involvement model (LPI), a five-level hierarchy model that depicts the physician's levels of competencies (from novice to expert) in addressing patient and family psychosocial needs. The levels of involvement are organized in a continuum from minimal to high involvement (provider centered focusing on medical issues, collaborative with information exchange advice, dealing with feelings and affect, proving basic psychosocial interventions, and high involvement at the individual and family therapy level). Table 5.4 summarizes examples of levels of involvement from different schools of thoughts in family science. The models include the level of family involvement (LFI) by Marvel and Morphew (1993), modified from the LPI model, and the parent and family life education model by Doherty (1995), adapted from the LFI model.

TABLE 5.4 **Levels of Health Care Professional Involvement Models**

Level	LPI (Doherty and Baird, 1986)	LFI, Modified (Marvel & Morphew, 1993)	Parent and Family Life Education Model (Doherty, 1995)
1	Physician centered	Minimal emphasis on family	Institution centered
2	Collaborative information exchange	Information and advice	Collaborative dissemination of information
3	Dealing with affect	Feelings and support	Working with family members' feelings and need for support
4	Basic psychosocial intervention	Brief, focused interventions	Psychoeducational
5	Individual or family therapy	Family therapy	Family therapy

Application of the LFI Framework

The LPI model has been applied in medical education and research to assess how physicians address psychosocial concerns with patients and families (Marvel et al., 1994). The model was revised in 1995 to become the LFI model, which was applied in clinical medicine to assess family-centered care (Marvel & Morphew, 1993) and in school psychology to conceptualize the competency levels of the school psychologists in developing family-school-community collaborations (Ho, 1997). In addition, the model has been useful to religious professionals' determination of interventions and areas of professional development (Hawley & Dahl, 2000). In 1995, Doherty, with input from parent and family educators, adapted the LFI model to parent and family education for facilitation of the acquisition of competencies in parenting or coparenting among parents, couples, or other family members. Other fields of study such as nursing have described their level of involvement with families by conceptualizing the unit of analysis of the family unit of care within the nurse–patient and –family partnership (Friedman et al., 2003). For instance, in pediatric and adult/geriatric health care, family is viewed as constant resource, with the individual as the unit of care and analysis. In primary and community health care nursing, the family is viewed as a sum of its parts whereby all family members are potential units of care and analysis. The unit of care includes family subsystems (e.g., dyads, triads, etc.) or the family as a whole. In other situations, such as public health nursing, the unit of care and analysis is the family subsystem within a society or community (Friedman et al., 2003). These different perspectives offer a framework for *family health* care professionals to delineate their level of involvement with families and the necessary skills required to intervene. For example, nurse interventions at the family systems level require advanced clinical and intervention skills (e.g., family therapy; Friedman et al., 2003). Likewise, family nurses require knowledge, attitudes, and skills in population-based public health nursing practice (Schoon et al., 2019).

Family and Professional Roles in the LFI Frameworks

The following are different levels of involvement in the LFI Frameworks:

Level 1

At this level, the role of the family in a health care system is limited. Family involvement is perceived from a supportive or legal perspective (Hennon et al., 2013). Families follow the organizational protocols that are individualistic and provider centered (Doherty, 1995; Doherty & Baird, 1986). The health care professional's role is to provide care focused on the client's/patient's medical complaint. There is limited input from the family. The needs of the index client or patient are given priority over the needs of the family or its subsystems.

Level 2

At this level, the role of the family in a health care system is collaborative in nature whereby the provider gives information and advice on a certain *family health* need (Hennon et al., 2013). The health care professional provides expertise and leadership during information and advising sessions. The interactions can take place at time of discharge during patient and family education or in a family-to-family educational setting in the health facility or community. Sharing feelings and support is limited. Information-giving sessions can occur in different formats, such as face-to-face or online (e.g., telehealth; Doherty, 1995). Professionals at this level are not equipped with the competencies to address feelings or the affective domain. However, they may have basic communication skills and skills for group processes (Hennon et al., 2013).

Level 3

At this level, families are encouraged to share feelings and support within an educational setting during their visit with the provider. Professional roles are similar to level 2, but the expertise includes family functioning knowledge and group counseling skills that include eliciting feelings and experiences from the family (i.e., brief counseling and coaching) and maintaining personal disclosures in discussions (Hennon et al., 2013). The interactions can take place at discharge during patient and family education or in a family-to-family educational setting in the health facility or community where normative family stressors are present or anticipated. Skills in understanding issues that need referral and the actual referral pathway are essential (Hennon et al., 2013).

Level 4

At this level, the role of the family is to be involved into an educational contractual agreement to address a family dysfunction or troubled dynamic that could be related to normative or non-normative family stressors within an at-risk or vulnerable family (Hennon et al., 2013). Professionals in this level assume roles in level 2 and 3 and include skills in assessment and planning for tailored, brief-focused intervention to assist in changing family functioning patterns to address problems before they become worse. Usually, interactions happen at the individual, subsystem, or family level. Level 4 involves an intersectional and multisectorial approach as providers engage collaboratively with other health care professionals and sectors to provide needed services to families (Hennon et al., 2013).

Level 5

At this level, the family has a contractual agreement to address significant problematic family patterns that need a skilled therapist (Hennon et al., 2013). The role of the professional is that of a skilled therapist with expertise in clinical therapeutic techniques. Usually, the therapeutic interactions can take place at the individual, subsystem, or family system levels and involve an extended series of family intervention sessions (Doherty, 1995).

Despite the LFI model's benefits in delineating professional roles, it has faced criticism for suggesting hierarchal professional boundaries and professional identity confusion for those in family professions, implying that therapy roles are superior to education and prevention roles (Myers-Walls et al., 2011). As a result, the domains of family practice (DFP) model (Myers-Wall et al., 2011) was developed to aid in understanding professional boundaries through the articulation of disciplinary "why, what, when, for whom, and how" with families to foster collaboration. The practical application of the model beyond delineation has been beneficial for providers to map holistic practical strategies to strengthening relationship skill building among low-income, at-risk families through collaborative targets within a community (Hall & Own, 2024). Thus, it is important for *family health* care professionals to understand their professional scope of practice and limitation to engage in meaningful and effective family-focused intervention and collaboration in an integrated and interprofessional whole health care system.

Collaborative and Integrated Interprofessional Family Health Care Teams

Family health disciplinary teams are necessary in any health care systems to solve complex health needs and conditions that affect individuals, families, communities and populations. Terminologies such as *multidisciplinary*, *interdisciplinary*, and *transdisciplinary* have been used to describe efforts made by different disciplines in the context of health care. Discipline in this case is referred to as the overarching field of work, such as health care, family science, law, and policy, while profession refers to roles achieved through education or professional training or trajectories, such as a doctors, nurses, and hygienists (Sell et al., 2022). Table 5.5 provides definitions of the three terminologies based on an extensive review of academic literature conducted by Cho and Pak (2006).

TABLE 5.5 Multidisciplinary, Interdisciplinary, and Transdisciplinary Definitions and Core Concept Components

Terminology	Definition and Description	Common Words	Key Concepts Components
Multidisciplinary	Draws on knowledge from different disciplines but stays within the boundaries of those fields The basic level of involvement of multiple disciplines that are working in parallel or sequentially, without challenging disciplinary boundaries	Additive: Serving or tending to increase	Who: The involved disciplines and/or professions How: The mode of collaboration Why: The aim and purpose What: The role of participants and disciplinary boundaries
Interdisciplinary	Analyses, synthesizes, and harmonizes links between disciplines into a coordinated and coherent whole Blurs disciplinary boundaries in order to generate new common methodologies, perspectives, knowledge, or even new disciplines	Interactive: Producing action on each other	
Transdisciplinary	Integrates the natural, social, and health sciences in a humanities context, and in so doing transcends each of their traditional boundaries	Holistic: Producing a material objective that has a reality other and greater than the sum of its constituent parts	

It is important to note that the term *multiple disciplinary* has been used to describe situations when involvement of different disciplines is not clear due to overlapping knowledge that is not integrated in each practice (Sell et al., 2022). Thus, a clear articulation of the nature of the collaboration by examining the key concept components for collaboration in interdisciplinary, multidisciplinary and transdisciplinary work is necessary (Cho & Pak, 2006; Sell et al., 2022). The components include who (involved disciplines and/or professions), why (aim and purpose), what (role of participants), how (mode of collaboration), and what (disciplinary boundaries). For example, *family health* professionals should know who is involved (Doekhie et al., 2017). Collaboration in such environments must include an aim and purpose among team members, which reflects the need to use or integrate knowledge, expertise, and methods from different team members to address a common problem. The mode of collaboration refers to the level of involvement, for example, articulating how different professions and disciplines contribute knowledge/expertise/perspectives and skills to meet a common goals and in a participatory manner.

Understanding the roles of the participants is also key. Each discipline and profession should be allowed to contribute their unique knowledge and skills and be ready to accept core responsibilities. It is important that there is a process of learning others' language, culture, and norms to develop knowledge that can facilitate the development of shared goals and solutions. Lastly, disciplinary boundaries should be adhered to depending on the level of involvement. For example, in multidisciplinary teamwork, professions with different backgrounds and skills share their perspectives. In interdisciplinary teams, collaboration crosses disciplinary and professional boundaries by integrating knowledge from different professions/disciplines. In transdisciplinary teams, boundaries are dissolved into holistic, collaborative paradigms. This approach not only involves sharing the assessment process, outcome selection (in collaboration with the family), intervention strategies, and implementing services, but also requires members to function as a cohesive unit by sharing knowledge and skills among members (Raver & Childress, 2015). There is a strong sense of shared responsibility for all team activities, functions, and roles. The regular and systematic sharing of knowledge and skills among diverse members of the team, including patients and families, is important in health care settings (Brand & Timmons, 2021). Likewise, it is important to note that when developing transdisciplinary teams, there needs to be investments in time and energy for effective collaboration to take place.

The LFI model has been useful in articulating the different levels of *family health* care professional collaboration. For instance, the model of competency levels in family-school-community collaborations (Ho, 1997) and the level of integration model (Getch & Lute, 2019) describe the level of *family health* professional collaboration and involvement of the family. Table 5.6 provides a summary of the collaborative community-based LFI model and integrated health care system model.

TABLE 5.6 **Levels of Health Care Professional Collaboration Models**

Level	Model of Competency Levels in Family-School-Community Collaborations (Ho, 1997)	Level of Integration Model (Getch & Lute, 2019)
1	Minimal collaboration with family	Minimal collaboration (coordinated care key element: communication)
2	Openness to engage families in collaborative ways	Basic collaboration at a distance (coordinated care key element: communication)
3	Systematic assessment and planned family–school partnerships for individual children	Basic collaboration onsite (co-located care key element: proximity)
4	Whole-school systematic assessment and planned family-school-community collaborations	Close collaboration onsite with some system integration (co-located care key element: proximity)
5		Close collaboration approaching an integrated practice (integrated care key element: practice change)
6		Full collaboration in a transformed/merged integrated practice (integrated care key element: practice change)

The model of competency levels in family-school-community collaborations focuses on the levels of collaboration within social environments (four levels), and the level of integration model focuses on involvement within integrated health care (six levels). Integrated health care is referred to as an "interprofessional health care approach characterized by a high degree of collaboration and communication among health professionals that involves sharing information and establishing shared comprehensive treatment plans to address the biological, psychological and social needs of the patient" (American Psychological Association, 2013, para. 2). Here's a descriptive analysis of the levels of involvement in collaborative practice using the LFI model:

- *Level 1*: At this level of collaboration, the family is a valued source of information and intervention. There is a clear understanding of the family as a microsystem. Providers are equipped with interviewing skills to conduct structured interviews. Knowledge of legal and ethical skills is essential. In terms of collaboration, there is minimum integration. Providers work at separate facilities and rarely communicate about cases.
- *Level 2*: At this level, team(s) are open to engage families in collaborative ways. Families and providers communicate assessment results. Providers offer to conduct needs assessments, offer advice, and make referrals. Collaboration is not integrated, but providers maintain separate facilities and separate systems while utilizing each other as resources. Communication may occur periodically and is generally driven by specific issues.
- *Level 3*: At this level, family is considered a necessary resource for the index client (e.g., a child in a school system). Provider skills needed include how to provide guidance and support, assessment of the family–school relationship, and developing family resources. In terms of integration/collaboration in a health care system space, providers are colocated in same facility but do not share practice space. Communication is regular, and referral is successful. Occasional patient discussion meetings occur. Providers feel part of the team. Providers' decisions still occur at the individual level.
- *Level 4*: At this level, providers use an ecological approach to address the needs of a whole system (e.g., school community). Providers demonstrate skills including designing, implementing, and evaluating well-developed family-school-community collaboration programs as well as interdisciplinary collaborative skills and leadership capacities. At this level of health system integration, there are promising initiatives of shared systems and providers work in close proximity. For example, the primary care front desk schedules all providers' appointments, and medical records are shared.
- *Level 5*: At this level, full integration is not yet completed, but providers function as a true team, with frequent communication. All providers have knowledge of the different roles team members need to play and have begun to change their own practice based on this knowledge.
- *Level 6*: At this level, there is the greatest amount of practice change into a single transformed or merged practice that applies the principle of whole health care.

Interprofessional Competency Frameworks

The concepts of interprofessional collaborative practice and interprofessional education have received much attention in the health care literature. Collaborative practice means that interprofessional teams from "multiple health workers from different professional backgrounds work together with 'persons' (i.e., patients, families, careers and communities) to deliver the highest quality of care across settings" (WHO, 2010b, p. 7). In interprofessional collaboration, providers from multiple health systems present themselves with clear roles and scopes of practice and have a shared understanding of the person/patient's priorities and needs (Reeves et al., 2018). Professionals come together to provide care for specific populations/health issues following a referral. For example, a primary care doctor works with a pharmacist at a local pharmacy or collaborates with a children's hospital. Such interprofessional collaboration improves access to health care, coordination of care between different sectors, and patient and family engagement in self-care and decision-making (Davidson et al., 2022), health, and health care costs (Smith et al., 2021), as well as team communication and job satisfactions (Labrague et al., 2022).

Within health care shortage contexts, it is also important to articulate how delegation plays out when implementing evidence-based task shifting and task-sharing strategies in interprofessional collaborative practice (Hoeft et al., 2018; Lange, 2021; Le et al., 2022). Task shifting is moving certain tasks when appropriate to other less skilled health workers to increase efficiency and affordability in the allocation of available human resources (WHO, 2007). On the other hand, task sharing is defined as the practice of delegating task(s) to health care workers beyond one's scope of practice, with the goal of increasing access to health care to underserved populations (WHO, 2007). Both task shifting and sharing requirements differ across countries and involve the training and ongoing educational support of health care workers (Yankam, 2023). An example of task shifting is delegating mental health assessment tasks to community health workers but making sure the delegated task is shared within a collaborative model with a mental health specialist or primary care physician. In this case, the specialist acts as the trainer, supervisor, and consultant in the collaborative relationship (Hoeft et al., 2018).

As indicated earlier, there are certain skills set that need to be acquired to work in a collaborative interprofessional and integrated health care systems. These skills are also called competencies, defined as "the abilities of a person to integrate knowledge, skills and attitudes in their performance of tasks in a given context" (WHO, 2022, p. iv). For *family health* care professionals to effectively and appropriately function and delegate roles in an interprofessional environment, they should become familiar with the competencies required for interprofessional practice. These competencies are usually "durable, trainable and, through the expression of behaviours, measurable" (WHO, 2022, p. iv). Interprofessional education and collaboration is one of the core competencies in health care today. The most common framework in the literature is the WHO (2010b) interprofessional education and collaborative practice. The framework sets standards for creating Interprofessional Education (IPE) competencies. The Interprofessional Education Collaborative (IPEC, 2023) has pioneered and disseminated evolving core competencies since

2011. The competencies have been embedded into both disciplinary undergraduate and graduate curricula as well as accreditation standards. The competencies are intended to prepare learners for lifelong learning and collaborative practice to improve *population health* outcome and health care service delivery. Table 5.7 lists the four IPEC competencies and sub-competencies as of 2023. Other IPE competencies from the literature consistent with the IPEC competencies are (a) patient-centered care, (b) interprofessional communication, (c) participatory leadership, (d) conflict resolution, (e) transparency of duties and responsibilities, and (f) teamwork (Vaseghi et al., 2022). *Family health* professionals are responsible for understanding their discipline-specific IPE competencies, which is beyond the scope of this book.

TABLE 5.7 **2023 IPEC Competencies**

Competency	Description	Sub-Competency
Values and Ethics	Work with team members to maintain a climate of shared values, ethical conduct, and mutual respect	VE1. Promote the values and interests of persons and populations in health care delivery, One Health, and *population health* initiatives. VE2. Advocate for social justice and health equity of persons and populations across the life span. VE3. Uphold the dignity, privacy, identity, and autonomy of persons while maintaining confidentiality in the delivery of team-based care. VE4. Value diversity, identities, cultures, and differences. VE5. Value the expertise of health professionals and its impacts on team functions and health outcomes. VE6. Collaborate with honesty and integrity while striving for health equity and improvements in health outcomes. VE7. Practice trust, empathy, respect, and compassion with persons, caregivers, health professionals, and populations. VE8. Apply high standards of ethical conduct and quality in contributions to team-based care. VE9. Maintain competence in one's own profession in order to contribute to interprofessional care. VE10. Contribute to a just culture that fosters self-fulfillment, collegiality, and civility across the team. VE11. Support a workplace where differences are respected, career satisfaction is supported, and well-being is prioritized.
Roles and Responsibilities	Use the knowledge of one's own role and team members' expertise to address individual and *population health* outcomes	RR1. Include the full scope of knowledge, skills, and attitudes of team members to provide care that is person-centered, safe, cost-effective, timely, efficient, effective, and equitable. RR2. Collaborate with others within and outside of the health system to improve health outcomes.

		RR3. Incorporate complementary expertise to meet health needs, including the determinants of health. RR4. Differentiate each team member's role, scope of practice, and responsibility in promoting health outcomes. RR5. Practice cultural humility in interprofessional teamwork.
Communication	Communicate in a responsive, responsible, respectful, and compassionate manner with team members	C1. Communicate one's roles and responsibilities clearly. C2. Use communication tools, techniques, and technologies to enhance team function, well-being, and health outcomes. C3. Communicate clearly with authenticity and cultural humility, avoiding discipline-specific terminology. C4. Promote common understanding of shared goals. C5. Practice active listening that encourages ideas and opinions of other team members. C6. Use constructive feedback to connect, align, and accomplish team goals. C7. Examine one's position, power, role, unique experience, expertise, and culture toward improving communication and managing conflicts.
Teams and Teamwork	Apply values and principles of the science of teamwork to adapt one's own role in a variety of team settings	TT1. Describe evidence-informed processes of team development and team practices. TT2. Appreciate team members' diverse experiences, expertise, cultures, positions, power, and roles toward improving team function. TT3. Practice team reasoning, problem-solving, and decision-making. TT4. Use shared leadership practices to support team effectiveness. TT5. Apply interprofessional conflict management methods, including identifying conflict cause and addressing divergent perspectives. TT6. Reflect on self and team performance to inform and improve team effectiveness. TT7. Share team accountability for outcomes. TT8. Facilitate team coordination to achieve safe, effective care and health outcomes. TT9. Operate from a shared framework that supports resiliency, well-being, safety, and efficacy. TT10. Discuss organizational structures, policies, practices, resources, access to information, and timing issues that impact the effectiveness of the team.

Occupational Challenges and Opportunities in Building and Strengthening a Whole Health Care Workforce Within 4HEALTHS

As part of being a helping professional in health care, there is usually a personal expectation of putting one's self-care and safety needs last while comforting and healing patients, families, populations, and communities. Unfortunately, if the expectations are not exercised or supported well in some contexts or situations the providers can experience occupational stress that may have a negative impact on one's health and well-being. Before, during, and after COVID-19, health care providers expressed a need for occupational interventions to mitigate and control occupational stress. The COVID-19 pandemic heightened the need for preparing a healthy and sustainable frontline health care workforce during emergencies (Sanchez-Taltavull et al., 2021). During the pandemic and other emergencies, a diverse health workforce is needed to provide care beyond the care of victims to include victim's families, vulnerable populations, communities, and public health systems. Access to a qualified health care workforce is a challenge due to an ongoing workforce shortage, which is worsened by workforce burnout. Thus, the ongoing need to build capacity and strengthen and sustain a strong, diverse, helping profession or health care workforce that is responsive to whole health care health systems is warranted. In this section, information drawn from a recent U.S Surgeon General's (2022) advisory on building a thriving health workforce, as well as other empirical evidence, is used to explore challenges and opportunities for building and strengthening a well-rounded workforce for whole health care.

Burnout and Burnout Disparities Among Health Care Providers

Burnout is "an occupational syndrome characterized by high degree of emotional exhaustion and depersonalization (i.e., cynicism), and low sense of personal accomplishment at work" (Office of the U.S. Surgeon General, 2022, p. 7). According to the National Academy of Medicine (2019), 35%–45% of U.S. nurses and physicians and 45%–60% of medical students and residents reported symptoms of burnout. Burnout consequences occur at various levels when health care providers feels like they cannot provide the best service for their patient and patients feel that they do not get the services they need. Figure 5.1 summarizes some of the common negative consequences of burnout among health care workers, including mental health, relationship, and chronic disease challenges at the individual level. Other consequences reported in the literature are risk for suicide or suicide attempts (Duthell et al., 2019).

In addition to burnout, health care providers may present with moral stress, moral injury, and compassionate fatigue. Health care providers experience moral distress and injury when they deal with the sufferings of others. Moral distress occurs from moral conflict and is referred to as occupation stress that occurs "when one knows the right thing to do, but institutional constraints make it nearly impossible to pursue the right course of action" (Jameton, 1984, p. 6). Moral injury, a concept that is common in the

Health worker burnout can have many negative consequences
"I can't provide the best care to my patients..."
"I can't get the care I need..."
Health Workers
· Insomnia, heart disease, and diabetes
· Isolation, substance use, anxiety, and depression
· Relationship and interpersonal challenges
· Exhaustion from overwhelming care and empathy
Patients
· Less time with health workers
· Delays in care and diagnosis
· Lower quality of care
· Medical errors
Health Care System
· Health workforce shortages and retention challenges
· Limited services available
· Risk of malpractice and decreased patient satisfaction
· Increased costs
Community and Society
· Erosion of trust
· Worsening population health outcomes
· Increased health disparities
· Lack of preparedness for public health crises
Office of the U.S. Surgeon General

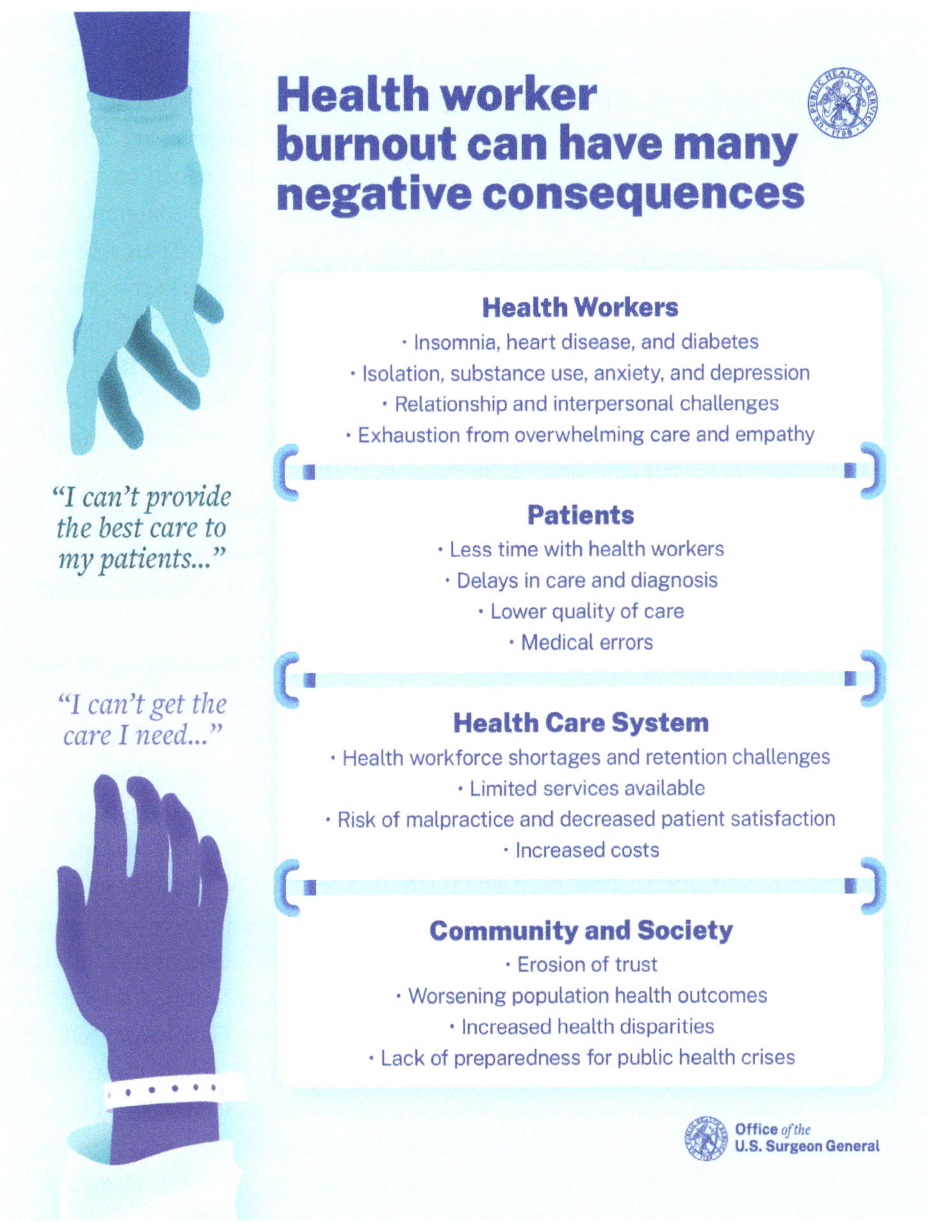

FIGURE 5.1 Common negative consequences of burnout among health care workers (Office of U.S Surgeon General, 2022)

military or war settings, was also coined during the COVID-19 pandemic to "represent an experience of the problem that results in a long-lasting change to an individual's sense of losing hope, trust, integrity" (p. 597). Both moral distress and injury deal with moral values or beliefs and result in psychological consequences of guilt, blame of self and others, anguish, and powerlessness that may lead to functional impairment (Čartolovni et al., 2021). A multidisciplinary concept of compassionate fatigue has also been defined in relation to burnout. It is described as a work-related stress common among health care providers that is considered a "cost of caring" that affects quality patient care due to one's loss of compassion (Sinclair et al., 2017). Health care providers who are not compassionate lack the interpersonal affective subjective feeling of witnessing another person's suffering and subsequent desire to offer help by showing caregiving behaviors that signal patterns of touch, posture, vocalization, commitment, and cooperation (Goetz et al., 2010). They demonstrate symptoms such as emotional exhaustion, physical exhaustion, insomnia, irritability, anxiety, depression, apathy, depersonalization, feelings of self-contempt, feelings of being untreated unfairly, poor job satisfaction, and chronic aches and pains, including headache, backache, and muscle tension. The difference between the term *compassionate care* and *empathy* or *sympathy* is that compassionate care is a practical care process that is provided by health care providers to decrease or relieve patients' pain, discomfort, or suffering (Tehranineshat et al., 2019). For example, a health care provider can show culturally compassionate care by communicating with their clients (patients and families) and exploring their concerns while placing themselves in clients' shoes to understand their situation and then collaboratively find alternative to ways to problem solve the suffering.

It is also important to understand disparities in burnout among health care providers. Data on burnout demonstrates that minority health care workers, females, immigrant health care workers, low-income health care workers, and health care workers in rural and tribal communities are at risk of structural vulnerabilities in the healthcare industry (Office of the U.S. Surgeon General, 2022). For instance, health care workers of color are more likely to experience low wages, unfair workload assignments, implicit bias, and microaggressions. During the pandemic minority workers were more likely to be assigned to care for patients with or suspected of COVID-19 and with inadequate personal protective equipment. Likewise, although immigrant health workers only comprised 18% of the health care workforce, more than one third died from COVID-19 in the 1st year of the pandemic, which indicates a disparity concern. Female health workers are more likely to present with burnout symptoms and disruptions of careers due to childcare responsibilities compared to their male counterparts. Minority workers and females are likely to experience the burden of the consequences related to low wages (Office of the U.S. Surgeon General, 2022). Rural health care workers and those who work with tribal communities are impacted with health care workforce shortages and lack of or poor health systems. Health care workers in tribal communities are severely impacted by lack of funding, lack of safe water, and food and housing insecurities (Office of the U.S. Surgeon General, 2022).

For health systems to provide whole health care, patients, families, populations and communities need healthy and competent health care providers at all levels of the 4HEALTHS. For example, at the *individual health*, providers need individual-level assessment and empowerment intervention programs. The individual assessment usually targets provider productivity performance, patient safety, and quality care. Empowerment programs target advocacy opportunities for positive changes and self-care management such a vaccination and positive health habits. The only drawback of such interventions is that they are short-lived, reactive, and not enough, as they do not address the systemic or organizational factors that have long-term impact.

A "whole of society" approach (Office of the U.S. Surgeon General, 2022) is a potential solution to systems-level challenges. In whole health care, patient- and family-centered care is important to make sure health care systems build capacity in patient, family, and community engagement beyond the biomedical model and include the biopsychosocial context. Thus, at the individual and *family health* level, providers need family members who check in, pay attention to warning signs of distress, and have knowledge of available resources. Workplace violence is also a real threat to health care providers (Chesire et al., 2022). Thus, providers can benefit from patients, families, and communities who are actively engaged in their care and are kind to health care workers. Health care quality and safety is an ethical win-win for clients and the care team.

In population and public health contexts, burnout affects service delivery in many ways. For example, at the organizational level of care, health care workers continue to be helpless when they try to address social determinants of health and are compounded with systemic issues of limited time and lack of patients and community trust. The focus on individual level care within silos using a biomedical approach is also a challenge. Figure 5.2 illustrates some of the common factors that contribute to societal, cultural, structural, and organization factors to burnout among health workers.

Moreover, the public health function of reassuring a competent workforce is a daunting task, especially in diverse local, national, and global contexts. It is difficult to standardize educational programs because of contextual needs and competing priorities. With these limitations, major challenges continue to exist. For example, there is still a lack of providers who are well prepared in *population health* and collaborative care that are needed to understand whole health care. If health system transformation is necessary to address workforce burdens such as burnout and its consequences on productivity and performance, there need to be changes in health care professional curricula and accreditation bodies to build capacity for a well-rounded public health workforce that can understand, advocate, and provide services in whole health care health system environments. For example, there is an urgent need of a workforce oriented toward health promotion and health protection skills in assessing and addressing social determinants of health, knowledge of effective prevention strategies, and the ability to communicate (using both traditional and non-traditional media) to engage an increasingly skeptical public.

In addition, although, metrics for *population health* provide avenues for determining needs for interdisciplinary teams for quality service delivery to populations at risk as well as those who are healthy to prevent them from being sick in the first place, traditional measures of productivity do not benefit providers. For example, metrics on time and finances and less emphasis on qualitative measures such as patients and families, as well as provider needs and satisfaction, are barriers to practice and likely to increase burnout. Likewise, with increased need for *population health* metrics comes with the burden of administrative tasks and documentation, resulting into more burnout. Such burdens should be evaluated periodically, and innovative, human-centered mitigation and response strategies should be redesigned with the end users: health care providers, patients, and families. Innovative workflow and usability issues with technology (e.g., electronic medical records) should also be revised. Likewise, innovative technologies for

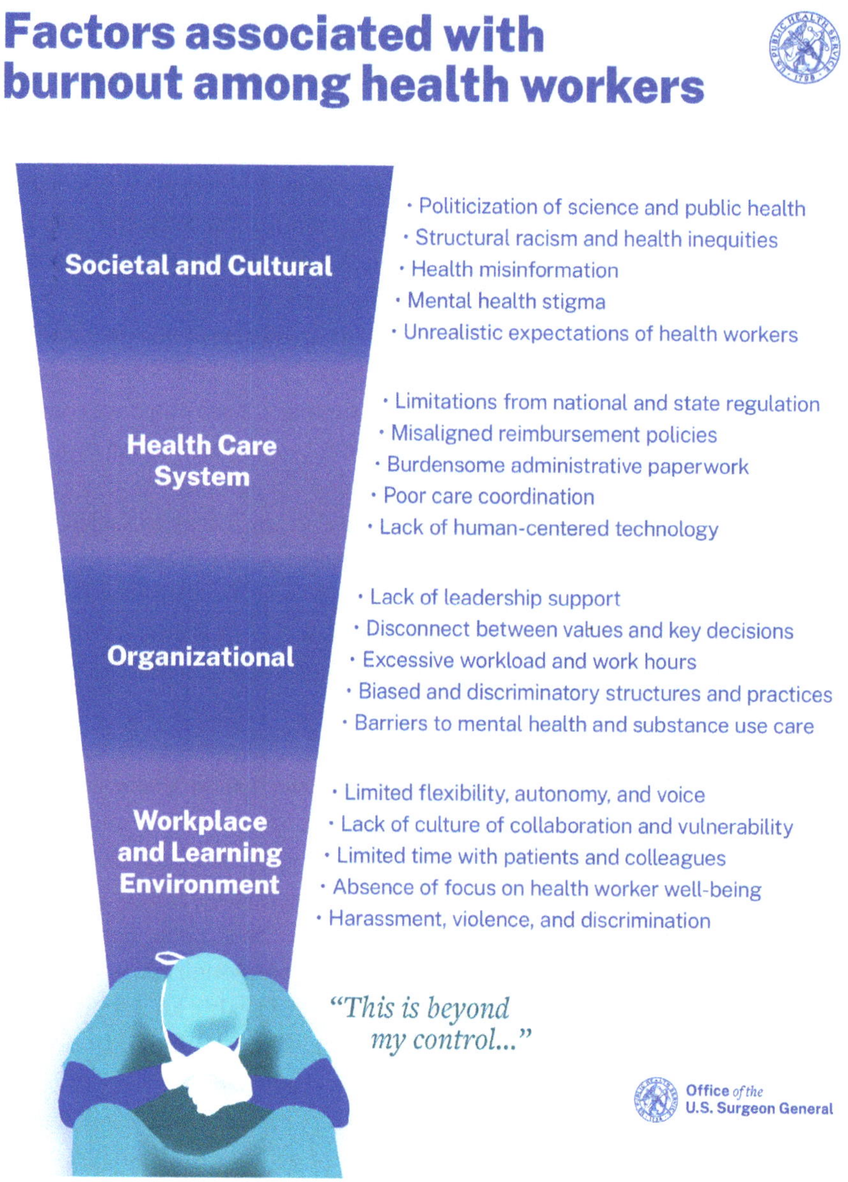

Factors associated with burnout among health workers

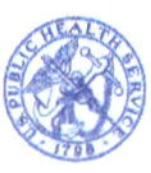

Societal and Cultural

- Politicization of science and public health
- Structural racism and health inequities
- Health misinformation
- Mental health stigma
- Unrealistic expectations of health workers

Health Care System

- Limitations from national and state regulation
- Misaligned reimbursement policies
- Burdensome administrative paperwork
- Poor care coordination
- Lack of human-centered technology

Organizational

- Lack of leadership support
- Disconnect between values and key decisions
- Excessive workload and work hours
- Biased and discriminatory structures and practices
- Barriers to mental health and substance use care

Workplace and Learning Environment

- Limited flexibility, autonomy, and voice
- Lack of culture of collaboration and vulnerability
- Limited time with patients and colleagues
- Absence of focus on health worker well-being
- Harassment, violence, and discrimination

"This is beyond my control..."

Office *of the* U.S. Surgeon General

FIGURE 5.2 Common societal, cultural, structural, and organization factors contributing to burnout among health workers (Office of the U.S. Surgeon General, 2022)

supervision and communication for telehealth advice and disease management, especially among the more vulnerable communities, should be in place. Health care systems should prepare the workforce to adapt to technologies that may mitigate burnout burdens. A growing field in health care is that of artificial intelligence.

In addition to the challenges and opportunities comes the need to have evidenced-based models of payment (reimbursement models) that not only capture physical needs (medical) but also psychological, spiritual, and social needs. These models should account for providers' time in prevention services and coordinated care teams beyond just procedures or a 15-minute visit. For such models to work, there must be compromises made in task-sharing and task-shifting policies for effective utilization of the health care workforce (Orkin et al., 2021; WHO, 2007). Schools and accreditation bodies should evaluate need and appropriate contexts to prepare a health care workforce that will meet the needs of diverse populations. Appropriate actions should be put forth to assess barriers and facilitators of health care worker expansions of disciplines' scopes of practice. This should include defining clear roles and responsibilities, strategies for delegation, and supervision (Orkin et al., 2021). At the implementation level, challenges related to discipline-specific workforce schedules and autonomy should also be reviewed collectively with those of other disciplines to facilitate appropriate teams and staff ratio per shift to meet the needs of a population of interest. It is critical that measures to ensure health care workers are supported by evidence-based legislation in the areas of training, equipment supply, adequate staffing, monitoring, and assessment of workplace illness and injury, access, and coverage of affordable mental health and substance use care are in place in public health systems. Punitive polices for a healthy workforce should be revised periodically. For example, policies on health care providers' mental and substance abuse can be reviewed to find way to help providers who are a potential fit to work but are affected by work distress–related substance abuse.

Overall, health care systems need to invest in good interprofessional leadership teams to lead the way to change the culture of the health care workforce. As part of transformative actions, leaders should advocate for peers and interdisciplinary team-based models that encourage completing tasks but also building a sense of belonging, collaboration, and support among key players (individual providers, their families, health care systems, their communities, and public health).

Conclusion

Assuring a competent and sustainable public health force is crucial to public health. Likewise, assuring a competent *family health* workforce is vital for whole health care and integrated care. This chapter introduced readers to the role of the health care workforce in *family health* and related challenges within a broader socioecological context that incorporates the 4HEALTHS framework. An emphasis is placed on the role of interprofessional competencies that cut across disciplines and professionals. In the next few chapters, family assessment and intervention and effective communication as core competencies in *family health* care are introduced.

Suggested Websites

U.S. Bureau of Labor Statistics: https://www.bls.gov/spotlight/2023/healthcare-occupations-in-2022/home.htm

Office of the U.S. Surgeon General, addressing health worker burnout: https://www.hhs.gov/sites/default/files/health-worker-wellbeing-advisory.pdf

WHO global health workforce statistics: https://www.who.int/data/gho/data/themes/topics/health-workforce

Suggested Readings

Doherty, W. J. (1995). Boundaries between parent and family education and family therapy: The Levels of Family Involvement model. *Family Relations: An Interdisciplinary Journal of Applied Family Studies, 44*(4), 353–358. https://doi.org/10.2307/584990

Doherty, W. J., & Baird, M. A. (1986). Developmental levels in family-centered medical care. *Family Medicine, 18*(3), 153–156.

Ho, B. S. (1997). The school psychologist's role based on an ecological approach to family-school-community collaborations. *The California School Psychologist, 2*(1), 31–38.

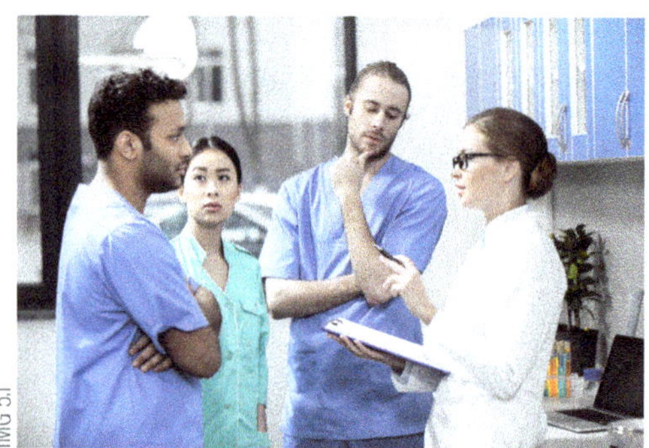

IMG 5.1

National Academies of Sciences, Engineering, and Medicine. (2023). A *population health* workforce to meet 21st-century challenges and opportunities: Proceedings of a workshop. National Academies Press. https://doi.org/10.17226/27232

World Health Organization. (2010). Framework for action on interprofessional education & collaborative practice. https://iris.who.int/bitstream/handle/10665/70185/WHO _HRH_HPN_10.3_eng.pdf?sequence=1

Reflection Questions

Think about how your interaction with the health care systems and reflect on the following questions:

1. What does interprofessional practice mean to you?
2. How many different disciplines or professionals have you met? Mention three.
3. Which of the three professionals in question 2 did you have a hard time understanding regarding their titles, roles, and responsibilities, and level of involvement with families? Why?

References

American Psychological Association. (2013). *Integrated health care*. https://www.apa.org/health/integrated-health-care

American Psychological Association. (2018). *Helping Professions*. https://dictionary.apa.org/helping-professions

Bell, J., & Breslin, J. M. (2008). Healthcare provider moral distress as a leadership challenge. *JONA'S healthcare law, ethics and regulation, 10*(4), 94–97.

Bogenschneider, K. (2014). *Family policy matters: How policymaking affects families and what professionals can do.* Routledge.

Brand, S., & Timmons, S. (2021). Knowledge sharing to support long-term condition self-management—Patient and health-care professional perspectives. *Health Expectations, 24*(2), 628–637.

Canadian Interprofessional Health Collaborative. (2010). *A national interprofessional competency framework*. University of British Columbia.

Čartolovni, A., Stolt, M., Scott, P. A., & Suhonen, R. (2021). Moral injury in healthcare professionals: A scoping review and discussion. *Nursing ethics*, *28*(5), 590–602.

Chesire, D. J., McIntosh, A., Hendrickson, S., Jones, P., & McIntosh, M. (2022). Dimensions of hospital workplace violence: Patient violence towards the healthcare team. *Journal of clinical nursing*, *31*(11–12), 1662–1668.

Choi, B. C., & Pak, A. W. (2006). Multidisciplinarity, interdisciplinarity and transdisciplinarity in health research, services, education and policy: 1. Definitions, objectives, and evidence of effectiveness. *Clinical and investigative medicine*, *29*(6), 351–364.

Davidson, A. R., Kelly, J., Ball, L., Morgan, M., & Reidlinger, D. P. (2022). What do patients experience? Interprofessional collaborative practice for chronic conditions in primary care: An integrative review. *BMC Primary Care*, *23*(1), 1–12.

Dickson, J. J. (2015). Supporting a generationally diverse workforce: Considerations for aging providers in the US healthcare system. *Journal of Best Practices in Health Professions Diversity*, *8*(2), 1071–1086.

Doekhie, K. D., Buljac-Samardzic, M., Strating, M. M., & Paauwe, J. (2017). Who is on the primary care team? Professionals' perceptions of the conceptualization of teams and the underlying factors: A mixed-methods study. *BMC family practice*, *18*, 1–14.

Doherty, W. J. (1995). Boundaries between parent and family education and family therapy: The Levels of Family Involvement model. *Family Relations: An Interdisciplinary Journal of Applied Family Studies*, *44*(4), 353–358. https://doi.org/10.2307/584990

Doherty, W. J., & Baird, M. A. (1986). Developmental levels in family-centered medical care. *Family Medicine*, *18*(3), 153–156.

Foldspang, L., Mark, M., Hjorth, L. R., Langholz-Carstensen, C., Poulsen, O. M., Johansson, U., ... & Rants, L. L. (2014). *Working environment and productivity: A register-based analysis of Nordic enterprises*. Nordic Council of Ministers.

Friedman, M. M., Bowden, V. R. & Jones, E. G. (2023). *Family Nursing. Research, Theory and Practice* (5th ed.). Prentice-Hall.

Froom, P., & Benbassat, J. (2000). Inconsistencies in the classification of preventive interventions. *Preventive Medicine*, *31*(2), 153–158.

Getch, S. E., & Lute, R. M. (2019). Advancing integrated healthcare: A step-by-step guide for primary care physicians and behavioral health clinicians. *Missouri Medicine*, *116*(5), 384–388.

Goetz, J. L., Keltner, D., & Simon-Thomas, E. (2010). Compassion: An evolutionary analysis and empirical review. Psychological Bulletin, 136(3), 351–374. https://doi.org/10.1037/a0018807

Gröne, O., & Garcia-Barbero, M. (2001). WHO European Office for Integrated Health Care Services. Integrated care: A position paper of the WHO European Office for Integrated Health Care Services. *Int J Integr Care*, *1*, e21.

Hall, L., & Ownby, C. (2024). The Domains of Family Practice Model: Delineation or collaboration. *National Council on Family Relations Networks*, *37*(1), 3–4.

Hawley, D. R., & Dahl, C. (2000). Using the levels of family involvement model with religious professionals. *Journal of psychology and theology*, *28*(2), 87–98.

Hennon, C. B., Radina, M. E., & Wilson, S. M. (2013). Family life education: Issues and challenges in professional practice. In G. Peterson & K. Bush (Eds.), *Handbook of Marriage and the Family*, (3rd ed. pp. 815–843). DOI:10.1007/978-1-4614-3987-5_33

Ho, B. S. (1997). The school psychologist's role based on an ecological approach to family-school-community collaborations. *The California School Psychologist*, *2*(1), 31–38.

Hoeft, T. J., Fortney, J. C., Patel, V., & Unützer, J. (2018). Task-sharing approaches to improve mental health care in rural and other low-resource settings: A systematic review. *The Journal of rural health*, *34*(1), 48–62.

Interprofessional Education Collaborative. (2023). *IPEC Core Competencies for Interprofessional Collaborative Practice: Version 3.*

Jameton, A. (1984). *Nursing Practice: The Ethical Issue*. Prentice Hall.

Labrague, L. J., Al Sabei, S., Al Rawajfah, O., AbuAlRub, R., & Burney, I. (2022). Interprofessional collaboration as a mediator in the relationship between nurse work environment, patient safety outcomes and job satisfaction among nurses. *Journal of nursing management, 30*(1), 268–278.

Lange, K. W. (2021). Task sharing in psychotherapy as a viable global mental health approach in resource-poor countries and also in high-resource settings. *Global Health Journal, 5*(3), 120–127.

Le, P. D., Eschliman, E. L., Grivel, M. M., Tang, J., Cho, Y. G., Yang, X., ... & Yang, L. H. (2022). Barriers and facilitators to implementation of evidence-based task-sharing mental health interventions in low-and middle-income countries: A systematic review using implementation science frameworks. *Implementation Science, 17*(1), 1–25.

Mantri S. (2008). Holistic medicine and the Western medical tradition. *American Medical Association Journal of Ethics, 10*(3), 177–180.

Marvel, M. K., & Morphew, P. K. (1993). Levels of family involvement by resident and attending physicians. *Family Medicine, 25*(1), 26–30.

Marvel, M. K., Schilling, R., Doherty, W. J., & Baird, M. A. (1994). Levels of physician involvement with patients and their families: A model for teaching and research. *Journal of Family Practice, 39*(6), 535–545.

Miller, B. D., & Wood, B. L. (1991). Childhood asthma in interaction with family, school, and peer systems: A developmental model for primary care. *Journal of Asthma, 28*(6), 405–414.

Minnesota Department of Health. (2019). *Public health interventions: Applications for public health nursing practice* (2nd ed.). https://www.health.state.mn.us/communities/practice /research/phncouncil/docs/PHInterventionsHandout.pdf

Myers-Walls, J. A., Ballard, S. M., Darling, C. A., & Myers-Bowman, K. S. (2011). Reconceptualizing the domain and boundaries of family life education. *Family Relations, 60*(4), 357–372.

Naslund, J. A., Shidhaye, R., & Patel, V. (2019). Digital technology for building capacity of non-specialist health workers for task-sharing and scaling up mental health care globally. *Harvard review of psychiatry, 27*(3), 181–192.

National Academies of Sciences, Engineering, and Medicine. (2023). *A Population Health Workforce to Meet 21st Century Challenges and Opportunities: Proceedings of a Workshop*. National Academies Press. https://doi.org/10.17226/27232

National Academies of Sciences, Engineering, and Medicine, Committee on Systems Approaches to Improve Patient Care by Supporting Clinician Well-Being. (2019). *Taking Action Against Clinician Burnout: A Systems Approach to Professional Well-Being*. National Academies Press. https://nam.edu/systems-approaches-toimprove-patient-care-by-supporting-clinician-well-being/

Neuman, B. (1982). *The Neuman's Systems Model: Application to Nursing Education and Practice*. Appleton-Century-Crofts.

Office of the U.S. Surgeon General. (2022). *Addressing Health Worker Burnout: The U.S Surgeon Generals' Advisory on Building a Thriving Health Workforce*. https://www.hhs.gov/sites/default/files/health-worker-wellbeing-advisory.pdf

Orkin, A. M., Rao, S., Venugopal, J., Kithulegoda, N., Wegier, P., Ritchie, S. D., ... & Upshur, R. (2021). Conceptual framework for task shifting and task sharing: an international Delphi study. *Human resources for health, 19*(61), 1–8-ttps://doi.org/10.1186/s12960-021-00605-z

Pratt, C. C. (1995). Family professionals and family policy: Strategies for influence. *Family Relations, 44* (1), 56–62.

Raver, S. A., & Childress, D. C. (2015). Collaboration and teamwork with families and professionals. In S. A. Raver & D. C. Childress (Eds.), *Family-Centered Early Intervention: Supporting Infants and Toddlers in Natural Environments* (pp. 120–130). Brookes Publishing Co.

Reeves, S., Xyrichis, A., & Zwarenstein, M. (2018). Teamwork, collaboration, coordination, and networking: Why we need to distinguish between different types of interprofessional practice. *Journal of interprofessional care, 32*(1), 1–3.

Sell, K., Hommes, F., Fischer, F., & Arnold, L. (2022). Multi-, inter-, and transdisciplinarity within the public health workforce: A scoping review to assess definitions and applications of concepts. *International Journal of Environmental Research and Public Health, 19*(17), 10902.

Schoon, P. M., Porta, C. M. & Scaffer, M. A (2019). *Population-based public health clinical manual: The Henry Street model for nurses* (3rd ed.). Sigma.

Sinclair, S., Raffin-Bouchal, S., Venturato, L., Mijovic-Kondejewski, J., & Smith-MacDonald, L. (2017). Compassion fatigue: A meta-narrative review of the healthcare literature. *International journal of nursing studies, 69*, 9–24.

Smith, S. M., Wallace, E., Clyne, B., Boland, F., & Fortin, M. (2021). Interventions for improving outcomes in patients with multimorbidity in primary care and community setting: A systematic review. *Systematic Reviews, 10*(1), 1–23.

Tehranineshat, B., Rakhshan, M., Torabizadeh, C., & Fararouei, M. (2019). Compassionate care in healthcare systems: A systematic review. *Journal of the National Medical Association, 111*(5), 546–554.

U.S. Bureau of Labor Statistics (2024, August, 29). *Healthcare Occupations.* https://www.bls.gov/ooh/healthcare/home.htm

van Diepen, C., Fors, A., Ekman, I., & Hensing, G. (2020). Association between person-centred care and healthcare providers' job satisfaction and work-related health: A scoping review. *BMJ open, 10*(12), e042658.

Vaseghi, F., Yarmohammadian, M. H., & Raeisi, A. (2022). Interprofessional collaboration competencies in the health system: A systematic review. *Iranian Journal of Nursing and Midwifery Research, 27*(6), 496–504.

World Health Organization. (2007). *Task shifting: Rational redistribution of tasks among health workforce teams: global recommendations and guidelines.* https://iris.who.int/bitstream/handle/10665/43821/9789?sequence=1

World Health Organization. (2010a). *Monitoring the building blocks of health systems: A handbook of indicators and their measurement strategies.* https://iris.who.int/bitstream/handle/10665/258734/9789241564052-eng.pdf

World Health Organization. (2010b). *Framework for action on interprofessional education and collaborative practice.* http://apps.who.int/iris/handle/10665/70185

World Health Organization. (2017, November, 30). *Protecting workers' healthhttps://www.who.int/news-room/fact-sheets/detail/protecting-workers'-health*

World Health Organization. (2019). *Classifying health workers: Mapping occupations to the international standard classification.* https://www.who.int/activities/improving-health-workforce data-and-evidence. https://cdn.who.int/media/docs/default-source/health-workforce/dek/classifying-health-workers.pdf?sfvrsn=7b7a472d_3&download=true

World Health Organization. (2022). *Global competency framework for universal health coverage.* https://iris.who.int/handle/10665/352710

World Health Organization (2024). *Health promotion and disease prevention through population-based interventions, including action to address social determinants and health inequity.* https://www.emro.who.int/about-who/public-health-functions/health-promotion-disease-prevention.html

Yankam, B. M., Adeagbo, O., Amu, H., Dowou, R. K., Nyamen, B. G. M., Ubechu, S. C., … & Bain, L. E. (2023). Task shifting and task sharing in the health sector in sub-Saharan Africa: Evidence, success indicators, challenges, and opportunities. *The Pan African Medical Journal, 46* (11). https://doi.org/10.11604/pamj.2023.46.11.40984

Figure credits

Fig. 5.1: The U.S. Surgeon General, https://www.hhs.gov/sites/default/files/health-worker-wellbeing-advisory.pdf, p. 9, 2022.

Fig. 5.2: The U.S. Surgeon General, https://www.hhs.gov/sites/default/files/health-worker-wellbeing-advisory.pdf, p. 12, 2022.

IMG 5.1: Copyright © 2017 Depositphotos/AlexFedorenko.

CHAPTER 6

Family Assessment in Family Health Care

I have been struck again and again by how important measurement is to improving the human condition.

—Bill Gates

Learning Objectives

By the end of this chapter, learners will do the following:

- Examine the basic key terminologies used to describe the meaning of family assessment in the context of *family health* care.
- Describe the importance of family assessment in *family health* care.
- Discuss different disciplinary theoretical foundations of family assessment.
- Explore three common comprehensive *family health* assessment tools in whole health care: *family health* history, the family genogram, and the family ecomap.
- Examine the challenges and opportunities of *family health* assessment within the 4HEALTH contexts.

Before you read on, consider the following questions:

- Is *family health* assessment important for generational health?
- Why is family assessment important in *family health* care?
- What is the best way to conduct a comprehensive *family health* assessment?
- Is there difference between a family assessment conducted during a standard point of care clinical setting versus one that is done in a research context?
- What is the nature of family assessment in the context of PFCC?

Notice that answers to these questions require a full acknowledgement and understanding of the role of *family health* and illness in *family health* care. The key concepts and constructs identified in Chapter 3 provide areas of foci for family assessment and intervention from a holistic approach that includes biopsychosocial, cultural, and policy considerations. Over the years, various models/strategies of family assessment have been developed across disciplines (Groteveant & Carlson, 1989). Some of the assessment strategies and tools have been tested, while others lack empirical validation. No one strategy/tool is claimed to be better than the other because of the complexity nature of the family. This chapter offers a discipline-neutral understanding of *family health* assessment and takes into consideration the diverse definitions of family and its structures, functions, and processes. This holistic point of view provides a better understanding of the family needs from a biopsychosocial perspective (physical and physiological clinical needs, psychological, social, and spiritual support). As mentioned in Chapter 5, family needs are usually met in diverse clinical settings, both traditional and nontraditional, facilitated by a diverse health care workforce depending on their level of competency and involvement. Thus, the discussions in this chapter draw concepts and methodologies from multiple disciplines to provide an overview of the importance of *family health* assessment. Challenges and opportunities for *family health* assessment within 4HEALTHS are also presented.

Importance of Family Assessment and Intervention in Family Health Care

As discussed in the previous chapters, acute and chronic illness as well as health exist in a social context that is best examined using biopsychosocial assessment strategies (Keitner, 2012). Hence, for health care systems to effectively build a culture of *family health*, there needs to be an investment in promoting the health of the family during both health and illness and not only during the illness of an individual family member across the life span. Similarly, if PFCC is to be effectively and appropriately practiced in real-life clinical settings, *family health* care professionals must continuously gather and exchange *family health* and illness information to facilitate interventions, follow-ups, and referrals (Bertakis & Azari, 2009). These provider expectations or competencies in family assessment and intervention are vital in building trusting relationships and improving health across multiple complex transitions during the *family health* and illness cycle and continuum of care (health promotion and disease prevention, early detections and early treatment, symptom management, rehabilitation, and palliative care). In *family health* care, family assessments are essential for determining *family health* needs and strengths, *family health* services to be delivered, and referral recommendations. Likewise, family involvement and engagement in family assessment is important in the provision of historical health information that will facilitate the design and implementation of effective family interventions (Josephson & AACAP Work Group on Quality Issues, 2007).

Defining Family Assessment

Family assessment is a core component for family-centered care and an important health care worker competency that guides clinical interventions and evaluation of clinical outcomes (Cook & Kenny, 2004). According to Merriam-Webster, the word *assessment* refers to the "the actions or instances of making judgments about something," in other words "appraising" something. From this definition, family assessment can be defined as actions or judgments made about how a family functions and relates. The actions of judgment are shared among the individual, family, and health care provider (Holman, 1983). In the family literature, different approaches have been used to define *family assessment* and the steps of conducting one. These approaches stem from various lenses, primarily using the systems, developmental, stress, and coping theoretical perspectives that bring a rich diversity to family subsystems foci (individual, dyad, etc.) (Carr, 2000).

Kaakinen et al. (2005) identify family nursing assessment in the context of the family nursing process that includes six steps: assessing the family story, analysis of the family story, design of a family plan of care/strategy, family intervention, family evaluation, and nurse reflection. The focus of this chapter is the first step of the nursing process, assessing the family story, which is referred to as family assessment and *family health* assessment. Conducting a family assessment helps providers and families identify areas for intervention (family deficits/problems) as well as strengths (family resources and competencies problems) that are instrumental for designing tailored interventions (Carr, 2000). During the family assessment, it is important for clinicians and providers to understand how the index patient(s) influences the family systems and subsystems, and vice versa (Keitner, 2012). Thus, assessing family interactional behaviors among family members in need of care and the provider is necessary (Josephson & AACAP Work Group on Quality Issues, 2007).

Unfortunately, to date, there is no global family assessment tool for clinical use in routine care (Carr, 2000). Methods used for conducting family assessments include interviews, self-reports of family history, and/or observational measures that may or may not be empirically validated. Family-orientated child and adolescent psychiatrists typically use face-to-face interviews compared to individually and/or biologically oriented clinicians who rely on information reported about the family (Josephson & AACAP Work Group on Quality Issues, 2007). Thus, it is important that *family health* practitioners and researchers alike become familiar with their practice area and the family assessment tools in use as the first step toward the implementation of family assessment in *family health* care.

Family Assessment Tools and Models From Multidisciplinary Theoretical Perspectives

Different principles, domains, and tools from multidisciplinary perspectives provide empirical-based and clinical-based domains of family assessment. The tools are variable in focus and are well established and mostly implemented in research environments. The purpose of this book is not to suggest any tools but to provide an awareness and knowledge of the importance of family measurements in *family health* care. For instance, in social work, Adel M. Holman (1983) describes the essential domains for understanding family assessment: articulating the family problem, family system, family environment, and family life cycle. Understanding a family's life stage of life and related tasks in a clinical setting is essential in evaluating the challenges faced or to be faced by the family when addressing health or illness statuses (Keitner, 2012). James Bray (1995) describes family assessment as a process that helps providers gather data on family composition, family process, family affect, family diversity, and ethnic variations. Gabor I. Keitner (2012), a psychiatrist, describes family assessment from a biopsychosocial process that incorporates an evaluation of patients' problems through the lens of the patients' social situations, interpersonal connections, and family functioning. Keitner (2012) identifies general principles of establishing connections with family for the first time when conducting family assessments. An emphasis is placed on assessing family relational factors that have an effect on health and illness such as presence of good communication, adaptability, clear rules, mutual support, open expression of appreciation, commitment to the family, family time together, good problem-solving skills, and extrafamilial social connections.

GENERAL PRINCIPLES FOR FAMILY ASSESSMENT

- Include as many family members as possible.
- Establish connection with all family members.
- Do not blame the family.
- Do not identify with the patient's perspective.
- Evaluate a wide range of family functions.
- Be sensitive to cultural and religious issues.

In marriage and family therapy, several empirical models of family assessment have been identified (Carr, 2000), such as the Beaver family systems model of family functioning (family competence and family style) developed by Beavers and Hampson (2000) and the circumplex model developed by Oslon (2000). The circumplex model conceptualizes three main family interaction variables for family assessment: family flexibility, cohesion, and communication skills. The Family Adaptability and Cohesion Evaluation Scale (FACES) is a well-known and widely used companion measure for the circumplex model (Olson, 2000; Olson et al., 2013). Another model is the McMaster model developed by Miller and colleagues (Miller et al., 2000), which conceptualizes family assessment by examining aspects of family functioning through six dimensions of family life: problem solving, communication, roles, affective responsiveness, affective involvement, and behavior control. Skinner et al.'s (2020) family assessment framework conceptualizes seven key dimensions: task accomplishment, role performance, communication, affective expression, involvement, control, values, and norms. Wilkinson et al. (1988) developed a comprehensives family assessment tool known as the Darlington family assessment. The tool consists of four main assessment targets and components: (a) *the child or children as individuals*: child health, child development, emotional disturbance, relationships, and conduct; (b) the *parenting system*: physical health, psychological health, marital partnership, parenting history, and parent-social; (c) *the parent–child relationships or parenting style*: care and control; and (d) *the family system as a whole* (family dynamics): closeness and distance, power hierarchies, emotional atmosphere, and rules and family development. Ellenwood and Jenkins (2007) pioneered a brief family interview tool for families with chronically ill members known as the Intervention-Based Family Assessment (IBFA). The IBFA is culturally sensitive nontraditional family therapy assessment and intervention approach for use in primary care settings that is different from the traditional approaches used in family therapist offices. The tool is intended to accomplish the following during the family assessment:

- help the family restore their level of functioning prior to the chronic illness
- help uncover the family rigid roles so that competency and respect are restored within the family system
- help the family understand how their own unique struggles with chronic illness are creating their presenting problems (e.g., confusion, depression)
- help the family begin to identify with their short- and long-term goals so that an appropriate level of life-long care can be established
- help identify the fears and concerns of each family member so that these can be freely discussed
- help promote a reestablishment and activation of core cultural and religious values, traditions, and beliefs
- help to engage extended families and health care agencies/personnel to aid in the care of the chronically ill member
- help to inform the marriage and therapist about ways to capitalize on the strengths of each family member so that appropriate interventions and networking with community agencies can be developed
- help to educate the family therapist on the family's knowledge of the chronic illness (Ellenwood & Jenkins 2007)

Table 6.1 provides the different key phases in IBFA and example questions that can be used in the family interview.

TABLE 6.1 Key Phases in Intervention-Based Family Assessment

Phases	Sample Assessment Questions
Phase I: Family Constellation and Participation	*Family constellation* • Who currently resides within your home? • Is there any member living outside of the home? *Individual family member's characteristics* • How would you describe each individual's strengths? • How would you describe each individual's weaknesses? *Family's participation in activities* • What type of hobbies or activities do you as a family participate in together or independently? • What type of hobbies or activities do you participate in with friends? • How frequently do you engage in these hobbies and/or activities?

<table>
<tr><td>Phase II: The Illness</td><td>Describe the medical diagnosis
• How do you see this diagnosis impacting on your chronically all members?
• What is your understanding of the prognosis?
• How did you acquire your knowledge of the medical condition?
• How did the onset of the chronic illness impact each family member</td></tr>
<tr><td>Phase III: Cultural-/ Religious-Based Practices</td><td>• What is your ethnicity?
• What religion do you practice, and how does this affect your willingness to seek medical or psychological treatment?
• What are family's cultural beliefs that would influence the care of the chronically ill person?</td></tr>
<tr><td>Phase IV: Family's Perceptions of The Illness</td><td>• How does each member take care of themselves in the areas of
▹ stress management (e.g., relaxion activities, exercising)?
▹ recreation (e.g., playing a sport)?
▹ pursuing personal interests (e.g., hobbies)?
▹ establishing support networks (e.g., seeking and responding to social invitations)?
▹ reserving family time (e.g., activities with spouse and children)?
▹ providing time for themselves?
• How does each family member express
▹ anger
▹ pain
▹ happiness
▹ joy
▹ grief
• How do the members perceive the impact of the illness on the family?
• What concerns does this family have for each other?</td></tr>
<tr><td>Phase V: Family's Level of Support and Future Plans</td><td>• Do you have support from your extended family (and with friends and community agencies)?
• If yes, describe how they support you.
• Do you feel comfortable seeking this support?
• What are your long-term plans for the care of your chronically ill family member?</td></tr>
<tr><td>Phase VI: Termination Phase</td><td>• When would be a good time to schedule another session?
• What location would be most convenient for you?
• Was this setting adaptable for your family?
• Knowing the needs of your chronically ill member, was this setting appropriate?
• Are there changes or suggestions that could make the next session more amenable to your family needs?</td></tr>
</table>

Audrey E. Ellenwood and Jeanne E. Jenkins, Selection from "Unbalancing the Effects of Chronic Illness: Non-Traditional Family Therapy Assessment and Intervention Approach," *The American Journal of Family Therapy*, vol. 35, no. 3, p. 271.

In medicine, Gabriel Smilkstein (1978) developed the Family APGAR, which has been used to assess family functioning and improve diagnosis and disease management with family in family practice (Takenaka, & Ban, 2016). The tool measures five constructs for family functioning: adaptability, partnership, growth, affection, and resolve (see Table 6.2).

TABLE 6.2 **Family APGAR Components**

Components	Definition	Example questions
Adaptation	Adaptation is the utilization of intra- and extrafamilial resources for problem solving when family equilibrium is stressed during a crisis.	How have family members aided each other in time of need? In what ways have family members received help or assistance from friends and community agencies?
Partnership	Partnership is the sharing of decision-making and nurturing responsibilities by family members.	How do family members communicate with each other about such matters as vacations, finances, medical care, large purchases, and personal problems?
Growth	Growth is the physical and emotional maturation and self-fulfillment that is achieved by family members through mutual support and guidance.	How have family members changed during the past years? How has this change been accepted by family members? In what ways have family members aided each other in growing or developing independent lifestyles? How have family members reacted to your desires for change?
Affection	Affection is the caring or loving relationship that exists among family members.	How have members of your family responded to emotional expressions such as affection, love, sorrow, or anger?
Resolve	Resolve is the commitment to devote time to other members of the family for physical and emotional nurturing. It also usually involves a decision to share wealth and space.	How do members of your family share time, space, and money?

Adapted from Gabriel Smilkstein, "The Family APGAR: A Proposal for a Family Function Test and Its Use by Physician," *The Journal of Family Practice*, vol. 6, no. 6.

Nurses have utilized diverse *family health* models and measurements in their practice to assess the health care function—a vital component of the family assessment in family nursing care (Sawin, 2016). Family assessment is viewed as an essential component of health care that facilitates the acknowledgment of major improvements and maintenance in health that occur primarily through commitments and modifications of places where family members, eat, play, learn, and live. The goal of the assessment is to improve health and help families adapt to illness, injury, or death. Maureen Leahey and Lorraine Wright pioneered one of the leading evidence-based and practice-based family nursing assessment clinical models known as the Calgary family assessment model (CFAM) in 1984 that incorporates family structural, developmental, and functioning and strength perspectives (Leahey, & Wright, 2016; Wright, & Leahey, 1984; see Table 6.3). Not all components of CFAM should be assessed in one meeting. The model guides the development of the 15-minute family interview that is easily adaptable in a busy clinical setting (Wright & Leahey, 1999). Table 6.4 displays the five ingredients (Wright & Leahey, 1999).

TABLE 6.3 **CFAM**

Component	Definition
Structural	Family structure, its members, the emotional bond between its elements compared to outsiders, and its context
Internal Structure	Family composition, gender and sexual orientation of members, rank or birth order of children, subsystems and limits
External Structure	Extended family and information on the origin and progeny of the family and wider systems that concern different social establishments and individuals with whom the family maintain some contact and who function as occasional support
Context	Ethnicity, race, social class, spirituality/religion, and environment
Developmental	Refers to the progressive transformation of family history over the life cycle phases: its history, life course/stages, family growth, birth and death, attachments
Functional	The way in which family members interact; the instrumental aspect of family functioning and the expressive aspect of family functioning
Instrumental	Routine activities of daily living
Expressive	The modes of communication, problem solving, beliefs, roles, rules, and alliances that can be explored

TABLE 6.4 **Key Ingredients for the 15-Minute Family Interview**

Key Ingredient	Definition	Examples
Manners	Core of common, everyday social behavior that has a benefit in instilling trusting relationships	Self-introductions: • always calling a patient by name • telling the patient your name • checking your attitude • explaining your role for that shift, • explaining a procedure before coming into the room with the equipment to do it, • if you tell the patient that you will be back at a certain time keeping that appointment, and being honest with the patient

Therapeutic Conversa-tions	The art of integrating task-oriented care with purposive and time-limited therapeutic listening conversations to promote healing and suffering. The process includes information giving and patient involvement in decision-making	Family involvement and engagement: • Families are routinely invited to accompany the patient to the unit/clinic/hospital. • Families are routinely included in the admission procedure. • Families are routinely invited to ask questions during the patient orientation. • Nurses acknowledge the patient's and family's expertise in managing health problems by asking about routines at home. • Nurses encourage patients to practice how they will handle different interactions in the future, such as telling family members and others that they cannot eat certain foods. • Nurses routinely consult families and patients about their ideas for treatment and discharge.
Family Genograms and Ecomaps	Drawing a quick genogram (and sometimes, if indicated, an ecomap) for all families, particularly for those families who will likely be part of their care for more than 3 days. [See details about these tools later in the chapter. This is an engagement strategy that helps the nurse to think family.]	Drawing a genogram and ecomap: The most essential information to obtain is data about ages, occupation/school grade, religion, ethnic background, migration date, and current health status of each family member. • Begin by asking easy questions (ages, current health) of the household family members. • Once this genogram information is obtained, if indicated, expand the data collection to obtain external family structure information in the form of an ecomap. • It may be useful to ask such questions as "Who outside of your immediate family is an important resource to you? Or is it a stress?" "How many professionals are involved in treating your husband's current heart problems?"
Therapeutic Questions	Key defining element in a therapeutic conversation to involve family in *family health* care in different contexts. Shows a willingness to learn from families and to work collaboratively.	Therapeutic questions: Use at least three questions depending on context: • Who of your family or friends would you like us to share information with and who not? (Indicates alliances, resources, and possible conflictual relationships.) • How can we be most helpful to you and your family or friends during your hospitalization? (Clarifies expectations, increased collaboration.)

		• What has been most/least helpful to you in past hospitalizations or clinic visits? (Identifies past strengths, problems to avoid, and successes to repeat.) • What is the greatest challenge facing your family during this hospitalization/ discharge/clinic visit? (Indicates actual/ potential suffering, roles, and beliefs.) • What do you need to best prepare you/ your family member for discharge? (Assists with discharge planning early.) • Who do you believe is suffering the most in your family during this hospitalization/ clinic visit/home care visit? (Identifies which family member is in the greatest need for support and intervention.) • What is the one question you would most like to have answered during our meeting right now (Wright, 1989)? I may not be able to answer this question at the moment, but I will do my best or will try and find the answer for you. (Identifies most pressing issue or concern.) How have I been most helpful to you in this family meeting? How could we improve?
Commending Family and Individual Strengths	Offering at least two compliments of behaviors observed or reported (i.e., commendations) to family members of individual or family strengths, resources, or competencies that the nurse observed or were reported to them. This approach offers the family members a new way of viewing themselves and finding way to move toward solutions to reduce potential or actual suffering.	An example of a commendation is: • "Your family is showing much courage in living alongside of your wife's cancer for 5 years." • A compliment would be "Your son is so gentle despite feeling so ill."

Source: Wright and Leahey (1999)

Marjorie Gordon (2007), a nurse theorist and scientist, developed a nursing assessment theory known as the Gordon's functional health pattern that utilizes a holistic structural approach for family assessment for individuals, families, and communities that is consistent with the nursing scope of practice. The model has been used to standardize nursing language in the electronic medical record (EMR; Rossi et al., 2023) to facilitate clinical reasoning and decision-making (Gengo e Silva Butcher & Jones, 2021). The model complements physicians' medical, social, and family history and a review of systems in the EMR (Gengo e Silva Butcher & Jones, 2021). The 11 functional health patterns captured in the assessments include health perception–health management, nutritional-metabolic, elimination, activity-exercise, sleep-rest, cognition-perception, self-perception–self-concept, roles-relationships, sexuality-reproduction, coping–stress tolerance, and values–beliefs patterns (Gordon, 2007). Table 6.5 summarizes these areas of family assessment.

TABLE 6.5 **Gordon's 11 Functional Health Patterns and Assessment Data**

Functional Health Patterns	Definition (Rossi et al., 2023)	Data Assessed From Tools Gengo e Silva Butcher & Jones, 2021)	Family Assessment Areas
Health Percep-tion–Health Management	Health/wellbeing and how health is managed	• Medication and/or treatment adherence • Current state of health or current symptoms; • History of smoking, alcohol, or other substances use; • Past medical history or problems; health-seeking behavior; • Allergies • Knowledge about disease or treatment. • Immunization status • The ability to make changes and adjustments to improve health or prevent injury	Family self-perception of health and well-being
Nutrition-al-Metabolic	Food and fluid consumption relative to metabolic need and local nutrient supply	• Type of diet, either recommended or not by a health care provider • Typical food or liquid intake or changes in typical intake • Weight/weight changes • Chewing/swallowing problems • Teeth/oral mucous membrane problems, and • Impaired skin integrity	Family patterns of food and fluid consumption
Elimination	Regularity of excretory function including strategies and devices used to assist/control	• Elimination problems. • Bowel and bladder patterns • Use of laxatives	Family elimination needs
Activity-Exercise	Activities of daily living, leisure, and recreation	• Exercise capacity/habits • Physical activity and limitations • Ability to perform activities of daily living, • Need for walking aids, • Recreation and leisure activities	Family physical exercise and leisure activities

Cognition-Perceptual	Cognitive and functional abilities, including adequacy of sensory models, experiences of pain	• Impaired speech • Visionhearing, taste, or smell status • The need for vision or hearing aids • Mmemory status, • Pain or discomfort, • Sensory perception,	Family perception of cognitive and functional abilities
Sleep-Rest	Sleep, rest, and relaxation practices	• Sleep habits/aids • Sleep quality, and difficulties getting to sleep or staying asleep	Family sleep quality and patterns
Self-Concept and Self-Perception	Self-presentation	• Perception about self (self-respect, self-esteem, or personal identity) • Perception about body image • Mood or personality	Family self-concept and perceptions about body images, mood, and personality
Sexuality-Reproductive Pattern	Sexual preferences and satisfaction; reproductive patterns	• Difficulties for or during intercourse • Sexualatisfaction, or concerns about sexual health • Gynecologic history • Intimate relationships	Family sexuality and intimacy
Coping-Stress Tolerance	Threshold and triggers for stress and effectiveness of coping strategies	• Coping mechanisms such as reactions to stressors or adjustment to stressors, stressors, and major changes in life	Family coping with stressful situations
Roles-Relationship	Role engagements and responsibilities within the family and society	• Responsibilities or role in the household and decision making across the life span • Occupation • Family structure or functioning, • Family relationship/ interactions.	Family role and power structure
Values-Belief	Life values, goals, or beliefs that guide choices and/or decisions	• Ethnic and cultural background • Spirituality, religion, faith, beliefs, and values	Family values/ belief systems

Consistent with Gordon's functional health patterns, Hooper et al. (2003) propose eight assessment domains for *family health* practices within health care function. These domains include family dietary practices, family sleep and rest practices, family physical activities, recreational practices that includes substance use and abuse, family self-care practices, environmental and hygiene practices, medically based preventative practices such as immunizations, screening, and use of alternative or complimentary therapies. Marilyn Friedman, a pioneer of family nursing, contributed knowledge to family assessment by developing the Friedman family assessment model (Friedman et al., 2003), which is based on structural-functional, systems, and developmental theories. She stresses the importance of assessing the family's internal and external environments during family assessment. Assessing the internal family environment, such as the family's involvement in health care activities, and external family environment, such as quality of the family–provider relationship and access to care, are essential in describing how well families perform the health care function (Friedman et al., 2003).

Other nursing scholars who have contributed to family assessment in health care, particularly in illness and crisis health care, are Karen Mischke-Berkey and Shirley Hanson (1991), who developed the family assessment and intervention model and Family Systems Stressors-Strength Inventory (FS3I). These models are based on the Neuman system and the family stress and coping models that emphasize family strength and the importance of including the family and provider perceptions on the family stressors during a *family health* assessment. Moreover, Katherine Knafl et al. (2021) pioneered the development of the Family Management Measure (FaMM) and family management style framework (FMSF), which are used to measure how families manage caring for a child or adult facing a health challenge. The FaMM consists of six scales: Child Daily Life, Condition Management Ability, Condition Management Effort, Family Life Difficulty, Parental Mutuality, and View of Family Impact.

Family Health History, Family Genogram, and Family Ecomap for Whole Health

There are several tools for family assessment in the literature. This section introduces the reader to the three most common comprehensive biopsychosocial family assessment tools, *family health* history, family genogram, and family ecomap, that have been used in clinical setting to identify individuals, families, and populations at risk in order to mitigate the related health consequences through different intervention targets, including the family. The family assessment tools provide areas of evaluation of biomedical context as well as the patient/client social context, the nature of the interpersonal connections, and family functioning (Gabor, 2012).

Family Health History

The CDC (2023) defines *family health* history "as a record of the diseases and health conditions in one's family that may be attributed to sharing of genes, healthy behaviors, living conditions in the environment" (para 1). Diseases such as cancer, heart disease, and diabetes are likely to be shared. Understanding a patient's *family health* history facilitates health care clinical decision-making as part of early detection and early treatment and ultimately improves overall patient and *family health* care. For example, *family health* history can help providers decide when to screen for chronic diseases (and which ones to screen for) and what behaviors to plan for lifestyle change. This has been very useful in delineating genetic, environmental, and lifestyle factors for risk stratification and engaging patients and providers in routine clinical care in the United States (Wu et al., 2019), especially in the science of precision medicine and precision health (CDC, 2022). Precision medicine, also known as personalized medicine, involves the determination of one's personal targets for unique disease risks and treatments, while precision health is "broader and includes precision medicine but also approaches that occur outside the setting of a doctor's office or hospital, such as disease prevention and health promotion activities" that can also be self-managed as well as public health managed (CDC, 2022, para. 2). The CDC recommends that providers help family gather and tract family history by offering the following tips to clients

- Use family gatherings to talk about health history.
- Look at death certificates and family medical records.
- Collect personal and medical information about parents, sisters, brothers, half-sisters, half-brothers, children, grandparents, aunts, uncles, nieces, and nephews: major medical conditions, causes of death, age at disease diagnosis, age at death, and ethnic background.
- Use a resource for tracking information in the U.S: Surgeon General's web-based tool called "My *Family Health* Portrait."

The American Medical Association recommends the following information be included in a family history:

- first-, second- and third-degree relatives
- age for all relatives (age at time of death for the deceased)
- ethnicity (some genetic diseases are more common in certain ethnic groups)
- presence of chronic diseases

Family Health Genogram

The family genogram is another useful clinical tool that provides a visual representation of the family structure, relationship, health status, and sociodemographic and economic status over three generations (Bray, 1995; Yehestial et al., 2000). The family genogram has been widely promoted as a useful tool for gathering, recording, and displaying the social context of the patients—a patient and family's medical and biopsychosocial status in family-oriented health care across disciplines (Campbell et al., 2002). The tool has been used in research environments as well (Varty et al., 2022). The tool originated in family therapy and has been adopted by other health care disciplines such as nursing and medicine in *family health* care practice. A family genogram in health care follows the typical format for a family therapy genogram interview, but with more emphasis on family illnesses, deaths, stress, and coping mechanisms of the patient and the family system (Larasati et al., 2020). The genogram interview is used as a therapeutic communication and intervention medium for family members to express emotions by telling "facts" and a medium for gathering health-related facts that can be used in developing medical or psychosocial directives, including boosting patients' morale and coping strength. As a psychoeducational tool, the genogram interview allows the provider/clinician and patient and family to discuss difficult topics in a nonjudgmental manner (Libbon et al., 2019). The best timing of administering a family genogram is during the comprehensive assessment upon the first visit/encounter with the healthcare system. Genograms are not static tools. They evolve as missing and new information is added during wellness visits and during complex and specialized encounters accordingly. The genogram provides an understanding of the patients' family members and caregivers and their influence and roles in health and illness, and helps plan effective health promotion and disease prevention and management measures (Libbon et al., 2019). Thus, understanding family strengths and resources is important during a focused or detailed family assessment (Josephson & AACAP Work Group on Quality Issues, 2007). Collecting a family genogram is a family affair; therefore, engaging the family is essential.

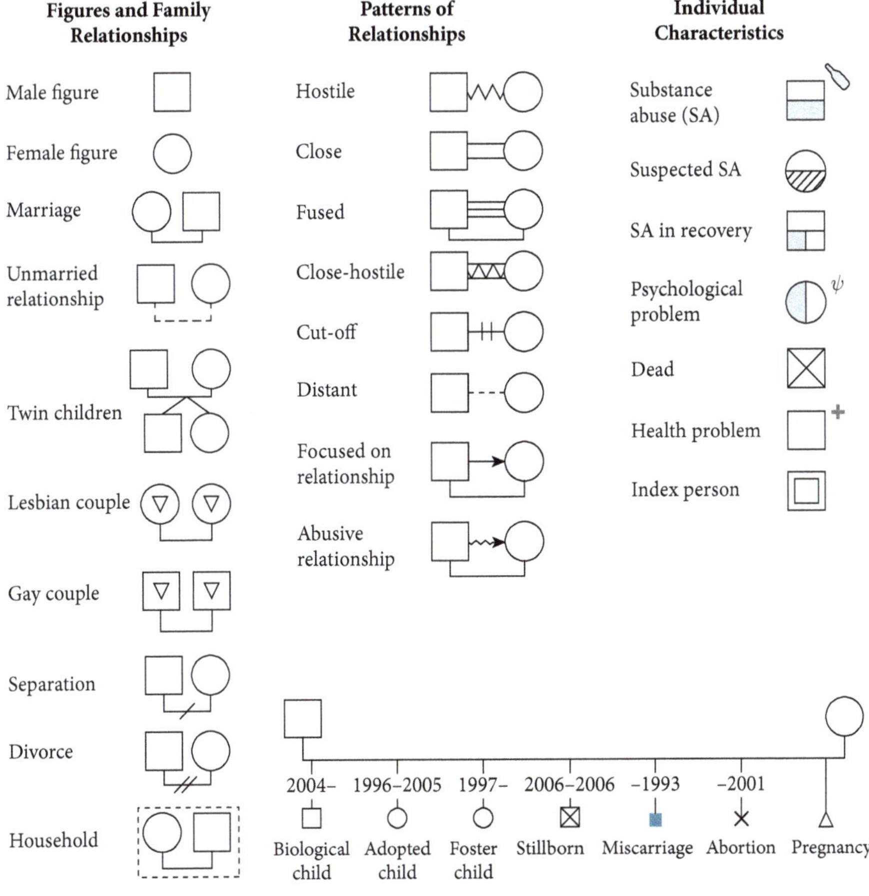

FIGURE 6.1 Example of symbols in a family genogram.

However, it is also important to note that the process can be done with or without the family present if needed (Libson, 2019). Various standardized symbols have been used when drawing family genograms (see examples in in Figure 6.1).

The following information should be included in the initial *family health* genogram:

- first-, second- and third-degree relatives
- age for all relatives (age at time of death for the deceased)
- ethnicity (some genetic diseases are more common in certain ethnic groups)
- presence of chronic diseases
- occupation
- family structures

Family Ecomap

The family ecomap, also known as an ecological map, is another visual clinical tool that represents the connections and strengths between an individual patient and their family as well as with their subsystems and reflects where they live, eat, age, worship, play, and age, such as the school, work, neighborhood, healthcare system, recreational systems, and related individuals/providers. This time-sensitive tool demonstrates the flow or lack of social, cultural and economic resources between the family and its subsystems (Campbell et al., 2002). The tool is helpful in determining the social determinants of health (SDOH), the effects of the SDOH on the patient and family, and how interprofessional teams can intervene to improve health outcomes (Kruger et al., 2024). Various standardized symbols have been used when drawing family genograms (see examples in in Figure 6.2 and 6.3). Box 2 provides basic steps that can be used to create as family ecomap.

Ethical Considerations in Family Health Assessment

It is essential to note that while family assessment may be promising, the issue of informed consent, autonomy, confidentiality, and privacy should always be upheld to protect patients and families. Before any family assessment, patients and families should be given adequate

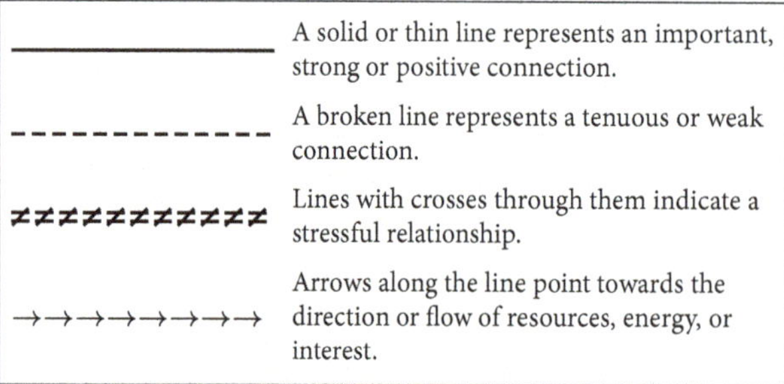

FIGURE 6.2. Examples of lines used in an ecomap (Kruger et al., 2024).

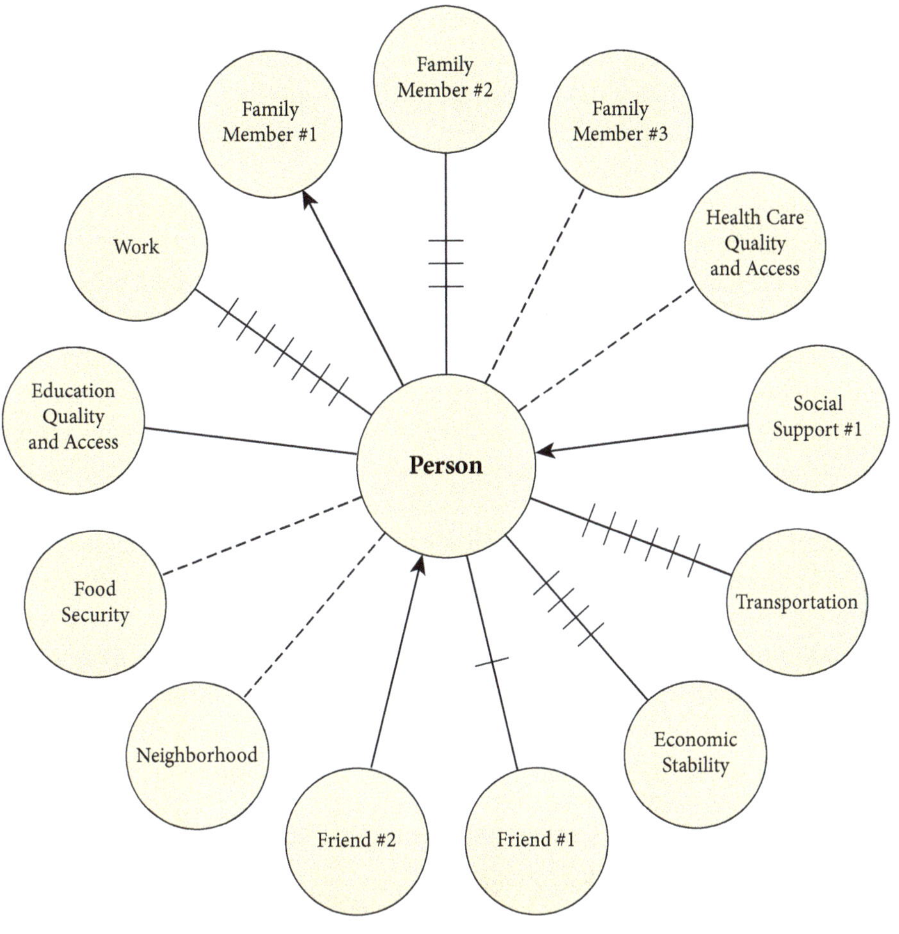

FIGURE 6.3 Example ecomap (Kruger et al., 2024).

information entailing and ensuring that they understand the process and implications to consent or not consent in the process. In addition, it is important to note that patients and families have the autonomy to make their own decision about what they want to share or not share. The provider's role is to educate about the process and benefits and acknowledge the patients and families' responsiveness. It is also important to assure the privacy of patient and family information in the home and in the clinic, especially with the increased digitalization of information and health records. Providers and as their patients and families must comply with privacy acts such as the U.S. Health Insurance Portability and Accountability Act (HIPAA).

Organizing Family Health Assessment for Holistic Whole Health Care

Although the three clinical tools, family history, *family health* genogram, and family ecomap, have been proposed in clinical practice, they have hardly been fully adapted into clinical practice and in patients' medical records, partly due to the massive data generated from the three different tools and lack of standardized measurement tools. Nevertheless, it is essential that clinicians and providers understand how to integrate the information generated from the three approaches into their practice to provide effective quality, safe, and timely care. Scholars in nursing have proposed a practical organization tool that captures a comprehensive three-generation blended approach to communicate holistic *family health* assessment (Olsen et al., 2004). The goal of this tool is to gather information in key areas that include risk factor identification, areas to inform patient and family clinical decisions, management, psychosocial support and education, risk reductions, health promotion and prevention, screening referrals, and disease management (Olsen et al., 2004). Furthermore, the family reasoning web framework has been used in the analysis of the family story. Eleven meaningful categories have been developed to guide clinicians in their decision-making process with the family (Kaakinen et al., 2015). These categories include family routines of daily living, family communication, family support and resources, family roles, family beliefs, family developmental stage, *family health* knowledge, family environment, family stress management, family culture, and family spirituality. Thematically, these 11 dimensions can be grouped into three major family measures: family structure, family function, and family processes. Table 6.6 provides the four areas of family measures and examples of questions that can be used to explore the constructs across the three family assessment tools (*family health* history, family genogram, and family ecomap). The analysis of the family story in relation to the dimensions can help the clinician identify family relational risk or protective factors that contribute to the patient's and family's health status (see Chapter 9).

TABLE 6.6 **Family Measures and Sample Questions Across *Family Health* History, Family Genogram, and Family Ecomap**

Family Assessment Concepts	***Family Health* History**	**Family Genogram**	**Family Ecomap**
Family Structure	Who makes up the family within the patient/family and across generations? Is the family traditional or nontraditional? What are the generational disease or health issue patterns across age and sex? Is their consanguinity (blood relationships)?	Who makes up the family within the patient/family and across generations? Is the family traditional or nontraditional? What is the nature and quality of the relationships and interactions?	Who makes up the family social network? What is the nature of the relationship and interactions between the patient/family and social networks? Does the family need resource or support?
Family Developmental Stage	Who makes the family and what are their developmental tasks to maintain health across generations?	Who makes the family and what are their developmental tasks to maintain health across generations. What is the nature of gender roles?	Who makes up the family and what is the nature of their developmental tasks? What services, support, and programs does the family need across the developmental stages?

Family Function	How is the reproductive function affected in health, illness, and death, and vice versa?	What is the nature and quality of the reproductive function?	What is the nature of the reproductive function in the family? What resources or support do the family have or not have to meet their reproductive needs?
	How is the socialization/behavioral control function affected in health, illness, and death, and vice versa?	What is the nature and quality of family socialization/behavioral control function?	What is the nature of the socialization/behavioral control function in the family? What resources or support do the family have or not have to meet their socialization/behavioral control needs?
	How is the affection function affected in health, illness, and death, and vice versa?	What is the nature and quality of the affection function?	What is the nature of the affection function in the family? What resources or support do the family have or not have to meet their affection function needs?
	How is the economic function affected in health, illness, and death, and vice versa?	What is the nature of the economic function?	What is the nature of the economic function in the family? What resources or support do the family have or not have to meet their economic function needs?
	How is the health care function affected in health, illness, and death?	How does the family meet their health care needs (physical, mental, social, spiritual)? What is the family's health literacy/knowledge?	What is the nature of the health care function in the family? What resources or support do the family have or not have to meet their health care function needs? What is the source(s) of *family health* literacy/knowledge?
Family Processes (Coping, Roles, Communication, Decision-Making, Routines and Rituals, Problem Solving)	How do health, illness and death affect family coping?	How does family cope with stress related to health, illness and death? What coping skills does the family have or need?	What resources or support do the family have or not have to cope with stress related to health, illness, and death?

	How do health, illness, and death affect family roles?	How are family roles affected by health and illness? Provider role, sick role, caregiver role? What caregiving skills does the family have or need? Do they need to adopt new family roles?	What resources or support do the family have or not have to adopt or enhance family and caregiving roles or skills to deal with health, illness, and death?
	How do health, illness, and death affect family communication?	How is family communication affected by health and illness?	What resources or support do the family have or not have to adopt or enhance family communication strategies to deal with health, illness, and death?
	How do health, illness, and death affect family decision-making?	How is the family making decisions about health and illness? What about the power structure?	What resources or support do the family have or not have to adopt or enhance family decision-making skills to deal with health, illness, and death?
	How do health, illness, and death affect family routines and rituals?	What are the family routines and rituals, and how do they influence heath, illness, and death (culture, beliefs, spirituality)? What are the family values and beliefs of illness and health, and how do they impact self-care and disease management?	What resources or support do the family have or not have to adopt or enhance family routines or rituals to deal with health, illness, and death?
	How do health, illness, and death affect family problem solving?	How does the family problem-solve in health, illness, and death?	What resources or support do the family have or not have to adopt or enhance family problem solving skills to deal with health, illness, and death?

Challenges and Opportunities of Family Health Assessment Within 4HEALTH

Family health assessment is an important aspect of whole health and whole health care. *Family health* assessment helps improve generational health. A commitment to person-centered care requires health care systems that invest in measures that capture persons/patients and families' holistic health needs to promote health and health equity. *Family health* assessment is an innovative strategy that can benefit precision medicine as it provides information about one's environment that can cause epigenetic changes and gene functions such as family stress and living conditions across the life span. Thus, to facilitate *family health* assessment in health care, it is important to take multilevel challenges and opportunities within the 4HEALTH into consideration.

At the *individual health* level, *family health* assessments facilitate clinician and provider encounters with their patients. Clinicians have the opportunity to improve patients' health or illness visits by investing their time and skills wisely in listening and acting on patients' stories and how their social contexts influence health, illness, or death, and vice versa. This broader approach can enhance the quality of the visit and patient and provider satisfaction, improve health care costs, and ultimately improve health outcomes by identifying physical, behavioral, and social targets for intervention. At the family level, *family health* assessments enable providers and clinicians to empower individual family members to engage in the health or the family system across the life span. At the population level, implementation of *family health* assessments facilitate health care systems to track measures of SDOH to inform interventions and outreach. Unfortunately, this approach may not be feasible if health care systems do not have the capacity and capability of designing and utilizing new or existing tools that capture *family health* data. For example, underutilization of *family health* history in clinical care settings is still a public health problem, especially among vulnerable populations (Khoury et al., 2022). Likewise, it is not feasible to have tools in place without clinicians and providers who have the skills and knowledge to conduct effective and thorough *family health* assessments. A diverse workforce is needed to facilitate *family health* data collection. Moreover, the process of developing reliable, valid, and time-sensitive measures is still evolving (Sawin, 2016). An emerging new initiative is the National Institute of Health's Patient-Reported Outcomes Measurement Information System (PROMIS) roadmap initiative, a highly reliable measure of patient-reported health status that will have future implications for *family health* assessment. The initiative recognizes the role of the healthcare system in addressing the need for common data elements of health measures beyond the biomedical and individual-centered measures (Sawin, 2016). Thus, at the public health level, it is important to prioritize a diverse health workforce that cannot only function within a biomedical model of care, but also a biopsychosocial model of care that will contribute to the implementation of genomic and precision medicine in health care (Khoury et al., 2022). Likewise, *family health* professionals who are equipped with public health principles are needed to assure the delivery of effective, ethical, and trustworthy community awareness and educational interventions that promote the use of *family health* history and family genograms and ecomaps in health care. This approach is essential in preparing a well-rounded, engaged, and informed consumer of *family health* assessments in whole health care.

Conclusion

This chapter reviewed the importance of *family health* assessment from a biopsychosocial perspective. The *family health* history, family genogram, and family ecomap are promising tools to help clinicians and providers understand the essence of the broader concept of health and *family health*. Of importance is the need of a diverse *family health* workforce that is ready to conduct comprehensive assessments of relational risks and protective factors and suggest family intervention targets to improve *population health* outcomes. The next chapters will introduce the role of effective communication and family interventions in *family health* care.

Suggested Websites

My *Family Health* Portrait: https://cbiit.github.io/FHH/html/index.html

Family Health History, The Basics: https://www.cdc.gov/genomics/famhistory/famhist_basics.htm#:~:text=Family%20health%20history%20is%20a,similar%20things%20in%20the%20environment

American Medical Association, Collecting a Family History: https://www.ama-assn.org/delivering-care/precision-medicine/collecting-family-history

International Family Nursing Association, Family Nursing Assessment and Intervention Map: https://internationalfamilynursing.org/2024/01/25/family-nursing-assessment-and-intervention-map/

IFNA, Practice Models for Nursing Practice With Families: https://internationalfamilynursing.org/resources-for-family-nursing/practice/practice-models/

Suggested Readings

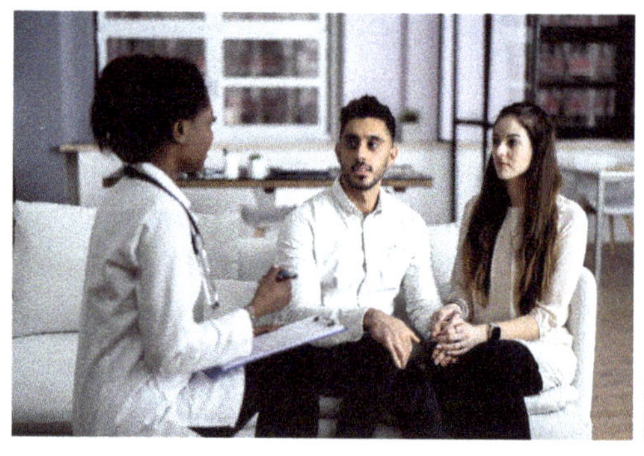

IMG 6.1

Campbell, T. L., McDaniel, S. H., Cole-Kelly, K., Hepworth, J., & Lorenz, A. (2002). Family interviewing: A review of the literature in primary care. *Family Medicine*, *34*(5), 312–318.

Keitner, G. I. (2012). Family assessment in the medical setting. *The Psychosomatic Assessment*, *32*, 203–222.

Kruger, J. S., Kim, I., Foltz-Ramos, K., & Ohtake, P. J. (2024). Utilizing an ecomap to visualize the impact of social determinants of health in an interprofessional forum. *Journal of Allied Health*, *53*(1), 61E–66E.

Libbon, R., Triana, J., Heru, A., & Berman, E. (2019). Family skills for the resident toolbox: The 10-min genogram, ecomap, and prescribing homework. *Academic Psychiatry*, *43*, 435–439.

Olsen, S., Dudley-Brown, S., & McMullen, P. (2004). Case for blending pedigrees, genograms and ecomaps: Nursing's contribution to the "big picture." *Nursing & Health Sciences*, *6*(4), 295–308.

Sawin, K. J. (2016). Measurement in family nursing: established instruments and new directions. *Journal of Family Nursing*, *22*(3), 287–297.

Reflection Questions

1. Do you or your family have a *family health* portrait or family genogram as part of your medical record? If not, why?
2. Do you think a *family health* genogram is important? Why?
3. What are possible barriers and facilitating factors that can influence the use of *family health* histories, genograms, and ecomaps in clinical practice? Briefly explain.

References

Beavers, R., & Hampson, R. B. (2000). The Beavers Systems Model of Family Functioning. *Journal of Family Therapy*, *22*(2), 128–143. https://doi.org/10.1111/1467-6427.00143

Bell, J. M. (2007). Distinguished Contribution to Family Nursing Award: Dr Marilyn M Friedman for Family nursing: Research, theory, and practice (1981, 1986, 1992, 1998, 2003). *Journal of Family Nursing, 13*(3), 287–289.

Campbell, T. L., McDaniel, S. H., Cole-Kelly, K., Hepworth, J., & Lorenz, A. (2002). Family interviewing: A review of the literature in primary care. *Family Medicine, 34*(5), 312–318.

Carr, A. (2000). Empirical approaches to family assessment. *Journal of Family Therapy, 22*(2), 121–127.

Centers for Disease Control and Prevention. (2022, May 17). *Precision health: Improving health for each of us and all of us.* https://www.cdc.gov/genomics/about/precision_med.htm

Gengo e Silva Butcher, R. D. C., & Jones, D. A. (2021). An integrative review of comprehensive nursing assessment tools developed based on Gordon's eleven functional health patterns. *International Journal of Nursing Knowledge, 32*(4), 294–307.

Halvorsen, K., Jensen, J. F., Collet, M. O., Olausson, S., Lindahl, B., Saetre Hansen, B., ... & Eriksson, T. (2022). Patients' experiences of well-being when being cared for in the intensive care unit—An integrative review. *Journal of clinical nursing, 31*(1–2), 3–19.

Haga, S. B., & Orlando, L. A. (2020). The enduring importance of *family health* history in the era of genomic medicine and risk assessment. *Personalized medicine, 17*(3), 229–239. https://doi.org/10.2217/pme-2019-0091

Josephson, A. M., & AACAP Work Group on Quality Issues. (2007). Practice parameter for the assessment of the family. *Journal of the American Academy of Child & Adolescent Psychiatry, 46*(7), 922–937. https://doi.org/10.1097/chi.0b013e318054e713

Kaakinen, J., Coehlo, D., Steele, R., Tabacco, A., & Hanson, S. (2015). *Family Health Care Nursing.* F. A. Davis.

Keitner, G. I. (2012). Family assessment in the medical setting. *The Psychosomatic Assessment, 32*, 203–222.

Kruger, J. S., Kim, I., Foltz-Ramos, K., & Ohtake, P. J. (2024). Utilizing an Ecomap to Visualize the Impact of Social Determinants of Health in an Interprofessional Forum. *Journal of Allied Health, 53*(1), 61E–66E.

Khoury, M. J., Bowen, S., Dotson, W. D., Drzymalla, E., Green, R. F., Goldstein, R., ... & Bunnell, R. (2022). Health equity in the implementation of genomics and precision medicine: A public health imperative. *Genetics in Medicine, 24*(8), 1630–1639.

Knafl, K. A., Deatrick, J. A., Gallo, A. M., & Skelton, B. (2021). Tracing the Use of the Family Management Framework and Measure: A Scoping Review. *Journal of family nursing, 27*(2), 87–106. https://doi.org/10.1177/1074840721994331

Larasati, T., Lipoeto, N. I., Mudjiran, Masrul, Hardisman, & Sutomo, A. H. (2020). "GENOGRAM physician involvement model": New approach for Indonesian physician involvement with family. *Korean J Fam Med., 41*(5), 325–331. https://doi.org/10.4082/kjfm.19.0017

Leahey, M., & Wright, L. M. (2016). Application of the Calgary family assessment and intervention models: Reflections on the reciprocity between the personal and the professional. *Journal of family nursing, 22*(4), 450–459.

Libbon, R., Triana, J., Heru, A., & Berman, E. (2019). Family skills for the resident toolbox: The 10-min genogram, ecomap, and prescribing homework. *Academic Psychiatry, 43*, 435–439.

Liossi, C., Hatira, P., & Mystakidou, K. (1997). The use of the genogram in palliative care. *Palliative medicine, 11*(6), 455–461.

McNellan, C. R., Gibbs, D. J., Knobel, A. S., & Putnam-Hornstein, E. (2022). The evidence based for risk assessment tools used in US child protection investigations: A systematic scoping review. *Child Abuse & Neglect, 134*, 105887.

Miller, I. W., Ryan, C. E., Keitner, G. I., Bishop, D. S., & Epstein, N. B. (2000). The McMaster approach to families: Theory, assessment, treatment and research. *Journal of family therapy, 22*(2), 168–189.

Berkey, K. M. & Hanson, S. M (1991). *Pocket guide to family assessment and intervention.* Mosby Year Book.

Olsen, S., Dudley-Brown, S., & McMullen, P. (2004). Case for blending pedigrees, genograms and ecomaps: Nursing's contribution to the "big picture." *Nursing & health sciences, 6*(4), 295–308.

Olson, D. H. (2000). Circumplex model of marital and family systems. *Journal of family therapy, 22*(2), 144–167.

Olson, D. H., Portner, J., & Lavee, Y. (2013). Family adaptability and cohesion evaluation scales III. In R. Sherman & N. Fredman (Eds.) *Handbook of measurements for marriage and family therapy* (1st Ed., pp. 180–185). Routledge.

Puskar, K., & Nerone, M. (1996). Genogram: A useful tool for nurse practitioners. *Journal of psychiatric and mental health nursing, 3*(1), 55–60.

Rogers, J., & Durkin, M. (1984). The semi-structured genogram interview. I: Protocol. II: Evaluation. *Family Systems Medicine, 2*(2), 176–187. https://doi.org/10.1037/h0091655

Rossi, L., Butler, S., Coakley, A., & Flanagan, J. (2023). Nursing knowledge captured in electronic health records. *International Journal of Nursing Knowledge, 34*(1), 72–84.

Sawin, K. J. (2016). Measurement in family nursing: Established instruments and new directions. *Journal of family nursing, 22*(3), 287–297.

Skinner, H., Steinhauer, P., & Sitarenios, G. (2000). Family assessment measure (FAM) and process model of family functioning. *Journal of Family Therapy, 22*(2), 190–210.

Smilkstein, G. (1978). The family APGAR: A proposal for a family function test and its use by physicians. *J fam pract, 6*(6), 1231–1239.

Takenaka, H., & Ban, N. (2016). The most important question in family approach: The potential of the resolve item of the family APGAR in family medicine. *Asia Pacific family medicine, 15*, 1–7.

Tomson, P. R. (1985). Genograms in general practice. *Journal of the Royal Society of Medicine, 78*(8), 34.

Watson, W. J., Poon, V. H., & Waters, I. A. (2014. *Genograms: Seeing Patients and Families.* https://tspace.library.utoronto.ca/bitstream/1807/124013/1/Genograms-Revised.pdf

Wilkinson, I., Barnett, M. B., Delf, L., & Pirie, V. (1988). Family assessment: Developing a formal assessment system in clinical practice. *Journal of family therapy, 10*(1), 17–32.

Wright, L. M., & Leahey, M. (1984). Nurses & families: A guide to family assessment & intervention. F.A. Davis.

Wright, L. M., & Leahey, M. (1999). Maximizing time, minimizing suffering: The 15-minute (or less) family interview. *Journal of Family Nursing*, 5, 259–273. https://doi.org/10.1177/107484079900500302

Wu, R. R., Myers, R. A., Sperber, N., Voils, C. I., Neuner, J., McCarty, C. A., ... & Orlando, L. A. (2019). Implementation, adoption, and utility of *family health* history risk assessment in diverse care settings: Evaluating implementation processes and impact with an implementation framework. *Genetics in Medicine, 21*(2), 331–338.

Yeheskel, A., Biderman, A., Borkan, J. M., & Herman, J. (2000). A course for teaching patient-centered medicine to family medicine residents. *Academic medicine, 75*(5), 494–497.

Figure credits

Fig. 6.1: Francine Shapiro, Florence W. Kaslow and Louise Maxfield, "Example of Standard Symbols in a Family Genogram," *Handbook of EMDR and Family Therapy Processes*, p. 79. Copyright © 2007 by John Wiley & Sons, Inc.

Fig. 6.2: Jessica S. Kruger, Isok Kim, Kelly Foltz-Ramos and Patricia J. Ohtake, "Utilizing an Ecomap to Visualize the Impact of Social Determinants of Health in an Interprofessional Forum," *Journal of Allied Health*, vol. 58, no. 1, p. 65. Copyright © 2024 by The Association of Schools Advancing Health Professions.

Fig. 6.3: Jessica S. Kruger, Isok Kim, Kelly Foltz-Ramos and Patricia J. Ohtake, "Utilizing an Ecomap to Visualize the Impact of Social Determinants of Health in an Interprofessional Forum," *Journal of Allied Health*, vol. 58, no. 1, p. 63. Copyright © 2024 by The Association of Schools Advancing Health Professions.

IMG 6.1: Copyright © 2022 Depositphotos/AndreyPopov.

CHAPTER 7

Person-Centered Relationships and Communication in Family Health Care

Effective communication is the cornerstone of patient-centered care.

—Cheri Clancy and Sandra Rutherford

Learning Objectives

By the end of this chapter, learners will do the following:

- Describe the key terminology related to effective communication and interactions in *family health* care.
- Describe the importance of evidence-based person–clinician and clinician–clinician interactions and communications in *family health* care.
- Discuss evidence-based and practice-based communication strategies that support patient-centered care decisions and information sharing in *family health* care.
- Describe the factors influencing person-centered relationships and communication in *family health* care within the 4HEALTH contexts.
- Demonstrate the use of patient-centered care and communication with individuals, caregivers and families, populations, and/or the public to support *family health* care.

Before you read on, consider the following questions:

- What would happen if your provider did a physical examination without asking you if you are okay with it?
- What if your health care professionals made their own assumptions about your treatment needs that turned out to be wrong because they did not understand what you were trying to communicate to them?
- What would happen if you got your medications from the pharmacy without written or verbal notice from your pharmacist or pharmacist assistant?
- What would happen if your adolescent child did not want a provider to tell you they are pregnant?

- What would happen if you were deaf and your provider did not have the tools to facilitate communication?
- What if you knew that your neighbor could access information about their care online but they did not have access to technology or the internet?
- What if you prefer a female health care provider and there is no one available?
- What if a health care provider was very rude to you?
- What if a provider had preconceived negative perceptions about your ethnic background—would you trust them?

Importance of Effective Communication and Relationships in Health Care Settings

As reflected in the questions, effective communication is the foundation of healthy relationships and interactions in any health care settings According to the Merriam-Webster online dictionary, *communication* can be defined as a process by which information is exchanged between individuals through a common system of symbols, signs, or behavior. Gutmman et al. (2021) describes communication as "reciprocal process of individuals sending and receiving precise and accurate information that forms and reforms one's attitudes, behaviors, and cognition influenced by internal and external factors" (p. e1465). Communication is a key element in developing trusting and caring interpersonal relationships (Honavar, 2018). Embedded within the Hildegard Peplau's middle-range nursing theory of interpersonal relations, provider–patient relationships can be viewed as therapeutic relationships that have professional communicative or linguistic characteristics in nature (Gastmans, 1998). According to the theory, the goal of the therapeutic relationship is two-folds: first to ensure survival of the patient/client and second to make sure that the patient/client understands the health problems in order to develop new behavior patterns (Black, 2014). In Peplau's theory, effective communication provides a sensory enrichment for interpersonal relations to evolve and grow through phases: orientation (formation of patient–nurse relationship), working (identification and exploitation) and resolution (Adams, 2017; Forchuk & Dorsay, 1995). Poor communication within the provider–patient relationship is considered a source of problems.

According to the U.S. Joint Commission International (2012), approximately 80% of sentinel events in health care are caused by communication errors. Communication inefficiency among providers has an estimated economic burden of $12 billion annually (Agarwal et al., 2010). The lack of effective communication can have negative consequences to patient safety and outcomes. For instance, poor written communication can lead to discontinuity of care, compromised patient safety, patient dissatisfaction, and inefficient use of valuable resources (Vermeir et al., 2015). In addition, communication that does not meet the needs of certain patients and their family can affect optimal patient health outcomes and engagement (Dooley et al., 2015). For instance, the lack of linguists and culturally qualified clinicians can jeopardize care for the deaf population (Wilson & Schild, 2014). Likewise, the lack of tailoring communication that is developmentally appropriate poses risks to patient safety and leads to provider stress (Thunberg et al., 2022).

Effective communication and teamwork, on the other hand, improves cost, resource utilization, safety, efficiency, patient satisfaction, and problem solving (Gharaveis et al., 2018). Greater practitioner empathy or communication of positive messages is believed to have positive outcomes in pain management (Howick et al., 2018). Positive patient–provider relationships are vital for improving access to primary care and health outcomes for underserved populations (Kamimura et al., 2020). Effective communication (verbal and nonverbal) between and health care providers and women has been associated with positive satisfaction with birth care (Ahmed, 2020).

Therapeutic Communication Processes, Mediums and Strategies

Communication Model

In health care, communication involves exchanges between two or more people in a given context. The exchanges can be verbal or nonverbal, assuming the role of a sender (the person who conveys the message) and the receiver (the person whom the message is sent to). Figure 7.1 displays a model of communication indicating how messages are shared between sender and receiver.

The exchanges of information happen in the contexts of interpersonal relationships between provider and provider, and provider and person (individuals, family, communities, and populations, public) across the care continuum. Within the relationships, providers can assume six fundamental communication tasks: fostering healing relationships, exchanging information, responding to patients' emotions, managing uncertainty, making informed decisions, and enabling patient self-management (Epstein & Street, 2007). Table 7.1 summarizes examples of the different communication tasks across the levels of prevention and cancer care continuum (Epstein & Street, 2007).

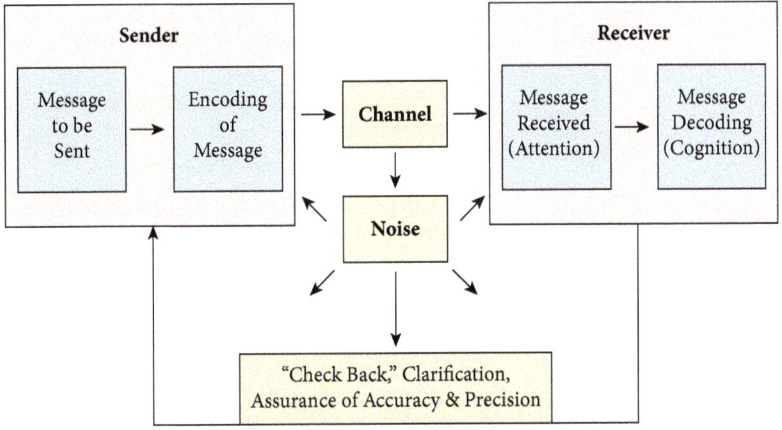

FIGURE 7.1 A communication model (Guttman et al., 2021, p. e1466).

TABLE 7.1 Examples of Communication Tasks Across the Cancer Care Continuum Phases

Level of Prevention	Cancer Continuum Phase	Examples of Communication Tasks
Primary Prevention	Prevention	Making decision about behavior change
Secondary Prevention	Screening	Exchanging information: Explaining the difference between a positive screening test and actual disease Managing uncertainty: Interpreting test results Fostering healing relationships: Establishing trust, understanding clinician limitations Enabling patient self-management: Eliminating disparities in access to and quality of care
	Diagnosis	Making decisions: Involving patients in decision-making Exchanging information: Improving patient knowledge about the diagnostic process Enabling patient self-management: Guiding the patient through the healthcare system Responding to emotions: Conveying empathy and taking action Recognizing indirect cue of distress Fostering healing relationships, making decisions: Activating patients to ask questions and participate in decisions
Tertiary Prevention	Treatment	Fostering healing relationships: Explaining and responding to unexpected complications Exchanging information: Dealing with adverse outcomes Offering both information and the skills to process the information Communicating with patients with low health literacy Enabling patient self-management Making decisions: Communicating evidence
	Survivorship	Fostering healing relationships: Lowering the level of patient anxiety Responding to emotions: Addressing fears of recurrence Enabling patient self-management Managing uncertainty: Interpreting survival estimates
	End of life	Exchanging information: Discussing treatment failure and transition to palliative care Fostering healing relationships: Accommodating patients' changing wishes for involvement in decision-making and increased family involvement Managing uncertainty: Helping the patient articulate end-of-life wishes

Mediums of Communication

Communication in health care settings takes place across the life span through different mediums known as modalities, channels, and devices (Oba & Berger, 2024). Communication modalities produce content and include speaking (oral), writing, sign language, and interpreter usage. Communication modalities, especially in low-resources settings, include letters and official memos (Dongyele et al., 2021). Communication channels are vehicles through which content is delivered, such as texting, phone calls, emails, social media, and face-to-face. Communication devices are equipment through which content can be produced and shared such as smartphones, smartwatches, or computers (Oba & Berger, 2024). Face-to face is the common channel through which communication happens between providers and health care consumers (Dongyele et al., 2021). Evolving information communication technology (ICT) strategies act as solutions to complexities linked to provider–patient communication (Baldwin et al., 2002). For example, ICT such as mobile phones are reported to improve emergency response, information management, access to health services, quality and safety of care, continuity of services, and cost containment in rural area (Chib, 2010). Likewise, ICT modalities such as internet, intranets, telephone, video conferencing, email, and short message service [SMS] have shown to facilitate support, medication management, education, and monitoring in a provide-patient-caregiver relationship (Gentles et al., 2010). Internet access for personal health records and telehealth use has gained traction in patient and family engagement (Randeree, 2009). In addition, the use of artificial intelligence (AI) has been considered in providing audit and feedback about providers' communication skills (Butow & Hoque, 2020). Secure messaging is also a new ICT channel for supporting information sharing in patient-centered communication (Hogan et al., 2018). Interventions that have employed secured electronic medical email messages have demonstrated a positive impact on patients' health behaviors (Goyder et al., 2015). Moreover, communication modalities through poster presentation are common in public health efforts (Saleh et al., 2013). Social media brings a new public health dimension to communicating about health issues and collaboration (Moorhead et al., 2013).

Person-Centered Care Communication

Peplau's interpersonal theory puts emphasis on the mastery of certain knowledge, skills, and attitudes (KSAs) related to the provider–patient relationship. The communication behavioral competencies include language use and counseling in human interactions, assessment, problem solving, teaching, and collaboration (Yamashita, 1997). In the health care literature, these skills are referred to as "soft skills": groups of skills that are transferable and nontechnical in nature (Daly et al., 2022). Other terminologies used to describe soft skills are people skills, interpersonal skills, social skills, transferable skills, life skills, emotional intelligence and behavioral skills, and noncognitive skills. Table 7.2 provides examples of soft skills required in health care settings (Touloumakos, 2020).

TABLE 7.2 **Examples of Soft Skills**

Soft Skill	Examples
Qualities	Emotional intelligence, including adaptability, flexibility, responsibility, courtesy, integrity, professionalism, and effectiveness and values such as trustworthiness and work ethic
Volitions, Predispositions, Attitudes	Good attitude, willingness to learn, hardworking, works well under pressure or uncertainty
Problem Solving and Decision-Making	Problem solving, decision-making, analytical thinking/thinking skills, creativity/innovation, manipulation of knowledge, critical judgment
Leadership	Leadership skills and managing skills as well as self-awareness, managing oneself/coping skills
Interpersonal Savvy/Skills	Social skills, and team skills, effective and productive interpersonal interactions
Communication	Elements of negotiation, conflict resolution, persuasion skills, and diversity as articulation work—orchestrating simultaneous interactions with people, information, and technology
Emotional Labor	Managing emotions related to service jobs
Aesthetics	Professional appearance
Others	Cognitive abilities or processes, ability to plan and achieve goals

Efforts to improve competencies in soft skills among medical students have received much attention in the literature (Jogerst et al., 2015; Joubert et al., 2006), partly because of existing patient mistreatments such as service denial, oppressive language, harsh words and rough examination among providers (Camara et al., 2020), lack of ideal models, and realities of practice (Rosenbaum, 2017). Likewise, demonstration of interdisciplinary communication competencies is increasingly becoming part of organizational quality and safety initiatives (Krautscheid, 2008; Sheldon & Hilaire, 2015). IPE competency skills include communication techniques, patient safety, diversity, team science, and cultural humility (Foronda et al., 2016). Skills in cultural humility entail providers' sense of self-reflection on one's own cultural beliefs, values, attitudes, and practice and being open and sensitive to others' differences (Brooks et al., 2019). In addition, skills to enhance confidence in dealing with aggression behaviors are also promoted (Baby et al., 2018).

Effective Communication Strategies

Many evidence-based strategies have been proposed in the literature to support person-centered care communication for different contexts. The following list is not exhaustive.

The Seven Cs of Communication Framework

Professor Scott Cutlip and Allen Center (1952) pioneered the seven Cs framework. The framework helps facilitate an understanding of the attributes of successful spoken and written communication (Hasan et al., 2022; Krishna, 2018). Table 7.3 summarizes the 7Cs of communication, with definitions and examples.

TABLE 7.3 **Attributes of Oral and Written Communication Messages**

Attributes	Definition	Examples
Clear	The message must be goal oriented and easy to understand.	Speak slowly and clearly, avoiding jargons and acronyms. Use spoken language/communication. Avoid technical communication. With written communication, use the one-paragraph, one-idea rule.
Concise	The message must be brief (succinct) and direct to help keep the user's focus.	Avoid being cyclic by avoiding wordy expressions and repetition; convey in least possible words without forgoing the other Cs of communication and eliminate adjectives or filler words/ phrases like "for instance," "actually," "kind of," "literally," "basically," or "I think that."
Concrete	The information must be exact and succinct, leaving no room for ambiguity.	Message should be specific. Ensure your message has important details and facts. Details should capture the intended audience.
Correct	The message should be accurate and written in the correct language, free of technical or grammatical problems, and timely. Correct messages enhance morale.	Provide accurate facts in the right contexts, use the right level of language, choose nondiscriminatory expressions, spell all names and titles correctly, and proofread messages.
Consideration	Consideration means understanding or to put yourself in the place of receiver while composing a message. The communication should be aimed to the intended audience while making sure both the recipient's thoughts and opinions are examined. The message must be objective and utilize language that shows respect for the recipient.	Ask yourself, "Why should my reader spend time reading this?" Foresee your audience's needs and their requirements, emotions, and problems. Show empathy. Focus on the "you" attitude instead of "I" or "we," "me" attitude.
Complete	Clarity is ensured by the completeness of the message. Message should comprise all the essential information for the target audience to help them make better choices.	Provide all the necessary information that answers the five Ws that make the message clear: who, what, when, where and why.
Courteous	Courteous communication is friendly, open, caring, and honest. The presenter must examine the receiver's ideas, skills, viewpoint, and background, to connect successfully. The sender must have a connection with and be involved with the target recipient in order to connect.	Using words and expressions that can lead to harmony and human bonding should be the eventual goal of the sender of the message. For example, use salutation when writing an email message. Avoid aggressive tones.

Active Listening

Active listening facilitates meaningful relationships and interactions with patients. It is an important component of the communication process. It involves therapeutic understanding of what the other person (sender) is communicating and feeling and then communicating that understanding back to them as the receiver (Mesquita & Carvalho, 2014). Table 7.4 lists three common attributes of the concept of active listening in health care (Shipley, 2010).

TABLE 7.4 **Common Attributes of the Concept of Active Listening in Health Care**

Attribute	Definition	Examples
Empathy	Being aware of, and sensitive to, the feelings, thoughts, and experiences of another	Pay attention to body language and while waiting to respond and taking the whole moment. Put yourself in the other person's shoes.
Being Nonjudgmental and Accepting	Understanding the whole person and recognizing that each patient is a unique individual with different beliefs, lifestyles, and culture	Keep an open mind to accept new ideas and keep your own thoughts and biases out of the way. Let a person explain their whole point before jumping to any judgments.
Reflection, Summarization, and Feedback	Processes that help patients to perceive that their message has been heard and understood	This is an actionable technique whereby you paraphrase the message back to the sender to ensure you understand correctly. Did you take away what the person wanted you to? If you need more information on a point someone is making, politely ask for more details. Like reflecting, summarizing the takeaways of a conversation in a clear manner can help both parties understand the next steps and reduce confusion. Sharing common experiences builds trusting relationships while also helping the speaker and the listener understand one another better.

Note: Examples are extracted from National Society of Leadership and Success (2023).

Motivational Interviewing

Motivational interviewing (MI) is a collaborative person-centered therapeutic strategy pioneered by Miller and Rollnick (1991, 2009). It is defined as a "directive, client-centered counselling style for eliciting behavior change by helping clients to explore and resolve ambivalence" (p. 105). MI is a collaborative, person-centered form of guiding to elicit and strengthen motivation for change. The strategy has been effectively used in the treatment of various lifestyle problems and diseases (Rubak et al., 2005) and in health care to improve clinicians' client communication and counseling skills (Brobeck et al., 2011; Söderlund et al., 2011). It is recommended in primary care settings as a potential patient activation and engagement strategy that could meet future needs of people at risk of developing chronic diseases and long-terms conditions (Anstiss, 2009). The major attributes of MI are readiness, ambivalence, and resistance. The principles of MI practices include expressing empathy, rolling with resistance, supporting self-efficacy, and developing discrepancies, and the MI methods include empathic listening skills, eliciting self-motivating statement (change talk), and responding to resistance (Rollnick & Miller, 1995). Table 7.5 provides MI attributes (concepts, principles, and methods).

TABLE 7.5 **MI Concepts, Principles and Methods**

MI Attributes	
MI Concepts	**Definition**
Readiness	A state of readiness to change along a continuum that fluctuates and can be influenced by others
Ambivalence	A doubtless normal and defining state endured by all that change is not made without inconvenience, even from worse to better
Resistance	A most active form of observable behavior that arises when the counselor loses demonstrable congruence with the client and therefore the behavior is amenable to change
MI Principles	
Expressing empathy	The fundamental principle that ensures that the counselor remains in step with the needs and aspirations of the client with reflective listening. It involves both simple summary statements, designed to ensure parity with the client, and more complex statements that enable the skilled counselor to gently highlight elements of the client's dilemma that might encourage resolution of ambivalence.
Rolling with resistance	This principle highlights the need to avoid nonconstructive conversations, which resembles a battle of wills.
Supporting self-efficacy	Developing a sense that "I can cope in this situation" and "I will do this in that difficult situation" will be of benefit to clients. It involves eliciting the inner conviction rather than imposing it from without. The client is encouraged to take charge of decision-making.
Developing discrepancies	A particular state of discomfort, termed discrepancy, that can arise from the contrast between what the person wants from life and the self-destructive nature of a problem.
MI Methods	
Empathic listening skills	Open questions, affirmation, summarizing, and reflective listening.
Eliciting self-motivating statements (change talk)	A nontechnical matter of eliciting statements and ignoring arguments for not changing but of giving the client time to express ambivalence free of distraction in an atmosphere in which the counselor's main task is to listen and understand. In the dialogue noted, reflective listening was used to do just this, and the last statement from the client is a self-motivating statement and an expression of concern about drinking.
Responding to resistance	Responding constructively to resistance, which can be viewed as damaged rapport, is particularly important in the early stages of an encounter, when the possibilities for miscommunication are so common.

Stephen Rollnick and William R. Miller, "What is Motivational Interviewing?" *Behavioural and Cognitive Psychotherapy*, vol. 23, no. 4.

ISBAR Framework

The Identify, Situation, Background, Assessment, and Recommendation framework, also known as ISBAR, is a structured, standardized framework for handover in clinical settings. ISBAR helps reduce errors and patient harm and improve continuity of care (Burgess et al., 2020). Handover tools are important in increasing awareness of communication and professional roles (Haddeland et al., 2022). The five elements of communication in the ISBAR framework are presented in Table 7.6.

TABLE 7.6 **The ISBAR Framework**

Elements of Communication	Examples
Introduction	Who are you, what is your role, where are you are, and why you are communicating?
Situation	What is happening now?
Background	What are the issues that led up to this situation?
Assessment	What do you believe is the problem?
Recommendations	What should be done to correct the situation?

Other essential communication skills include goal-setting techniques such as the SMART framework (CDC, 2018), as well as skills in ethical communication, such as the "one-to-five" method (Fischer-Grönlund et al., 2021; see Table 7.7).

SMART Goals

- Specific. Goals/objectives should provide the "who" and "what" of the clinical–patient communication and interaction activities:
  - ▷ Use only one action verb since objectives with more than one verb imply that more than one activity or behavior is being measured.
  - ▷ Avoid verbs that may have vague meanings to describe intended outcomes (e.g., "understand" or "know") since it may prove difficult to measure them. Instead, use verbs that document action (e.g., "At the end of the therapeutic session, the provider and patient will list three things do d as part of the follow-up implementation plan").
  - ▷ Remember, the greater the specificity, the greater the measurability.
- Measurable
  - ▷ The focus is on "how much" change is expected. Goals/objectives should quantify the amount of change expected.
  - ▷ It is impossible to determine whether objectives have been met unless they can be measured.
  - ▷ The objective provides a reference point from which a change in an expected behavior can clearly be measured.

- Attainable
  - ▹ Objectives should be attainable within a given time frame and with available program resources.
- Realistic
  - ▹ Objectives are most useful when they accurately address the scope of the problem and programmatic steps that can be implemented within a specific time frame.
  - ▹ Objectives that do not directly relate to the program goal will not help toward achieving the goal.
- Time-Phased
  - ▹ Objectives should provide a time frame indicating when the objective will be measured or a time by which the objective will be met.
  - ▹ Including a time in the objectives helps in planning and evaluating the goal/objective.

TABLE 7.7 **One-to-Five Ethical Communication Process**

Steps	Description of Context	Example of Questions
Story about the situation	The participants narrate and share an ethically difficult situation form clinical practice.	Can you please narrate an ethically difficult situation from your clinical work? Does someone need further clarification? Can you please share your personal experience of the situation? What do you experience as difficult? Can you tell us more about it? What do you all think about this situation?
Reflections and dialogue of emotions involved	The participants share experiences and emotions expressed in relation to the dilemma.	How did you feel? What in this situation arouses these feelings?
Formulation or problem/dilemma	The participants identify the value conflict and reflect on the ethical dimensions	What is ethically difficult in this situation? How can you formulate the problem/dilemma? What is the ethical conflict in your story? What is at stake?
Analysis	Various perspectives of the situation are highlighted to promote a broadened understanding of the ethically difficult situation in the group.	How can you understand or explain this situation? Which perspectives are involved? Which values, principles, or norms are at stake? Could it be in this way? What could it be due to?
Choice of action or approach	A common interpretation and reinterpretation of the value conflict.	How can you act? How can you relate?

Health care professionals in *family health* care should also master skills in establishing boundaries within a patient–provider relationship (Manfrin-Ledet et al., 2015) and interdisciplinary teams (Liberati et al., 2016). In terms of public health, the WHO framework suggests the following six principles for effective communication, which are applicable to the local and national contexts:

- Accessible
  - ▹ Make information available online.
  - ▹ Identify effective channels.
  - ▹ Ensure accessibility.
- Actionable
  - ▹ Move audiences to action.
  - ▹ Start behavior change campaigns.
  - ▹ Communicate in emergencies.
- Credible
  - ▹ Have technical accuracy.
  - ▹ Be transparent.
  - ▹ Coordinate with partners.
  - ▹ Speak as "one WHO."
  - ▹ Utilize the WHO brand.
- Relevant
  - ▹ Know the audience.
  - ▹ Listen to the audience.
  - ▹ Tailor the message.
  - ▹ Motivate the audience.
- Timely
  - ▹ Communicate early.
  - ▹ Communicate at the right time.
  - ▹ Build the conversation.
- Understandable
  - ▹ Use plain language.
  - ▹ Tell real stories.
  - ▹ Make it visual.
  - ▹ Use familiar languages.

Barriers to Person-Centered Therapeutic Communication and Relationships in Family Health Care

There are many barriers to communication in health care settings (Guttman et al., 2021). Some of the barriers are tailored toward a systems-level uptake of evidence-based patient-centered communication, and relationships can be categorized within the 4HEALTH contexts.

For instance, within the individual and *family health* levels, the focus should be on finding effective ways to facilitate health literacy among vulnerable populations. Low health literacy and English as a second language has an impact on how individuals and families seek and access health care services and how they participate in decision-making practices. Lack of resources such as health information technology can impact provider–physician relationships, especially when the world is moving toward technology. Family relationship and caregiving experiences can also influence clinical provider relationships, especially with families that are going through stressful emotions. In addition, provider involvement with families should take into account how family communication practices may influence the relationship/interaction and communication.

At the population level, time management is a common communication barrier (Kiwanuka et al., 2019). Providers should be strive to advocate for patient-centered care health care systems that provide more time to listen to the patients and build relationships (O'Hare, 2018). Systems-level changes on how providers are incentivize and documentation and medical billing need to change to help make care more patient centered (Berwick, 2009). Interprofessional boundaries are intended to strengthen providers' ability to care for patients. However, if not used properly, they can make it difficult to fully grasp and acknowledge patients' suffering (Dalal et al., 2017).

In addition, systems-level changes should stem from a clear understanding of the types and characteristics of health systems service delivery: task oriented, process oriented or person centered. Utilizing the PC4 model as a framework (Kwame & Petrucka, 2021), patient-centered care entails the highest point of care whereby communication between the provider and patient and their family is collaborative and mutual; the care uses different mediums of communications and tasks based on care and context (see Figure 7.2). Tasked oriented is the lowest level, whereby the clinician is focused on completed the medical task with minimum patient engagement (Kwame & Petrucka, 2021). Process oriented is an intermediate state that indicates a risk of skipping back to task-oriented approaches or moving toward patient-centered care. Providers focus on understanding care conditions with minimum encouragement to let patients and families express their thoughts and needs. Testing for such a model is beneficial for system-level changes.

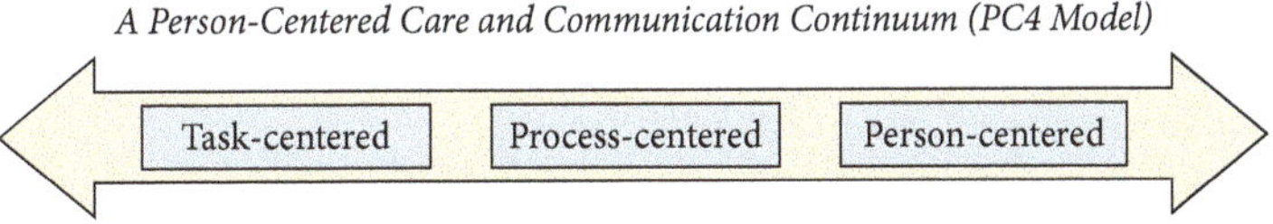

FIGURE 7.2 A person-centered care and continuum (PC4 model).

Task-shifting strategies in interprofessional practices should be evaluated using the PC4 framework to provide clear expectations of providers' time commitment for person-centered communication. Communication in public health has gained recognition because of the importance of communication and interpersonal theories in changing human behavior (Rimal & Lapinski, 2009). This window of opportunity is vital for promoting effective communication to protect individuals, families, communities, and populations. Health care systems should make sure providers have culturally competent communication skills to promote equity and eliminate health disparities among populations of interest (Mor-Anavy et al., 2021). Effective health communication between health care providers and clients using methods such as teach-back and shared decision-making can promote informed decisions among vulnerable populations (those with low health literacy and English as a second language), which is instrumental to health and well-being (Office of Disease Prevention and Health Promotion, n.d.a.). Furthermore, making electronic health information accessible and easy to understand is vital for promoting health and well-being. Table 7.8 displays some useful Healthy People 2023 health communication indicators and targets (Office of Disease Prevention and Health Promotion, n.d.b.) that have implications for public health workforce education (communication and cultural competencies), research in health disparities, communication access disparities, and access to health information technology (Bernhardt, 2004). The data demonstrate a need for continuous research to assess the impact of training among providers for promoting evidence-based and practice-based evidence communication. Several immediate and intermediate health outcomes that can be used to track outcomes have been proposed (Levinson et al., 2010; see Figure 7.3).

TABLE 7.8 **Sample Health People 2023 Objectives and Targets**

Health Communication: General	**Tracking Progress**
Increase the number of state health departments that use social marketing in health promotion programs.	Developmental
Increase the health literacy of the population.	Research
Increase the proportion of adults who talk to friends or family about their health.	Getting worse
Health care	
Increase the proportion of adults whose health care provider checked their understanding.	Little or no detectable change
Decrease the proportion of adults who report poor communication with their health care provider.	Little or no detectable change
Increase the proportion of adults whose health care providers involved them in decisions as much as they wanted.	Little or no detectable change
Increase the proportion of adults with limited English proficiency who say their providers explain things clearly.	Developmental
Health IT	
Increase the proportion of adults offered online access to their medical record.	Target met or exceeded

Increase the proportion of people who can view, download, and send their electronic health information.	
Increase the proportion of adults who use IT to track health care data or communicate with providers.	Target met or exceeded
Increase the proportion of people who can view, download, and send their electronic health information.	Developmental

Notes: Baseline only: No data is available beyond the initial baseline data, thus, no information on progress made.Target met or exceeded: Target set at the beginning of the decade is achieved. Improving: Progress is made towards meeting our target. Little or no detectable change: No progress has been made or lost ground. Getting worse: Further from meeting our target than we were at the beginning of the decade. Developmental objectives represent high-priority public health issues that are associated with evidence-based interventions but don't yet have reliable baseline data. Source: Office of Disease Prevention and Health Promotion, Office of Assistant Secretary for Health, U.S Department of Health and Human Services (n.d.a., n.d.b.)

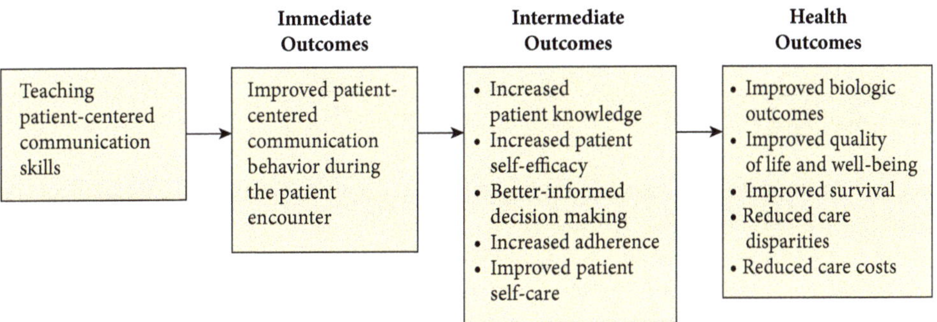

FIGURE 7.3 Link between teaching patient-centered communication skills and various outcomes (Levinson et al., 2010).

Conclusion

This chapter discussed the importance of effective *family health* care professional–person relationships and communications in influencing *population health* outcomes. The different mediums and tools of communication were described. For health professionals who are thinking families, the awareness of the multilevel barriers to the uptake of evidence-based communication and relationship strategies is essential for future implementation of person-centered care health care systems. System-level changes are needed for effective implementation. The next chapter will discuss the policy-making process and advocacy in *family health* care.

Suggested Websites

Agency for Healthcare Research and Quality: Strategy 2, Communicating to Improve Quality: https://www.ahrq.gov/patient-safety/patients-families/engagingfamilies/strategy2/index.html

Healthy People 2030, Health Communication: https://health.gov/healthypeople/objectives-and-data/browse-objectives/health-communication

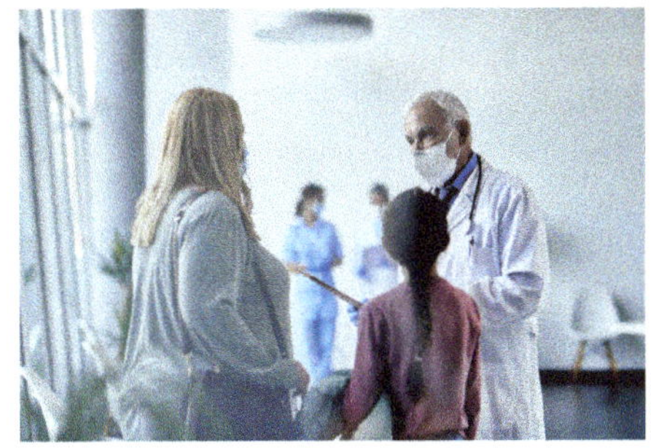

IMG 7.1

The Institute for Healthcare Communication (IHC): https://healthcarecomm.org/about-us/
WHO Principles for Effective Communication: https://www.who.int/about/communications/principles

Reflection Questions

1. How can you build trust between patient and providers across diverse individual and families?
2. What skills do you think health care professional need to work on?
3. If you were a health care system leader, what would you change at the systems level to increase more time for providers to build relationships with their patients?
4. What medium of communication do you think would work best for your needs?
5. How can you show empathy?

References

Adams, L. Y. (2017). Peplau's contributions to psychiatric and nursing knowledge. *Journal of Mental Health and Addiction Nursing, 1*(1), e10–e18.

Agarwal, R., Sands, D. Z., & Schneider, J. D. (2010). Quantifying the economic impact of communication inefficiencies in U.S. hospitals. *Journal of healthcare management / American College of Healthcare Executives, 55*(4), 265–282.

Ahmed, H. M. (2020). Role of verbal and non-verbal communication of health care providers in general satisfaction with birth care: A cross-sectional study in government health settings of Erbil City, Iraq. *Reproductive Health, 17*(35),1–9. https://doi.org/10.1186/s12978-020-0894-3

Anstiss, T. (2009). Motivational interviewing in primary care. *Journal of Clinical Psychology in Medical settings, 16*, 87–93.

Baby, M., Gale, C., & Swain, N. (2018). Communication skills training in the management of patient aggression and violence in healthcare. *Aggression and Violent Behavior, 39*, 67–82.

Baca, M. (2011). Professional boundaries and dual relationships in clinical practice. *The Journal for Nurse Practitioners, 7*(3), 195–200.

Baldwin, L. P., Clarke, M., Eldabi, T., & Jones, R. W. (2002). Telemedicine and its role in improving communication in healthcare. *Logistics Information Management, 15*(4), 309–319.

Bernhardt J. M. (2004). Communication at the core of effective public health. *American Journal of Public Health, 94*(12), 2051–2053. https://doi.org/10.2105/ajph.94.12.2051

Berwick, D. M. (2009). What "patient-centered" should mean: Confessions of an extremist: A seasoned clinician and expert fears the loss of his humanity if he should become a patient. *Health affairs, 2*(1), w555–w565.

Black, B. P (2014). *Professional nursing: Concepts and challenges*. Elsevier.

Brobeck, E., Bergh, H., Odencrants, S., & Hildingh, C. (2011). Primary healthcare nurses' experiences with motivational interviewing in health promotion practice. *Journal of Clinical Nursing, 20*(23-24), 3322–3330.

Burgess, A., van Diggele, C., Roberts, C., & Mellis, C. (2020). Teaching clinical handover with ISBAR. *BMC Medical Education, 20*, 1–8.

Butow, P., & Hoque, E. (2020). Using artificial intelligence to analyse and teach communication in healthcare. *The Breast, 50*, 49–55.

Brooks, L. A., Manias, E., & Bloomer, M. J. (2019). Culturally sensitive communication in healthcare: A concept analysis. *Collegian, 26*(3), 383–391.

Camara, B. S., Belaid, L., Manet, H., Kolie, D., Guillard, E., Bigirimana, T., & Delamou, A. (2020). What do we know about patient-provider interactions in sub-Saharan Africa? A scoping review. *Pan African Medical Journal, 37*(1).

Centers for Disease Control and Prevention. (2018). *Writing SMART objectives.* https://www.cdc.gov/healthyyouth/evaluation/pdf/brief3b.pdf

Chib, A. (2010). The Aceh Besar midwives with mobile phones project: Design and evaluation perspectives using the information and communication technologies for healthcare development model. *Journal of Computer-Mediated Communication, 15*(3), 500–525.

Cutlip, S. M., & Center, A. H. (1952). *Effective public relations: Pathways to public favor.* Prentice Hall.

Dalal, A. K., Bates, D. W., & Collins, S. (2017). Opportunities and challenges for improving the patient experience in the acute and postacute care setting using patient portals: The patient's perspective. *Journal of Hospital Medicine, 12*(12), 1012–1016. https://doi.org/10.12788/jhm.2860

Daly, S., McCann, C., & Phillips, K. (2022). Teaching soft skills in healthcare and higher education: A scoping review protocol. *Social Science Protocols, 5*(1), 1–8.

Dongyele, M., Ansong, D., Osei, F. A., Amuzu, E. X., Mensah, N. K., Kwame Owusu, A., ... & Newton, S. (2021). Communication Medium Used by Clients and Health Professionals in Accessing and Providing Healthcare in Low Resource Setting: A Descriptive Cross-Sectional Study. *Advances in Public Health, 2021*, 1–7.

Dooley, J., Bailey, C., & McCabe, R. (2015). Communication in healthcare interactions in dementia: A systematic review of observational studies. *International Psychogeriatrics, 27*(8), 1277–1300.

Epstein, R. M., & Street, R. L, Jr. (2007) *Patient-Centered Communication in Cancer Care: Promoting Healing and Reducing Suffering.* National Cancer Institute.

Fischer-Grönlund, C., Brännström, M., & Zingmark, K. (2021). The "one to five" method—A tool for ethical communication in groups among healthcare professionals. *Nurse Education in Practice, 51*, 102998.

Fischer, H. R., Houchen, B. J., & Ferguson-Ramos, L. (2008). Professional boundaries violations: Case studies from a regulatory perspective. *Nursing Administration Quarterly, 32*(4), 317–323.

Forchuk, C., & Dorsay, J. P. (1995). Hildegard Peplau meets family systems nursing: Innovation in theory-based practice. *Journal of Advanced Nursing, 21*(1), 110–115.

Foronda, C., MacWilliams, B., & McArthur, E. (2016). Interprofessional communication in healthcare: An integrative review. *Nurse education in practice, 19*, 36–40.

Gastmans, C. (1998). Interpersonal relations in nursing: A philosophical-ethical analysis of the work of Hildegard E. Peplau. *Journal of advanced nursing, 28*(6), 1312–1319.

Gentles, S. J., Lokker, C., & McKibbon, K. A. (2010). Health information technology to facilitate communication involving health care providers, caregivers, and pediatric patients: A scoping review. *Journal of medical Internet research, 12*(2), e1390.

Gharaveis, A., Hamilton, D. K., & Pati, D. (2018). The impact of environmental design on teamwork and communication in healthcare facilities: a systematic literature review. *HERD: Health Environments Research & Design Journal, 11*(1), 119–137.

Guttman, O. T., Lazzara, E. H., Keebler, J. R., Webster, K. L., Gisick, L. M., & Baker, A. L. (2021). Dissecting communication barriers in healthcare: A path to enhancing communication resiliency, reliability, and patient safety. *Journal of patient safety, 17*(8), e1465–e1471.

Goyder, C., Atherton, H., Car, M., Heneghan, C. J., & Car, J. (2015). Email for clinical communication between healthcare professionals. The Cochrane database of systematic reviews, 2015(2), CD007979. https://doi.org/10.1002/14651858.CD007979.pub3

Haddeland, K., Marthinsen, G. N., Söderhamn, U., Flateland, S. M., & Moi, E. M. (2022). Experiences of using the ISBAR tool after an intervention: A focus group study among critical care nurses and anaesthesiologists. *Intensive and Critical Care Nursing, 70*, 103195.

Hasan, N., Pandey, M. K., Ansari, S. N., & Purohit, V. R. (2022). An Analysis of English Communication Skills. *World Journal of English Language, 12*(3), 194–202.

Hogan, T. P., Luger, T. M., Volkman, J. E., Rocheleau, M., Mueller, N., Barker, A. M., ... & Bokhour, B. G. (2018). Patient centeredness in electronic communication: Evaluation of patient-to-health care team secure messaging. *Journal of medical Internet research*, *20*(3), e82.

Howick, J., Moscrop, A., Mebius, A., Fanshawe, T. R., Lewith, G., Bishop, F. L., ... & Onakpoya, I. J. (2018). Effects of empathic and positive communication in healthcare consultations: A systematic review and meta-analysis. *Journal of the Royal Society of Medicine*, *111*(7), 240–252.

Jogerst, K., Callender, B., Adams, V., Evert, J., Fields, E., Hall, T., ... & Wilson, L. L. (2015). Identifying interprofessional global health competencies for 21st-century health professionals. *Annals of global health*, *81*(2), 239–247.

Joint Commission Center for Transforming Healthcare. (2012). *Joint Commission Resources Hot topics in health care—transitions of care: The need for a more effective approach to continuing patient care.*

Kamimura, A., Higham, R., Rathi, N., Panahi, S., Lee, E., & Ashby, J. (2020). Patient–provider relationships among vulnerable patients: The association with health literacy, continuity of care, and self-rated health. *Journal of patient experience*, *7*(6), 1450–1457.

Kiwanuka, F., Shayan, S. J., & Tolulope, A. A. (2019). Barriers to patient and family-centred care in adult intensive care units: A systematic review. *Nursing open*, *6*(3), 676–684.

Krautscheid, L. C. (2008). Improving communication among healthcare providers: Preparing student nurses for practice. *International Journal of Nursing Education Scholarship*, *5*(1).

Krishna, D. K. (2018). Decoding 7cs in effective communication. *International Journal of Communication*, *28*(1–2), 37–46.

Kwame, A., & Petrucka, P. M. (2021). A literature-based study of patient-centered care and communication in nurse-patient interactions: Barriers, facilitators, and the way forward. *BMC nursing*, *20*(1), 158.

Levinson, W., Lesser, C. S., & Epstein, R. M. (2010). Developing physician communication skills for patient-centered care. *Health affairs*, *29*(7), 1310–1318.

Liberati, E. G., Gorli, M., & Scaratti, G. (2016). Invisible walls within multidisciplinary teams: Disciplinary boundaries and their effects on integrated care. *Social Science & Medicine*, *150*, 31–39.

Manfrin-Ledet, L., Porche, D. J., & Eymard, A. S. (2015). Professional boundary violations: A literature review. *Home Healthcare Now*, *33*(6), 326–332.

Mesquita, A. C., & Carvalho, E. C. D. (2014). Therapeutic listening as a health intervention strategy: An integrative review. *Revista da Escola de Enfermagem da USP*, *48*, 1127–1136.

Miller, W. R., & Rollnick, S. (1991). *Motivational interviewing, preparing people to change addictive behavior.* Guilford Press.

Miller, W. R., & Rollnick, S. (2009). Ten things that motivational interviewing is not. *Behavioural and cognitive psychotherapy*, *37*(2), 129–140.

Moi, E. B., Söderhamn, U., Marthinsen, G. N., & Flateland, S. (2019). The ISBAR tool leads to conscious, structured communication by healthcare personnel. *Sykepleien Forskning*, *14*(74699), e-74699 DOI: 10.4220/Sykepleienf.2019.74699en.

Moorhead, S. A., Hazlett, D. E., Harrison, L., Carroll, J. K., Irwin, A., & Hoving, C. (2013). A new dimension of health care: Systematic review of the uses, benefits, and limitations of social media for health communication. *Journal of medical Internet research*, *15*(4), e1933.

Mor-Anavy, S., Lev-Ari, S., & Levin-Zamir, D. (2021). Health literacy, primary care health care providers, and communication. *HLRP: Health Literacy Research and Practice*, *5*(3), e194–e200.

National Society of Leadership and Success (2023, January). *Effective Communication*. National Society of Leadership and Success. https://www.nsls.org/blog/best-practices-for-effective-communication.

Oba, D., & Berger, J. (2024). How communication mediums shape the message. Journal of Consumer Psychology, 34(3), 406–424.

Office of Disease Prevention and Health Promotion. (n.d.a.). *About the Objectives. Healthy People 2030. U.S. Department of Health and Human Services*. https://health.gov/healthypeople/objectives-and-data/about-objectives

Office of Disease Prevention and Health Promotion (n.d.b.). *Health Communication.* Healthy People 2030. U.S. Department of Health and Human Services. https://health.gov/healthypeople/objectives-and-data/browse-objectives/health-communication

O'Hare, A. M. (2018). Patient-centered care in renal medicine: Five strategies to meet the challenge. *American Journal of Kidney Diseases, 71*(5), 732–736.

Rimal, R. N., & Lapinski, M. K. (2009). Why health communication is important in public health. *Bulletin of the World Health Organization, 87*(4), 247–247a.

Rollnick, S., & Miller, W. R. (1995). What is motivational interviewing? *Behavioural and cognitive Psychotherapy, 23*(4), 325–334.

Rubak, S., Sandbæk, A., Lauritzen, T., & Christensen, B. (2005). Motivational interviewing: A systematic review and meta-analysis. *British journal of general practice, 55*(513), 305–312.

Rosenbaum, M. E. (2017). Dis-integration of communication in healthcare education: Workplace learning challenges and opportunities. *Patient education and counseling, 100*(11), 2054–2061.

Saleh, S. M., Azahari, M. H. H., Ismail, A. I. H., & Yaacob, H. (2013, December). Diabetes healthcare awareness in Malaysia: Communication medium through poster in socioeconomic patterns. In *2013 International Conference on the Modern Development of Humanities and Social Science* (pp. 361–364). Atlantis Press.

Sheldon, L. K., & Hilaire, D. M. (2015). Development of communication skills in healthcare: Perspectives of new graduates of undergraduate nursing education. *Journal of Nursing Education and Practice, 5*(7), 30., 1–37 https://doi.org/10.5430/jnep.v5n7p30

Shipley, S. D. (2010, April). Listening: A concept analysis. *Nursing forum, 45*(2), 125–134).

Söderlund, L. L., Madson, M. B., Rubak, S., & Nilsen, P. (2011). A systematic review of motivational interviewing training for general health care practitioners. *Patient education and counseling, 84*(1), 16–26.

Thunberg, G., Johnson, E., Bornman, J., Öhlén, J., & Nilsson, S. (2022). Being heard—Supporting person-centred communication in paediatric care using augmentative and alternative communication as universal design: A position paper. *Nursing inquiry, 29*(2), e12426.

Touloumakos, A. K. (2020). Expanded yet restricted: A mini review of the soft skills literature. *Frontiers in psychology, 11*, 568111

Vermeir, P., Vandijck, D., Degroote, S., Peleman, R., Verhaeghe, R., Mortier, E., ... & Vogelaers, D. (2015). Communication in healthcare: A narrative review of the literature and practical recommendations. *International journal of clinical practice, 69*(11), 1257–1267.

Wilson, J. A. B., & Schild, S. (2014). Provision of mental health care services to deaf individuals using telehealth. *Professional Psychology: Research and Practice, 45*(5), 324–331. https://doi.org/10.1037/a0036811

Woodhall, L. J., Vertacnik, L., & McLaughlin, M. (2008). Implementation of the SBAR communication technique in a tertiary center. *Journal of Emergency Nursing, 34*(4), 314–317.

World Health Organization. (n.d.). *WHO principles for effective communications.* https://www.who.int/about/communications/principles

Yamashita, M. (1997). Family caregiving: Application of Newman's and Peplau's theories. *Journal of Psychiatric and Mental Health Nursing, 4*(6), 401–405.

Figure credits

Fig. 7.1: Oren T. Guttman et al., "A Communication Model," *Journal of Patient Safety*, vol. 17, no. 8, p. 1466. Copyright © 2021 by Wolters Kluwer Health.

Fig. 7.2: Abukari Kwame and Pammla M. Petrucka, "A person-Centered Care and Continuum (PC4 Model)," BMC Nursing, vol. 20, p. 7. Copyright © 2021 by Springer Nature.

IMG 7.1: Copyright © 2022 Depositphotos/ZigicDrazen.

CHAPTER 8

Intersectorial and Multisectorial Approaches and Family Health Care

When you need to innovate, you need collaboration.

—Marissa Mayer

Learning Objectives

By the end of this chapter, learners will do the following:

- Define the following concepts: intersectorial approach, multisectorial approach, sector and stakeholder.
- Describe the role of intersectorial and multisectorial approaches in *family health* care.
- Articulate the benefits of an Era 3.0 Health System Transformation Framework in optimizing a family-centered intersectorial and multisectorial perspective.
- Identify the barriers and enablers of intersectorial and multisectorial collaboration in health and health systems.
- Examine the potential challenges and opportunities for family-focused intersectorial and multisectorial approaches within the "4HEALTHS" context namely: *individual health*, *family health*, *population health*, and public health.

Before you read on, consider the following questions:

During the Covid-19 pandemic or during any emergency that you have encountered in your lifetime…

- What kind of stakeholder groups (e.g., government, civil society, and private sector) were involved in the emergency?
- What sectors (e.g., health, environment and economy, safety, transportation, etc.) were involved in the emergency?
- How were individuals, families and communities involved?
- Why should families be at the center of the emergency plans?
- What benefits did you observe from the multisectorial engagement and collaboration?

Definition of Intersectorial and Multisectorial Approach

Intersectorial (IA) and multisectorial (MSA) approaches are common concepts and actions in the field of public health, health policy, and politics that still lack consensus and conceptualization on their definitions. The terms are rooted in evidence-based research on inequitable health outcomes that calls to action the engagement of sectors outside health sector (Trowbridge, Tan, Hussain, Osman, & Di Ruggiero, 2022). Broad terms such as "joint-working," "cross-sectoral," approach, and "integrated approach" have been used interchangeably for IA and MSA (The Primary Health Care Performance Initiative, 2015–2022). According to Dubois, St-Pierre, and Veras (2015), intersectorial action (IA) or collaboration is referred to as a "recognized relationship between part or parts of the health sector and part or parts of another sector, that has been formed to take action on an issue or to achieve health outcomes in a way which is more effective, efficient or sustainable than could be achieved by the health sector working alone," p. 2937). Moreover, Trowbridge and colleagues (2022) defined IA as the "alignment of strategies and resources between actors from two or more policy sectors to achieve complementary objectives" (p. 2022). Similar to IA, Multisectorial approach (MSA) is referred to "deliberate collaboration among various stakeholder groups (e.g., government, civil society, and private sector) and sectors (e.g., health, environment, and economy) to jointly achieve a policy outcome" (Salunke & Lal, 2017, p. 163). By deliberate it means that parties involved in MSA are ready to build relationships and networks that aim at addressing shared goals (The Primary Health Care Performance Initiative, 2015–2022). Both IA and MSA address broad health systemic issues within the six building blocks of health systems (i.e., leadership/governance, finances, health information technology, service delivery, health care workforce and access to essential medication). Thus, the main targeted shared goals of IA and MSA is to achieve process outcomes such as "effective community engagement, improved community-wide collaboration, increased interorganizational trust, or goal alignment" that will result into improved "community and systems-level outcomes" (*Population Health* Innovation Lab (2024a, p. 3).

IA and MSA require multistakeholder and multisector partnerships on shared goals of interest (Trowbridge, et al., 2022). By definition the concept of stakeholder can be broadly referred to as someone (an influencer) who can have an effect on an effort or maybe affected by an effort of their representative firm/agency/entity/organization because they hold knowledge of interest of that firm/agency/entity/organization (Darškuvienė, & Bendoraitienė, 2013). On the other hand, the Meriam online dictionary, describes the word "sector" as a noun to be "a sociological, economic, or political subdivision of a society" which demonstrates a division of some kind. Multi means "more than one." Multisectorial groups are usually variable depending on the intended goal of the collaboration. The stakeholders can be for profit on nonprofit as well a non-governmental or public-private governmental (Ro & Chan, 2022). In health care, common sectors include public, private and public-private health sectors are engaged in service delivery. The private sector refers to non-state stakeholders or organization neither owned nor directly controlled by the government such as for profit and not-for-profit organizations (Klinton, 2020; WHO, 2024). Using service delivery as an example, the actors/stakeholders within the private sectors may include supply chain of health products, pharmaceutical, manufactures of health products and equipment, health insurance providers' private institutions and educational centers, etc. Types of industry such as health, housing and transportation, education, health, social work, agriculture, public administration, and the environment have been used to reflect various sectors. The civil society is also one of the great intersectorial and multisectorial stakeholders in the health sector. The term describes stakeholders ranging from various agencies government and private agencies including "charitable societies, churches, neighborhood organizations, social clubs, civil rights lobbies, parent-teachers associations, unions and trade associations" (Brown, Khagram, Moore & Frumkin, 2000, p. 8).

The Role of Intersectorial and Multisectorial Approach in Family Health Care

The delivery of person-centered care to achieve optimal individual and family well-being requires substantial investment and commitment in transformed health care systems that support initiatives such as the "whole government approach" or "Health in All Policies." (Kusano, 2014). For instance, the initiative the "whole-of-government (WoG)" approach to health is focuses on "integrated policies and programmers that are intended to achieve "shared or complementary interdepended goals" within public service agencies to improve *population health*" (The Primary Health Care Performance Initiative, 2015–2022, para 2). The focus of such initiatives is to engage and support intersectorial and multisectorial collaboration between the health sector and non-health sectors as well as public and private sectors. An approach that engages the broader society also known as the "whole of society" is essential in supporting the engagement of key stakeholders such as individuals family, communities, associations, the civil society and private sectors that are beyond the public services (Ortenzi, Marten, Valentine, Kwamie, & Rasanathan, 2022).

Overall, intersectorial (IA) and multisectorial (MSA) collaborative approaches that integrates services with other *sectors* can have positive impact on individual, family, community and *population health* outcomes. Such collaborative approaches take into account the contributions of the social, economic and political determinants on health (Mondal, Van Belle, & Maioni, 2021) that if ignored can increase health inequalities (Salunke, & Lal, 2017). As discussed in previous chapters, the increased need of addressing related social and social needs in patient- and family-centered care for quality, safety and improved health outcomes is essential. It is difficult to improve or support the *family health* functions without addressing the conditions where the family lives, learns, play, works, socializes and ages from an IA and MSA across clinical settings. The work pioneered in the field of pediatrics has accelerates the need to develop clinical-based models that identify and integrate measures to address social factors through a multisectorial approach (Castrucci, & Auerbach, 2019). The clinical models support the National Academies of Science, Engineering, and Medicine (NASEM) 2019 consensus report on integrating social care into the delivery of health care. Figure 8.1 depicts an example of family- focused multisectorial and multistakeholder conceptual framework. For example, the *family health* and illness issue of childhood obesity

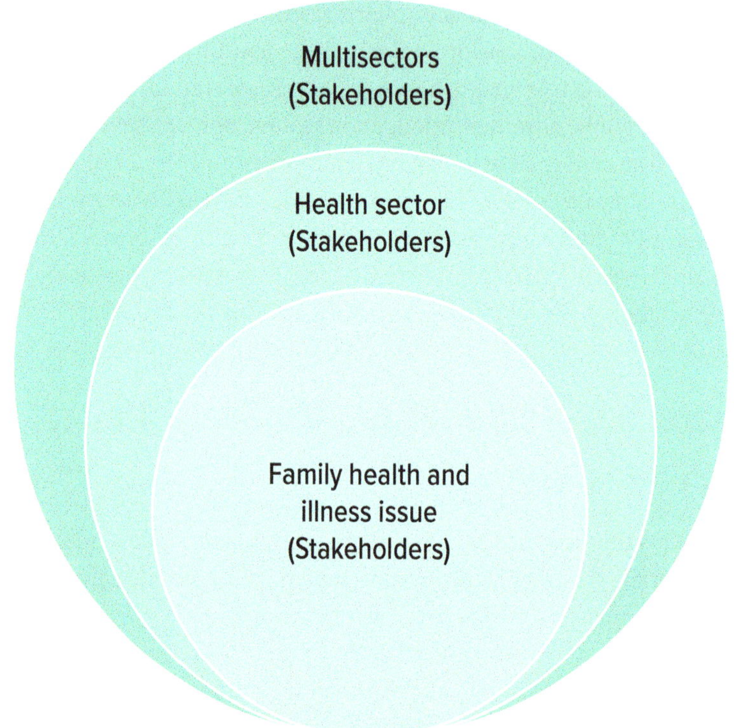

FIGURE 8.1 Conceptual Framework for MSA approach framework

can be viewed from this MSA approach beyond the health sector by examining how the control and management needs of the child and family affected by obesity (*Family health and illness issue*), can be met by health interventions directed to the individual, family, population and community and health system (*Health sector*). The figure also depicts the contextual influence of other sectors that can influence child and family behavioral change to combat the obesity epidemic such as the engagement of the economic sector (budget on obesity control to support children and families) and recreational and built in environment (access to age appropriate programming) (Multisectors). The key stakeholders could be individuals and family members (*Family health and illness issue),* primary care, alternative complementary medicine specialty, pharmacy *(Health Sector),* Community organic food store, citizen health advocate group, housing department *(Multisector).*

Era 3.0 Health Systems Transformation Framework and Family-Centered Intersectorial and Multisectorial Perspectives

For a family-centered intersectorial and multisectorial approach and collaboration to work, there needs to be transformative changes at the health systems levels. In the United States, Halfon, Long, Chang, Hester, Inkelas and Rodgers (2014) conceptualize a trajectory of three eras of health and health care operating systems (see Table 8.1) and proposed an era 3.0 health systems transformation framework that can guide large-scale health system reform to optimize health and wellbeing (see Table 8.2). The trajectory of the health and health operation systems across three eras namely, era 1.0 (1850s–1960s), 2.0 (1950s to 2000), and 3.0 (2000 going forward), demonstrate transformed concept of health, the goal of health system, the model of health, focus of services, organizational operation model, financing, role or provider/organization, and the role of the individual community.

TABLE 8.1 **Three Eras of Health and Health Care-Three Operating Systems**

	First Era-1.0: Medical Care And Public Health Services (1850s To 1960s)	**Second Er-2.0: Health Care System (1950s To Present Day)**	**Third Era-3.0: Health System (2000 Going Forward)**
Definition of Health Causation	Absence of acute disease	Reduction of chronic disease	Creating capacities to achieve goals, satisfy needs, fortify reserves
Goal of Health System	Improve life expectancy	Reduce disability	Optimize health
Model of Health and Disease	Biomedical	Biopsychosocial	Life-course health development
Primary Focus of Services	Diagnose and treat acute conditions	Prevent and manage chronic disease	Promote and optimize health of individuals and populations
Organizational Oper-ational Model	Clinics and offices linked to hospitals	Accountable care organizations and medical homes	Community-account-able health develop-ment systems
Dominant Payment Mechanisms	Indemnity insurance; fee-for-service	Prepaid health bene-fits. capitation	Health trusts and management of balanced portfolio of financing vehicles
Role of Health and Health Care Provid-er/Organization	To protect from harm, cure the sick, and heal the ill	To prevent and control risk, manage chronic disease, and improve quality of care	To optimize health and well-being
Role of Individual and Community	Inexperienced patient	Activated partner in care	Co-designers of health

Neal Halfon et al., Selection from "Applying A 3.0 Transformation Framework To Guide Large-Scale Health System Reform," *Health Affairs*, vol. 33, no. 11, p. 2004.

The 3.0 era emphasizes optimal health and a life course health development beyond the usual biopsychosocial model. There is also an emphasis on community accountable models and responsive financial models. The framework proposes the involvement of multiple actors and organizations including engaged patient and family in shared leadership, policy development and decision-making as co-designer beyond just being active partners in care. This approach is beneficial to *family health* and person/patient-centered care.

The transformation of the health care systems across the three eras can be analyzed from the lens of the health systems characteristics from sick care systems (Era 1.0), to a coordinated health care system (Era 2.0) and lastly, the community-integrated health system (Era 3.0) (see Table 8.2). The later system captures the need for MSA. A community-integrated health system demonstrates the following key characteristics: population and community outcomes, community-integrated health care with public health and other sectors/partners, integrated whole health care, coordinated and collaborative health technology system, high continuous improvement learning systems and a focus on social determinants of health (see Table 8.2).

TABLE 8.2 **U.S. Health System Transformation**

Health System Characteristic	Era 1.0: Sick Care System	Era 2.0: Coordinated Health Care System	Era 3.0: Community-Integrated Health System
Objective	Acute care and infectious disease	Patient-centered care; coordinating episodes of care across levels of care and managing chronic conditions	Population and community health outcomes; optimizing the health of populations over the lifespan and across generations.
Organization Of Services	Independent health care providers; hospital clinics, primary care providers, and specialists operate separately	Systems of health care, such as accountable care organizations and medical homes; teams of health care providers accept collective responsibility for quality outcomes and overall cost of care	Community-integrated health system integrated health care networks partner with police health and community organizations to both reduce community health risk factors and provide coordinated illness care.
Care Process	Little coordination between inpatient and outpatient medical care; dominated by an acute care treatment model	Coordinated care to better manage medical risk at each level (primary, secondary. and tertiary) of the health care delivery system	Integrated health, psychosocial services, and wellness care designed to optimize and maintain health and well-being across the life course.
Payment Methodology	Fee-for-service; rewards volume of services	Value-based payments; health care providers rewarded for better patient outcomes, better patient experience of care, and lower total cost of care	Recognize value with long-term time horizons and capture multisector financial impacts outside of health care cost; sustainable financing alternatives such as population-based global budgets; single budget for a broad scope of health care services, combined with incentives.
Health Information Technology	Separate paper medical records exist but are not connected	Electronic health care information exchanges connect various provider networks	Health and medical information follows the person; there is connectivity between the health and human service systems; and actors have access to real-time data on quality, costs, and outcomes for individuals and populations.

Quality of Care	Large variations in quality and low transparency	Consistent quality: using standard quality outcomes and improvement processes through collaborative learning	High and continuously improving quality through a learning health system.
Population Health Improvement	Not addressed	Focused on health of patients/clients only	Focused on health outcomes for geographically defined population, including upstream socioeconomic and developmental correlates of health.

Financing—which is a barrier and facilitator of intersectorial and multisectorial collaboration (McGuire, et al. 2019) is also captured through multisector financial impact and alternative payment model proposals. Examples of proposed transformed financial strategies that capture multisectorial impact outside the health sector costs include global budgets, single budget combined with incentives. Such payment reforms include co-financing or risk-based contracting or health trusts through different sectors (Halfon, et. al., 2014). Co-financing in this case, involves sharing revenues or purchases across the different sectors, hence a health gain for non-health sectors (McGuire et al, 2019). Co-financing mechanism can be conceptualized in different ways. Table 8.3 summarizes an example of types of financial mechanisms for co-financing multisectorial initiatives in the literature and their definitions.

TABLE 8.3 **Type of Financial Mechanisms for Co-financing**

Financial mechanism	**Definition**
Revenue Collection	
1. Pooled funds	At least two budget holders make contributions to a single pool for spending on pre-agreed services or interventions. This can be done at various levels (national, regional, local) and accessed in different ways (i.e., grants or regular budgetary system).
2. Aligned budgets	Budget holders align resources, identify own contributions towards pre-specified common objectives. Joint monitoring of spending and performance, but management remains separate.
3. Structural integration	Full integration of cross-sector responsibilities, finances, and resources under single management or a single organization.
Purchasing	
1. Joint or lead commissioning	Separate budget holders jointly identify a need and agree on a set of objectives, then commission services and track outcomes. The commissioning itself can be done through a joint authority board or through one agency taking commissioning responsibility.
2. Cross-charging	The mechanism whereby a cross-sector financial penalty is incurred for the non-achievement of a pre-specified target. Cross-charging compensates sectors who incur an external cost from another sectors poor performance.
3. Transfer payments	Sectoral budget holders make service revenue or capital contributions to bodies in other sectors to support additional services or interventions in this other sector.

Factors Influencing Intersectorial, and Multisectorial Collaboration in Family Health Care

Barriers and Enablers

Overall implementing transformative health systems requires dismantling pre-Covid-19 public health systems that rely on traditional silos of health care delivery and facilitating comprehensive, participatory, multidisciplinary approaches to address social determinants (Rifkin, Fort, Patcharanarumol, & Tangcharoensathien, 2021). Although efforts to implement intersectorial (IA) and multisectorial (MSA) approaches are underway, there is still underutilization of these initiatives in health care. Understanding the barriers and enablers is essential for successful implementation and uptake. Various implementation barriers and facilitators have been reported in the literature (e.g., Amri, Chatur, & O'Campo, 2022; van Rensburg, & Brooke-Sumner, 2023; Mondal, Van Belle, & Maioni, 2021). For instance, Alhassan, and colleagues (2021); concluded that agenda and goal alignment among partners, quality of relationships, were enabling factors while different goals, poor partnership structure, constitution and processes were barriers to implementation of a MSA. Table 8.4 lists some of the related barriers and enablers.

TABLE 8.4 **Barriers and Facilitating Factors Influencing Implementation Uptake of Intersectorial and Multisectorial Approaches and Collaboration**

Barriers	Facilitators
Power struggles/dynamics. Differences in commitment and professional authority between sectors/organizations Lack of formal agreements between sectors Persistent structural barriers such a stigma, racism Not framing the issue beyond health Not targeting sustainability and intersectoral actions/goals Lack of role clarity, accountability, information-sharing, engaging the public, and understanding the local political context Lack of coordination Difficult in cultural shift to embrace acceptance of new organizational culture with more tolerance for uncertainties Budget cuts	Equal power relations and mutual respect Setting up new formal structures such as interdepartmental committees, and working groups with experts, academics and community leaders Trust among involved partners Ensuring funding, human resources, and technological support Strong leadership and accountability mechanisms Availability of technological support Policy frames, encourage a diversity of perspectives Motivation for those involved based on shared values, trust, and frequent communication Access to emergent networks that are informal but high functioning in solving practical problems through increased communication between actors.

Moreover, McGuire, et al. (2019) articulated specific barriers and enablers on implementation and continuation of co-financing model in MSA collaboration across nine conceptual themes (see Table 8.5).

TABLE 8.5 **Barriers and Enablers to Uptake, Implementation and Continuation of Co-financing Models**

Themes	Barriers	Facilitators
Conceptual Buy-In	Actor resistance due to perceived risk, ambiguities and threats	Favorable political climate, client, actor and public support
Model Design, Planning Framing and Implementation	Unclear terms and unmatched partnership	Effective planning Context level for implementation
Organizational Resources and Capacity	Inadequate or incongruent resources	Matched Partnership
	Differences in human resources and ways of working	Adequate Expertise and Capacity
	Leadership	Leadership
	Time	Time
Relational and Organizational Culture	Non-constructive relational and work dynamics	Established positive relational and work dynamics
Evidence, Output Data Monitoring and Evaluation	Insufficient result focused practices	Set targets
Finance and Accounting Practices	Unmatched methods and capacity to adapt to needs	Financial control

Barriers and Facilitators of Person and Family-Centered Intersectorial and Multisectorial Approach within the 4HEALTHS Contexts

The following section presents challenges and opportunities that may facilitate a family -centered intersectorial (IA) and multisector collaboration (MSA) within the 4HEALTHS.

Individual and Family Health

As mentioned in the previous chapters, individuals and families make up communities, populations, and thus remain to be key players in health development in public health (Barnes, Hanson, Novilla, Magnusson, Crandall, & Bradford, 2020). For instance, families continue to play a key role in prevention through healthy child development (primary prevention) and caregiving (secondary and tertiary prevention) across the life span (Hanson, et al., 2019; Ho, Mahirah, Ho, & Thumboo, 2022). Unfortunately, a common and priority player in health care systems is primarily the individual patient and not the family or household, despite the mounting evidence of the complexity of health and health behaviors (Hanson, et al., 2019). Without effective engagement of the individual and family in public health it will be difficult to address the social determinants of health using a multidisciplinary and multi-sectorial collaborative lens. If the family cannot fulfil its functions because of lack of involvement and having a voice in the decision-making process during program planning, implementation and evaluation, it will be difficult to achieve optimal health in any health care system. Thus, successful family-focused multisectorial collaboration need *family health* professionals who "think family," involve, and empower families to be the best ongoing learner, advisor, co evaluator and leader (Hanson, 2019).

Population Health

An enabling environment that incorporates family-focused multisectorial partnerships is one that has an impact on the health of individuals and families in their community (i.e., where they live, play, worship, learn, grow/age and heal). The community as well as health systems within a community play a key role in meeting the medical, behavioral, social, and environmental needs of the individuals and families and population. In order for the health sector and non-health sectors to meet the social determinants of health within a community of interest an integrated care delivery system that combines primary care and public health is warranted to provide for a better understanding *population health* (American Academy of Family Physicians (AAFP), 2024a). A partnership beyond the health care systems (primary care and other practice partners) to include individuals and families, community leaders, educators and advocates is essential. These partners ensure the right resources are available at the right time, and that they reflect people's needs and priorities. For example, when working with low income families in a community responsive care environment, it is vital that *family health* care professional meet the needs of the family through meaningful and trusting community collaborative programs that cut across sectors/organizations (American Academy of Family Physicians, 2024b). For example, use community peer-to-peer support groups instead of regular coaching interventions within the primary healthcare system.

In addition, it is also vital that new multisectoral community business models for *population health* improvement are put in place beyond calls for improving health disparities (Kindig, & Isham, 2014). The business models should provide accountability, commitment, supportive polices and infrastructures that acknowledges the presence of multiple determinants of health that are beyond the patients' experiences and cost of their health care (Kingdig & Isham, 2014). Such business model will provide opportunities to assess contextual key stakeholders' capability and opportunities both formal and informal to address the determinants beyond the healthcare system. For example, in the community business model, stakeholders should commit resources depending on their mission and level of control (shared or limited) (Kingdig & Isham, 2014). An example of a community-based initiative is the Accountable Communities of/for Health (ACHs)—an evolving community strategy for implementing health-focused and community-based multisector collaborative (MSCs) in the U.S. (Brunton, et al., 2021). This model provides infrastructure, prioritization of integrated, high-impact interventions; and adaptation in local context. Key players in the Accountable Communities of/for Health (ACH) model include health care, housing, social services, public health, employment training, and economic development (*Population Health* Innovation Lab, 2024b).

Public Health

The Covid-19 pandemic was a worldwide test on a recovery and efficiency of public and private health systems in meeting the need of individuals, families, communities and populations. It was obvious that mutlisectoral approach to health was and continues to be needed to strengthen and build resilient health systems during time of normalcy and emergencies (Hellevik, Mustafa, Zhang, Shirsat, & Saikat, 2023). Missed opportunities in evidence-based public health strategies especially among populations at-risk were evident. One of the set-backs was the ongoing traditional health care budget allocation which is tailored toward preventable diseases (75%) vs less than 5% spent on prevention and public health (Mays, 2016). Hence, in order to foster effective patient-and family centered care for *population health* improvement, public health must ensure that there is collective actions of multiple sectors both government and private as well as individuals and families. Utilizing multisectorial approaches may reduce public health waste and insufficiency that has been linked to fragmentation of services, variability in practice, resources strained, limited reach, limited public health visibility and understanding, limited evidence-base and slow innovation and adaptation. A strong family-centered leader is also needed. The leader should leverage the benefits of non-traditional multisectorial partnership with shared visions of health that responds to local and contextual public health priorities and strategies such as the Healthy People 2023 strategy in the U.S. (Gillen & Denubila-Griffin, 2024). It is also important to make sure that the public health function of data gathering, sharing and application of evidence is accomplished through MSA collaborative strategies and measures (Amri, Chatur, & O'Campo, 2022). A lack of a well-trained workforce in population and public health principles and strategies has been reported as a barrier in assessment and monitoring in multisectorial practice (Armstrong, Doyle, Lamb & Waters, 2006). Hence, it is essential that public health efforts be tailored towards building and supporting a skilled workforce that is equipped to strengthen and support multisectorial partnerships to improve health.

Moreover, as indicated earlier in the chapter, funding for MSA work is challenge. However, the evidence also indicates the benefits of unrestricted grants not tied to near-term deliverables (*Population Health* Innovation Lab, 2024c). The benefits of this strategy include support on a range of outcomes, maintenance of sustainable partner connections, and provision of short-term collaborative measures such as levels of commitment, partnership values, and system structural changes (*Population Health* Innovation Lab (2024c). Continues improvement measures should also take place among MSA teams to strengthen collaboration. Lastly, creating champions to develop and support policy initiatives that support MSA is an essential public health service (World Health Organization, 2023). With the lack of or limited *family health* in current public health strategies, the champions should also advocate for a *Family Health* in Public Health perspective as part of MSA policy initiatives (Barnes et al., 2020.).

Conclusion

The purpose of this chapter was to introduce the reader to intersectorial and multisectorial collaboration in *family health* care and its potential to improve the quality of *family health* care through holistic and integrated health and non-health care systems. In particularly, the chapter demonstrates the importance of situating person/patient- and family-center care at the center of *population health* and public health for future effective multisectorial programming to address the social determinants of health. A number of barriers, facilitators and oportunties are noteworthy. The complexities of barriers and enablers shared provide many windows of opportunities that can be capitalized by *family health* professionals when working directly or indirectly in multisectorial teams at various levels of interventions.

Suggested Websites

Population Health Innovation Lab:
https://pophealthinnovationlab.org/aligning-brief-series/
The Association of State and Territorial Health Officials:
https://www.astho.org/topic/toolkit/building-non-traditional-public-health-multisector-partnerships/
University of Kansas Free Community Tool Box, online resource:
https://ctb.ku.edu/en/table-of-contents/participation/encouraging-involvement/identify-stakeholders/main

Suggested Readings

World Health Organization (31 August, 2023). Working together for equity and healthier populations: sustainable multisectoral collaboration based on health in all policies approaches. https://www.who.int/publications/i/item/9789240067530

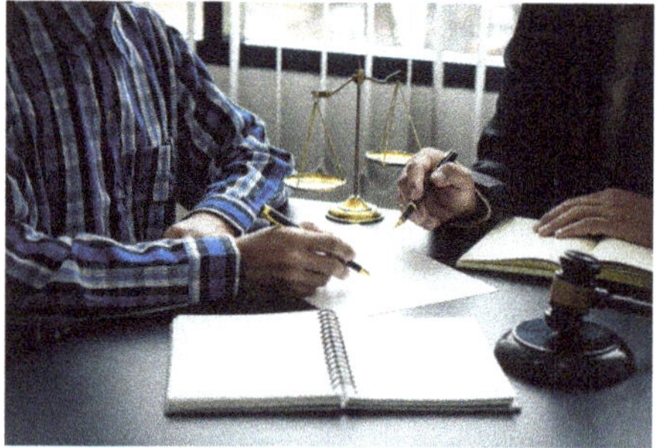
IMG 8.1

Reflection Question

Think about the following questions:

1. What does multisectorial mean to you? Why?
2. Do you think illness and health are multisectorial issue? Why?
3. What are possible barriers and facilitating factors of multisectorial collaboration? Briefly describe identify 2 barriers and 2 enablers and discuss how they influence mutlisectorial collaboration.

References

Alhassan, J. A. K., Gauvin, L., Judge, A., Fuller, D., Engler-Stringer, R., & Muhajarine, N. (2021). Improving health through multisectoral collaboration: enablers and barriers. *Canadian journal of public health, 112*(6), 1059–1068.

American Academy of Family Physicians (2024a). *Integration of Primary Care and Public Health* (Position Paper). https://www.aafp.org/about/policies/all/integration-primary-care.html

American Academy of Family Physicians (2024b). *Poverty and Health.* (Position Paper) https://www.aafp.org/about/policies/all/poverty-health.html

Amri, M., Chatur, A., & O'Campo, P. (2022). Intersectoral and multisectoral approaches to health policy: an umbrella review protocol. *Health research policy and systems, 20*(1), 21. https://doi.org/10.1186/s12961-022-00826-1

Armstrong, R., Doyle, J., Lamb, C., & Waters, E. (2006). Multi-sectoral health promotion and public health: the role of evidence. *Journal of public health, 28*(2), 168–172.

Barnes, M. D., Hanson, C. L., Novilla, L. B., Magnusson, B. M., Crandall, A. C., & Bradford, G. (2020). Family-centered health promotion: perspectives for engaging families and achieving better health outcomes. *INQUIRY: The Journal of Health Care Organization, Provision, and Financing, 57,* 0046958020923537.

Brown, L. D, Khagram, S., Moore, M. H. & Frumkin, P. (2002, July). *Globalization, Ngos and Multi-Sectoral Relations* Available at http://dx.doi.org/10.2139/ssrn.253110

Brunton, C., Duong, T. C., Jacobs, F., Levi, J., Meadows, P., Midura, B., Sim, S. Thomason, & Weiss, A. F. (2021, April, 6). Multisector Partnerships Such As ACHs: How Can They Improve *Population Health* And Reduce Health Inequities?. *Health Affairs Forefront.* DOI: 10.1377/hblog20210406.792026

Darškuvienė, V., & Bendoraitienė, E. (2013). The stakeholder concept analysis. *Organizacijų vadyba: sisteminiai tyrimai, 68,* 41–52.

Dubois, A., St-Pierre, L., & Veras, M. (2015). A scoping review of definitions and frameworks of intersectoral action. *Ciência & Saúde Coletiva, 20,* 2933–2942.

Gillen C. & Denubila-Griffin, M. (2024, March 27). Leveraging Healthy People 2023 to Build Non-Traditional Multisector Partnerships. ttps://www.astho.org/topic/toolkit/building-non-traditional-public-health-multisector-partnerships/

Hanson, C. L., Crandall, A., Barnes, M. D., Magnusson, B., Novilla, M. L. B., & King, J. (2019). Family-focused public health: supporting homes and families in policy and practice. *Frontiers in public health, 7,* 434838. https://doi.org/10.3389/fpubh.2019.00059

Halfon, N., Long, P., Chang, D. I., Hester, J., Inkelas, M., & Rodgers, A. (2014). Applying a 3.0 transformation framework to guide large-scale health system reform. *Health Affairs, 33*(11), 2003–2011.

Hellevik, S., Mustafa, S., Zhang, Y., Shirsat, A., & Saikat, S. (2023). Multisectoral action towards sustainable development goal 3. d and building health systems resilience during and beyond COVID-19: Findings from an INTOSAI development initiative and World Health Organization collaboration. *Frontiers in Public Health, 11,* 1104669. https://doi.org/10.3389/fpubh.2023.1104669

J van Rensburg, A., & Brooke-Sumner, C. (2023). Intersectoral and multisectoral approaches to enable recovery for people with severe mental illness in low- and middle-income countries: A scoping review. *Global mental health (Cambridge, England), 10,* e19. https://doi.org/10.1017/gmh.2023.10

Kindig, D. A., & Isham, G. (2014). *Population health* improvement: a community health business model that engages partners in all sectors. *Frontiers of Health Services Management, 30*(4), 3–20.

Ho, Y. C. L., Mahirah, D., Ho, C. Z. H., & Thumboo, J. (2022). The role of the family in health promotion: a scoping review of models and mechanisms. *Health promotion international, 37*(6), daac119.

Kusano, Y. (2014). Nursing Perspectives on Person-and People-Centered Integrated Care for All. *International Journal of Person Centered Medicine, 4*(3), 163–166.

Klinton, J. (2020). *The Private Health Sector: An Operational Definition*. Geneva. https://www.who.int/docs/default-source/health-system-governance/private-health-sector-an-operational-definition.pdf

Mays, G. P. (2016). "Understanding the Value of Multi-Sector Partnerships to Improve *Population Health*" (2016). *Health Management and Policy Presentations*. 127. https://uknowledge.uky.edu/hsm_present/127

McGuire, F., Vijayasingham, L., Vassall, A., Small, R., Webb, D., Guthrie, T., & Remme, M. (2019). Financing intersectoral action for health: a systematic review of co-financing models. *Globalization and health, 15*, 1–18.

Mondal, S., Van Belle, S., & Maioni, A. (2021). Learning from intersectoral action beyond health: a meta-narrative review. *Health policy and planning, 36*(4), 552–571.

National Academies of Sciences, Medicine Division, Board on Health Care Services, & Committee on Integrating Social Needs Care into the Delivery of Health Care to Improve the Nation's Health. (2019). *Integrating social care into the delivery of health care: Moving upstream to improve the nation's health.* https://nap.nationalacademies.org/catalog/25467/integrating-social-care-into-the-delivery-of-health-care-moving

Ortenzi, F., Marten, R., Valentine, N. B., Kwamie, A., & Rasanathan, K. (2022). Whole of government and whole of society approaches: call for further research to improve *population health* and health equity. *BMJ Global Health, 7*(7), e009972. https://doi.org/10.1136/bmjgh-2022-009972

Population Health Innovation Lab (2024a, April 2). *Population Health Through Multisector Collaboration.* https://pophealthinnovationlab.org/wp-content/uploads/2023/04/AS4H_Brief1.pdf

Population Health Innovation Lab (2024b, April 2). Accountable Communities of/for Health: Transforming Health Systems through Dedicated Multisector Collaboration. *Brief* 2 https://pophealthinnovationlab.org/wp-content/uploads/2023/05/AS4H_Brief2.pdf

Population Health Innovation Lab (2024c, April 2). *Recommendations for Practitioners, Funders, and Policymakers Seeking to Improve Population Health Through Multisector* Collaboration https://pophealthinnovationlab.org/wp-content/uploads/2023/05/AS4H_Brief6.pdf

Rifkin, S. B., Fort, M., Patcharanarumol, W., & Tangcharoensathien, V. (2021). Primary healthcare in the time of COVID-19: breaking the silos of healthcare provision. *BMJ global health*, 6(11), e007721. https://doi.org/10.1136/bmjgh-2021-007721

Ro, M. J., & Chan, N. L. (2022). Multilevel and Multisector Approaches to Health. In S. C. Kwon C.Rrinh-Shevrin, N. S. Ilam & S.S Yi (Eds.) *Applied Population Health Approaches for Asian American Communities*, (2 nd Ed, pp163–178).

Salunke, S., & Lal, D. K. (2017). Multisectoral approach for promoting public health. *Indian journal of public health, 61*(3), 163–168. https://doi.org/10.4103/ijph.IJPH_220_17

The Primary Health Care Performance Initiative (2015-2022). *Multi-Sectoral Approach* https://www.improvingphc.org/improvement-strategies/governance/multi-sectoral-approach

Trowbridge, J., Tan, J. Y., Hussain, S., Osman, A. E. B., & Di Ruggiero, E. (2022). Examining intersectoral action as an approach to implementing multistakeholder collaborations to achieve the sustainable development goals. *International Journal of Public Health, 67*, 1604351. https://doi.org/10.3389/ijph.2022.1604351

World Health Organization. (2024, April, 2). *What is the private health sector?* https://www.emro.who.int/uhc-health -systems/access-health-services/private-health-sector.html

World Health Organization (2023, August 31). *Working together for equity and healthier populations: sustainable multisectoral collaboration based on health in all policies approaches.* https://www.who.int/publications/i/item/9789240067530

Figure credit

IMG 8.1: Copyright © 2021 Depositphotos/saiarlawka9@gmail.com.

CHAPTER 9

Evidence-Based Family-Level Interventions in Family Health Care

Design is not just what it looks like and feels like. Design is how it works.

—Steve Jobs

Learning Objectives

By the end of this chapter, learners will do the following:

- Analyze the concepts relevant to family-level interventions in *family health* care.
- Identify the typologies of family-level interventions across the continuum of health care and family life stages.
- Support the use of current evidence-based and practice-based family-level interventions to make clinical reasoning in *family health* care.
- Explore the cultural, race/ethnicity, gender, and ethical considerations in designing and implementing family-level interventions in *family health* care.
- Examine the potential challenges and opportunities for family-level interventions in *family health* care within the 4HEALTHS contexts.

Before you read on, consider the following questions:

- What is the meaning of evidence-based practice intervention?
- What is the meaning of practice-based evidence intervention?
- What is an evidence-based family-level intervention in the context of health, illness, and health care?
- What are the settings of implementing family-level interventions in health care?
- What are the population targets for evidenced-based family-level interventions in health care?
- Do family-level interventions versus medical care have an impact on health?
- What kinds of family-level interventions work best to improve family outcomes?
- Who is qualified to administer family-level interventions in health care?
- What is intervention research?

The Importance of Family-Level Interventions and Intervention Research in Family Health Care

Individuals and families across the life span constantly interact with health care systems (including a diverse health care workforce, health care plans, and health care organizations) along the continuum of care for wellness checks, health education, patient and family education, screenings, acute and chronic disease management, and/or rehabilitation. The different points of persons-system health care interactions are part of what is referred to the "patient experience." Patient experience is an integral component of health care quality that includes the value of getting timely care, easy access to information, and good communication with providers (Agency for Healthcare Research and Quality, 2023). The interpersonal nature of relationships or interactions such as patient-family-clinician relationships that take place during decision-making provide a backdrop for understanding intervention targets for enhancing the major quadruple aims for optimizing health care systems: improved patients, family and provider experiences, *population health*, and health care costs (Bodenheimer & Sinsky, 2014). As mentioned in previous chapters, family-level targets are often overlooked in population and health equity measures (Weiss-Laxer et al., 2020).

In this chapter, the points of "intervening" with the family following a family assessment are introduced. According to Merriam-Webster's online dictionary, i*ntervention* means "the act or an instance of intervening such as the act of interfering with the outcome or course especially of a condition or process (as to prevent harm or improve functioning), educational *intervention*, surgical *interventions* for cardiovascular disease." When intervening with families, the key term *family intervention* is commonly used, especially in the mental health literature (American Psychological Association, 2024). For example, according to the American Psychological Association (2024), family interventions "exist to improve outcomes for person with the disorder or illness by improving family engagement and effectiveness in handling the challenges associated with the problem" (para. 1). In acute care settings, family nurses define family nursing interventions as time-limited, collaborative in nature, initiated and/or facilitated by nurses, and directed at either the individual or the family to solve problems (Eustace et al., 2015). Martire et al. (2004), describe family-focused intervention as "non-medical interventions that are psychologically, socially or behaviorally oriented that involve members of the patient's family or both the patient and family members" (p. 601). In this chapter, the term *family health intervention* (FHI) is used synonymously to refer to family interventions, family systems interventions, family-focused interventions, family-based interventions, and family-oriented interventions derived from family-level intervention research in the contexts of health and illness.

Typology of Family Health Interventions in Family Health Care

Health and illness (acute and chronic) have a familial nature, and prevention is effective when there is positive family engagement and functioning. Thus, FHIs are an essential component of *family health* care. As mentioned in previous chapters, patients/persons in persons-centered care do not exist in a vacuum. They exist within different social systems, including family-level systems. Family level in this case encompasses the "collective measures of *family health* behaviors and processes or pathways or performing interventions with multiple family members (2 or more family members)" (National Institute of Health, 2019, para. 1). Family members can be caregivers or friends and related sub-systems depending on how *family* is defined. Family systems are diverse in nature and present with health- and illness-related problems at different life stages.

Levels of Prevention in FHI

Although there is still criticism surrounding Neuman's theory in terms of conceptual clarity (August-Brady, 2000), the application of Neuman's middle-range theory of "prevention as intervention" in conceptualizing FHIs remains undeniable. This approach is consistent with the level of prevention in preventative science, mentioned earlier in the book. The theory postulates the points of entry of the individual and family into health care systems and the type of the interventions or actions needed to address the individual and family problems/stressors. According to the theory, *family health* care providers deliver FHIs at the primary, secondary, and tertiary prevention levels (Fawcett & Neuman, 1992; Hanson et al., 2019). Types of FHIs vary and range from engagement, coaching, education, and empowerment to skill-developing strategies. Primary prevention intervention modalities strengthen the family's defense and resistance mechanisms by employing strategies that prevent family stressors and reduce risk factors related to health and illness (Fawcett & Neuman, 1992). Primary prevention strategies that target changes in health practices and awareness of *family health* risks and protective factors provide increased protection to the family. For example, among families at risk for child abuse, child maltreatment public health awareness campaigns and family strengthening programs would be a primary prevention strategy. The goal is to prevent child abuse from occurrence in the first place. Secondary prevention intervention modalities protect and strengthen the family's basic structure by employing strategies that provide appropriate screening and early treatment of presenting symptoms to attain optimal family system stability or wellness and energy conversation (Fawcett & Neuman, 1992). Examples of secondary prevention for families at high risk for child abuse may include screening for child abuse at the point of care, parent and family education, and training in child abuse prevention and home visits. The goal is to assess and reduce the immediate impact of child abuse. Tertiary prevention intervention modalities protect the family by promoting reconstitution or return to wellness following a treatment plan (Fawcett & Neuman, 1992).

Examples for tertiary prevention include family case management, referrals to in-home services, counseling, and rehabilitation/replacement. In this case, the provider intends to provide strategies to the family that will help the family rebuild itself or reduce the impact of the child abuse and prevent its reoccurrence. Table 9.1 provides an overview of the typology of the levels of prevention and examples of key *family health* interventions provided by diverse *family health* care professionals.

TABLE 9.1 **A Typology of the Stage of *Family Health*, Levels of Prevention, and Family Interventions**

Level of Prevention	Examples	Strategies
Primary	Patient and family education Parent and family life education Family education and support Home visits (e.g., nurse-family partnership) Family engagement Family-provider interactions and relationship	Teaching health promotion Ensuring strong start of children Teaching anticipatory guidance
Secondary	Family interviewing Family support Family psychoeducation Family case management Family engagement Family-community coalitions Family-provider interactions and relationship	Screening Crisis prevention Community-based coalitions to identify needs and implement programming to address risk and protective factors Encouraging maintaining and/or adopting household health practices that are vital in addressing existing chronic conditions such as heart disease, cancer, diabetes, and disability
Tertiary	Family case management Family therapy Cognitive behavioral therapy Family support Family engagement Family grief therapy	Relatives, friends, and the family's social support network, such as neighbors and church

Common Risks and Protective Factors Addressed by FHIs

FHIs in health care address multiple familial risks and protective factors throughout different transition points in the individual and family life span across the health and illness continuum of care. FHIs address the biopsychosocial, developmental, cultural, and spiritual family systems' relational dynamics and processes (Fawcett & Neuman, 1992). In illness and health encounters, family members are interested in interventions that can help them make sense of the new situation and new role as caregiver (Davidson et al., 2010). The different forms of FHIs in Table 9.1 are designed for individual and families who are healthy and those who are living with a chronic condition (e.g., mental disorders, substance abuse problems) across various settings, life spans, and care continuums (Chelsa, 2010). It is important to remember that in FHIs, the family unit is viewed as a resource and a priority group that needs both preventative and curative services across the life course (Barnes et al., 2020).

The ultimate goal of FHIs is to retain, attain, or maintain stability of family systems' health function (health, well-being, and resiliency) during health and illness encounters. FHIs improve family members' understanding of the condition and health outcomes such as physiological/physical, social, mental, and spiritual outcomes and communication, family cohesion, and connectedness outcomes. Likewise, FHIs that strengthen family cohesion increase the family's capability of managing changed stressful situations (Wolffbrandt et al., 2024). The family strengths perspective identifies and builds on positive attributes by displaying qualities of commitment, appreciation and affection, positive communication, time together, a sense of spiritual well-being, and ability to cope with stress and crisis (Sittner et al., 2007).

Some of the common family relational risks and protective factors are shown in Table 9.2. Common family stressors may include health, illness, developmental life changes, death, relationship stressors, family events (e.g., vacations), and changes in family routines such as cultural and religious practices and expectations (Fawcett & Neuman, 1992). Stressors outside the family unit may include socioeconomic status, political climate, work changes, and neighborhood and community safety.

TABLE 9.2 **Family Relational Risk and Protective Factors**

Family Relational Risk Factors	Family Relational Protective Factors
High interpersonal conflict	Good communication
Low relationship satisfaction	Adaptability
Poor problem-solving skills	Clear rules
High levels of criticism and blame	Mutual support
Intrafamilial hostility	Open expression of appreciation
Poor family organization	Commitment to the family
Inconsistent family structure	Spending time together
Family perfectionism and rigidity	Good problem-solving skills
Low family cohesion and closeness	Extrafamilial social connections
Lack of extrafamilial support system	

Mechanism of Actions and Delivery Modes

Understanding the factors influencing *family health* (e.g., behaviors and attitudes), the underlying process and mechanism of actions, is crucial in the development and implementation of FHIs (Wäsche et al., 2021). The term *mechanism of action* has been used in medicine to describe "how a drug or other substance produces an effect in the body. For example, a drug's mechanism of action could be how it affects a specific target in a cell, such as an enzyme, or a cell function, such as cell growth" (National Cancer Institute, 2024, para. 1). Mechanism of action in an FHI can be referred to as the theoretical or empirical accounting of why and how a particular change in the individual family member, the family system, or its subsystem occurred as a consequence of taking part in an intervention (Gitlin et al., 2000). Knowing the mechanism of action of an FHI may provide information about how it affects *family health* and how it can be adopted for diverse families and populations. The process of adoption of intervention in real-life applications, and vice versa, is important in implementing evidence-based practice (Glasgow et al., 2003). The Calgary family intervention model (CFIM) in family nursing posits three mechanism of actions based on family functioning domain: cognitive, affective, and behavioral (Wright & Leahey, 1994). The cognitive domain's mechanism of actions includes teaching new activities with rationales to increase knowledge (*family health* literacy). The affective domain entails changing the family's beliefs and perceptions of a family event and encounter, and the behavioral domain includes encouraging behavioral changes through structured actions that ensure success and improved self-efficacy. Affective focused FHIs include psychoeducational family therapy approaches involving the restructuring of family interaction patterns and giving basic information about the illness and its course, cause, treatment, and prognosis (Binumon et al., 024). Relational-focused FHIs address family relationships or family functioning by changing family processes such as communication and problem solving (Knafl et al., 2016). Despite the CFIM model's benefits, it has been criticized for its limited use in family dynamic contexts (Mileski et al., 2022). During structural family dysfunctions, family interventions are designed to bring harmony to new family adaptations and relationships. Likewise, the limited utility of *family health* systems in health promotion practice hampers the collection of robust evidence on mechanisms of actions in *family health* (Barnes et al., 2020).

FHIs facilitate healthy relationships and family processes such as effective caregiver role, management of stress and coping, problem solving, and communication impact individual and *family health* promotion, disease prevention, early detection and treatment, and rehabilitation outcomes. The benefits of FHIs have been reported on both individual and family functioning, such as improved communication, increased cohesiveness, and improved problem solving abilities (Campbell, 2003; Weihs et al., 2002), and that the family context is a potent factor influencing illness course in chronic conditions (Chesla, 2010). FHIs improve health through health education and the adoption of healthier behaviors (Arnason et al., 2021). FHI targets incorporate interpersonal relationships with the family unit or its sub-systems such as dyads (parent–child, patient–physician) or triads (patient-family-provider). For example, FHIs that improve parent–child relationships are also likely to improve mental, emotional, and behavioral (MEB) health issues among Latinx youth (Pineros-Leano et al., 2023). It is important to note that family therapeutic assessments/interviews (Tharinger et al., 2007) and conversations (Gervais et al., 2020) are important FHIs with the benefit of determining family resources and support (Ellenwood & Jenkins, 2007). Likewise, family conversations are helpful in finding meaning and hope (Persson & Benzein, 2014). In nursing the "15-minute interview" has received much attention in the family nursing literature (Bell, 2012; Leahey & Wright, 2016).

There has been significant family research conducted on FHIs in critical care such as the intensive care unit (Naef et al., 2022), whereby family members (i.e., family caregivers) experience high levels of stress and uncertainly about their loved ones (Alfheim et al., 2019). Families in this situation often report acute psychobiologic impact such as anxiety, depression, trauma system avoidance, and high cortisol levels (a biomarker of stress; Turner-Cobb et al., 2016). The most important needs in the ICU include accessing information about the patient, visiting the patient, hope, talking with a doctor each day, and being assured that the best care is being given to the patient (Jacob et al., 2016).

Recommended FHIs in ICU settings include family presence, family caregiver support, family communication with family members (routine interdisciplinary family conferences), family consultation, family meetings, family navigations, and spiritual support and family-related operational interventions for environmental issues (e.g., noise, hygiene practices, and sleep surface to reduce sleep deprivation; Davidson et al., 2017). ICU rounds that incorporate family members improve communication and satisfaction among clinicians (Allen et al. ,2017). The family's need for communication has also been reported among emergency department family members (Hsiao et al., 2017).

FHIs can be delivered in various modes or formats that include face-to-face, individual family or groups of families, health information technology applications (e.g., behavior monitoring tools, decision aids, health information portals), and social media elements. For example, face-to-face educational interventions to improve cognition include definition, type, risk factors, symptoms, treatment, prevention, differentiation from other diseases, coping strategies, communication skills, prognosis, and the role of the family caregiver. Educational interventions can be administered in an online format (Utz et al., 2023). FHIs may also take place in nontraditional health care settings such as the home, clinic, community, and faith-based organizations. In these situations, *family health* care workers work with families to assess, prevent, treat, and manage physical and biopsychosocial problems depending on their scope of practice and professional values/philosophies as well as level of involvement skills. Thus, understanding the characteristics of the health care team involved with families is essential (Jensen, 2015). Table 9.3 provides a summary of different FHI targets.

TABLE 9.3 **Targets of FHI**

Family Life Stage	**Prenatal Period**	**Birth and Neonatal Period**	**Early Years: 0–3 Years**	**3–6 Years**	**Preteens and Teens: 7–18 Years**	**Young Adults: 19–26 Years**	**Adult: 27–49 Years**	**Late Adult: 50–64 Years**	**Elderly: 65 and Older**
Family Health Interventions (Primary, Secondary, and/or Tertiary)	Pregnancy preventions	Prenatal care	Early childhood interventions	Middle childhood interventions	Early, middle, and late adolescence interventions	Early adulthood interventions	Middle adulthood interventions	Late adulthood interventions	Elderly interventions
Setting	Examples: Home, school, work, community, health care systems (acute and chronic care), policy-making settings (e.g., jurisdictions)								
Family Health Care Providers	Trained biopsychosocial and cultural *family health* providers across the life span. Examples of providers: fertility specialist, OB/GYN, pediatrics, child life specialist, family medicine, family nurse practitioner, internal medicine, acute care nurses, hospice nurse, psychologist, family life educator, family therapist								

Family Outcomes

In terms of family outcomes, Wright and Leahey's (2016) domains of family functioning have been utilized in family nursing research, namely the cognitive, affective, and behavioral domains. The cognitive domain includes outcome measures on family understanding, capability, and coping. The affective domain outcome measures include family caring and individual and family emotional well-being. Finally, the behavioral domain outcomes measures include family interactions within and outside family, and individual and family behavior behaviors such as nutritional practices, health beliefs and practices, physical activity/exercise, preventative screenings, health care access and utilization, and social resource access and utilization. Reported outcomes measured in the ICU FHIs include improved parental confidence and competence in their caregiving role and improve parental psychological health; reduced anxiety, depression, post-traumatic stress, parental stress, and generalized stress; improved family satisfaction with care; and reduced depression (Davidson et al., 2017). Outcomes related to finding meaning and purpose are also common among patients managing chronic illness such as HIV (Wacharasin, 2010).

Adaptation and Implementation of Evidence-Based Family Health Interventions

Evidence-based practice is crucial in health care because it leads to higher quality care, improved patient outcomes, reduced costs, and greater provider satisfaction than traditional approaches to care (Melnyk et al., 2010). The adaptation, implementation, and maintenance of evidence-based FHIs in the context of patient-centered care is not easy, especially when there is still limited empirical evidence on the family-level influences on health (Wäsche et al., 2021), lack of family intervention research using experimental and quasi-experimental designs (Östlund & Persson, 2014), and lack of understanding what matters to the patient and their family, especially among families of color or low-income families (Ho et al., 2022; Sigurdson et al., 2020) and those who suffer race and racism beyond culture. To proactively be able to improve quality of care and patient and family experience, *family health* care providers should understand the importance of evidence-based practice and implementation science in shortening the knowledge-practice gaps in *family health* (Leahey & Svavarsdottir, 2009). The available family-level research in health care has shed light on evidence that is instrumental in patient-centered care models. Patient-centered models shift health care systems from disease-focused to patient-focused care with the goal of promoting health and well-being (Yu et al., 2023). A person-/patient-centered care model emphasizes the biopsychosocial and cultural intervention targets of *individual health* promotion and disease prevention and management (Smith et al., 2013).

Evidence-based FHIs have been tested and proven effective (to some degree) in changing targeted cognitive, affective, and relational behaviors (e.g., family engagement, *family health* literacy, family caregiving, family well-being, family processes and functions) through outcome evaluations in settings that influence views of chronic disease management, screening, health promotion, and disease prevention. There has been growth in empirical family research and evidence-based FHIs to improve certain health conditions (e.g., mental health and mental disorders, cancer, pregnancy and childbirth, diabetes, being overweight and obese) and population groups (e.g., infants, children and adolescents, people with disabilities, parents of caregivers, and older adults). Evidence-based mental health FHIs are common and have been reported to reduce episodes of psychosis (Claxton et al., 2017). Patient and family engagement interventions has been on the rise with increased interest in person-centered care. Some basic assumptions in evidence-based FHIs include the following:

- Family is a central core structure that the community is built in.
- Family psychosocial practices, behaviors, and traditions impact family members and the community as whole.
- The family interacts with the community through psychosocial relationships.
- The physical health of the family as a system is greater than the sum of the health of individual family members but is affected by the health of individual family members and the roles they play.
- The health experience of each family member has an impact on the health of the other family members as well as the overall health of the family (Neuman & Fawcett, 1992).
- Each family member's own health may be affected by whether their needs are met and by the actions of the health care team (Davidson, 2009).
- Intervening with family should be culturally sensitive to avoid harming clients and failing to meet the needs of diverse enthnoracial communities (Maiter, 2009).

Implementation of FHI

Translation of evidence-based FHIs requires a good grasp of the status of family intervention research in closing both the primary research-theory-practice gap as well as the secondary real-life application gaps within the contexts of health and illness. The primary gaps are closed through basic intervention research studies. By definition, an intervention research study tests phenomenon of interest by action of interventions through causal mechanism sand learning from actions to improve practice and health outcomes (Hawe & Potvin, 2009). This kind of research captures the value of what Melnyk and Morssion-Beedy (2012) call the "so what factor" of research with high-impact potential to positively bring change and improve family outcomes in real-world settings. For example, according to Knafl et al. (2016), a review of FHI efficacy studies demonstrated intervention effects in improving knowledge of disease conditions, disease management and medication adherence, child health outcomes, and family functioning. Community-based focused interventions that incorporating guided role-playing exercises and relational and psychoeducational components in a home setting demonstrated short-term

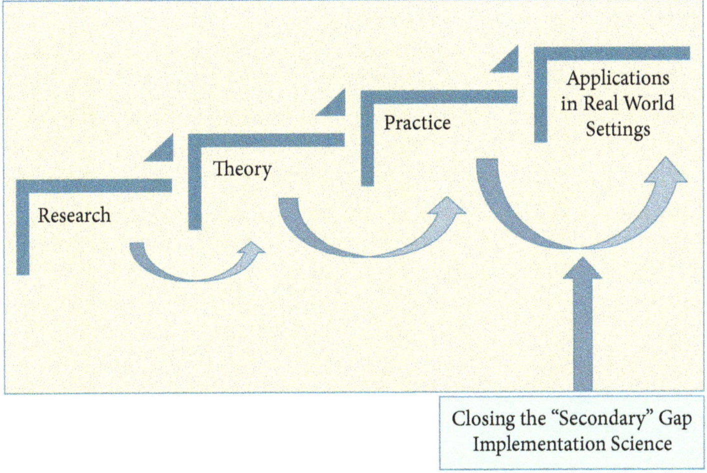

FIGURE 9.1 Envisioning a nursology research-therapy-practice-application model of implementation science (Eustace & Fawcett, 2019).

positive effects for support of families of children living with chronic conditions (Nur et al., 2023). Implementation science—a science that focuses on generating knowledge about the "research-theory-practice-application" gap between evidence-based interventions (i.e., effective interventions) and how these interventions work or are applied (i.e., implementation strategies) in the real world (usual/routine settings; i.e., hospital, home, community, etc.)—helps close gaps in knowledge translation (see Figure 9.1). These kinds of studies focus on effectiveness and are still rare in family studies.

Family health care professionals should be able to find the best evidence available using different evidence-based strategies and integrate the evidence into their practice. For example, skills in searching the evidence and determining levels of evidence is crucial. Translation of evidence into practice requires the *family health* care professional to have skills in identifying and implementing evidence-based practice (see Table 9.4).

TABLE 9.4 **Steps in Evidence-Based Practice**

Step		Examples
1	Cultivate a spirit of inquiry.	Start asking questions that lay the groundwork: "In families with women who are at risk for breast cancer, how does spousal support to promote breast health awareness compared with usual care affect access and utilization of clinical breast examination?" Or, "In families living with diabetes, how does family assessment compared with individual assessment influence the family's appraisal of familial risks?"
2	Ask clinical questions in PICOT format.	Inquiries in this format take into account patient population of interest (P), intervention or area of interest (I), comparison intervention or group (C), outcome (O), and time (T).

3	Search for the best evidence.	The search for evidence to inform clinical practice is tremendously streamlined when questions are asked in PICOT format.
4	Critically appraise the evidence.	Once articles are selected for review, they must be rapidly appraised to determine which are most relevant, valid, reliable, and applicable to the clinical question.
5	Integrate the evidence with clinical expertise and patient preferences and values.	Research evidence alone is not sufficient to justify a change in practice. Clinical expertise, based on patient assessments, laboratory data, and data from outcomes management programs, as well as patients' preferences and values, are important components.
6	Evaluate the outcomes of the practice decisions or changes based on evidence.	Monitoring and evaluating any changes in outcomes are important to spot flaws in implementation and identify more precisely which patients are most likely to benefit.
7	Disseminate results.	Sharing one's experiences with colleagues and other consumers is important. This leads to needless duplication of effort and perpetuates clinical approaches that are not evidence based. Examples of dissemination initiatives are rounds in your institution, presentations at local, regional, and national conferences, and reports in peer-reviewed journals, professional newsletters, and publications for a general audience.

In addition, understanding the type of available evidence is also essential. Melnyk and Morrison-Beedy's (2012) progression trajectory is a useful diagram for *family health* care providers and scholars to utilize when evaluating the status of the level of family-level interventions (see Figure 9.2).

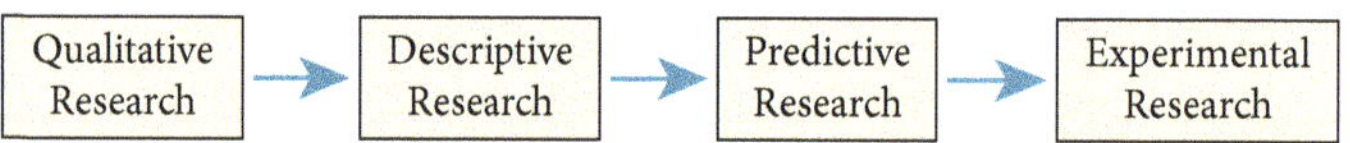

FIGURE 9.2 Qualitative research, descriptive research, predictive research, and experimental research (Melynk & Morrison-Beedy, 2012, p. 2).

Decision-making using the best evidence to answer family-level clinical questions depends on the ability to utilize and analyze a related hierarchy of evidence in one's profession. In this chapter, three hierarchies of evidence are presented, one for nursing and health care professions, another from family medicine, and one from family therapy (see Table 9.5).

TABLE 9.5 **Hierarchy Evidence Guide for Nursing and Health Care Professionals**

	Evidence Level	**Types of Evidence**
Research Evidence	Level I	Experimental study, randomized controlled trial (RCT) Explanatory mixed-methods design that includes only a level I quantitative study Systematic review of RCTs, with or without meta-analysis
	Level II	Quasi-experimental study Explanatory mixed-methods design that includes only a level II quantitative study Systematic review of a combination of RCTs and quasi-experimental studies, or quasi-experimental studies only, with or without meta-analysis
	Level III	Nonexperimental study Systematic review of a combination of RCTs, quasi-experimental and nonexperimental studies, or nonexperimental studies only, with or without meta-analysis Exploratory, convergent, or multiphasic mixed-methods studies Explanatory mixed-methods design that includes only a level III quantitative study Qualitative study Systematic review of qualitative studies with or without meta-synthesis
Nonresearch Evidence	Level IV	Opinion of respected authorities and/or nationally recognized expert committees or consensus panels based on scientific evidence; includes clinical practice guidelines Consensus panels/position statements
	Level V	Based on experiential and nonresearch evidence; includes scoping reviews, integrative reviews, literature reviews, quality improvement and program or financial evaluation, case reports, and opinions of nationally recognized expert(s) based on experiential evidence

Adapted from "Appendix D," *Johns Hopkins Evidence-Based Practice for Nurses and Healthcare Professionals: Model and Guidelines*, ed. Deborah Dang et al., p. 1.

In medicine, Ebell et al. (2004) proposed a framework to guide health providers' evidence in patient-centered care known as the strength of recommendation taxonomy (SORT). Through SORT, evidence for effective interventions is selected based on three major attributes: (a) strength of recommendation (A, B, or C, 2); level of evidence (level 1: good quality patient-centered evidence; level 2: limited quality patients centered evidence; and level 3: other evidence), and (c) consistency or nonconsistency among study findings (see Reading 9.1). A SORT algorithm for determining the strength of a recommendation (Ebell et al., 2004) based on a body of evidence for an individual study is provided in Reading 9.2 and Reading 9.3, respectively.

In general, only key recommendations for readers require a grade of the "Strength of Recommendation". Recommendations should be based on the highest quality evidence available. For example, Vitamin E was found in some cohort studies (Level 2 study quality) to have a benefit for cardiovascular protection, but good-quality randomized trials (Level 1) have not confirmed this effect. It is therefore preferable to base clinical recommendations in a manuscript on the level 1 studies.

Strength of Recommendation	Definition
A	Recommendation based on consistent and good quality patient-oriented evidence *
B	Recommendation based on inconsistent or limited quality patient-oriented evidence *
C	Recommendation based on consensus, usual practice, opinion, disease-oriented evidence,* and case series for studies of diagnosis, treatment, prevention, or screening.

Use the table below to determine whether a study measuring patient-oriented outcomes is of good or limited quality, and whether the results are consistent or inconsistent between studies:

	Type of study		
	Diagnosis	**Treatment / Prevention/ Screening**	**Prognosis**
Study Quality			
Level 1 Good quality patient-oriented evidence	• Validated clinical decision rule • Systematic Review (SR)/meta-analysis of high quality studies • High quality diagnostic cohort study **	• SR/meta-analysis of RCTs with consistent findings • High quality individual randomized controlled trial (RCT) + • All or none study ++	• SR/meta-analysis of good quality cohort studies • Prospective cohort study with good follow-up
Level 2 Limited quality patient-oriented evidence	• Unvalidated clinical decision rule • SR/meta-analysis of lower quality studies or studies with inconsistent findings • Lower quality diagnostic cohort study or diagnostic case-control study **	• SR/meta-analysis of lower quality clinical trials or of studies with inconsistent findings • Lower quality clinical trial + • Cohort study • Case-control study	• SR/meta-analysis of lower quality cohort studies or with inconsistent results • Retrospective cohort study or prospective cohort study with poor follow-up • Case-control study • Case series
Level 3 Other evidence	Consensus guidelines, extrapolations from bench research, usual practice, opinion, disease-oriented evidence (intermediate or physiologic outcomes only), and case series for studies of diagnosis, treatment, prevention, or screening.		

	Consistency Across Studies
Consistent	• Most studies found similar or at least coherent conclusions (coherence means that differences are explainable) • or • If high quality and up-to-date systematic reviews or meta-analyses exist, they support the recommendation.
Inconsistent	• Considerable variation among study findings and lack of coherence or • If high quality and up-to-date systematic reviews or meta-analyses exist, they do not find consistent evidence in favor of the recommendation

* Patient-oriented evidence measures outcomes that matter to patients: morbidity, mortality, symptom improvement, cost reduction, quality of life. Disease-oriented evidence measures intermediate, physiologic, or surrogate endpoints that may or may not reflect improvements in patient outcomes (i.e.blood pressure, blood chemistry, physiological function, and pathological findings)

** High quality diagnostic cohort study: cohort design, adequate size, adequate spectrum of patients, blinding, and a consistent, well-defined reference standard

+ High quality RCT: allocation concealed, blinding if possible, intention-to-treat analysis, adequate statistical power, adequate follow-up (>80%).

++ An all-or-none study is one where the treatment causes a dramatic change in outcomes, such as antibiotics for meningitis or surgery for appendicitis, which precludes study in a controlled trial.

READING 9.1 "The Strength of Recommendation Taxonomy." (Mark H. Ebell et al., Selection from "Strength of Recommendation Taxonomy (SORT): A Patient-Centered Approach to Grading Evidence in the Medical Literature," *The Journal of the American Board of Family Practice*, vol. 17, no. 1, p. 62.

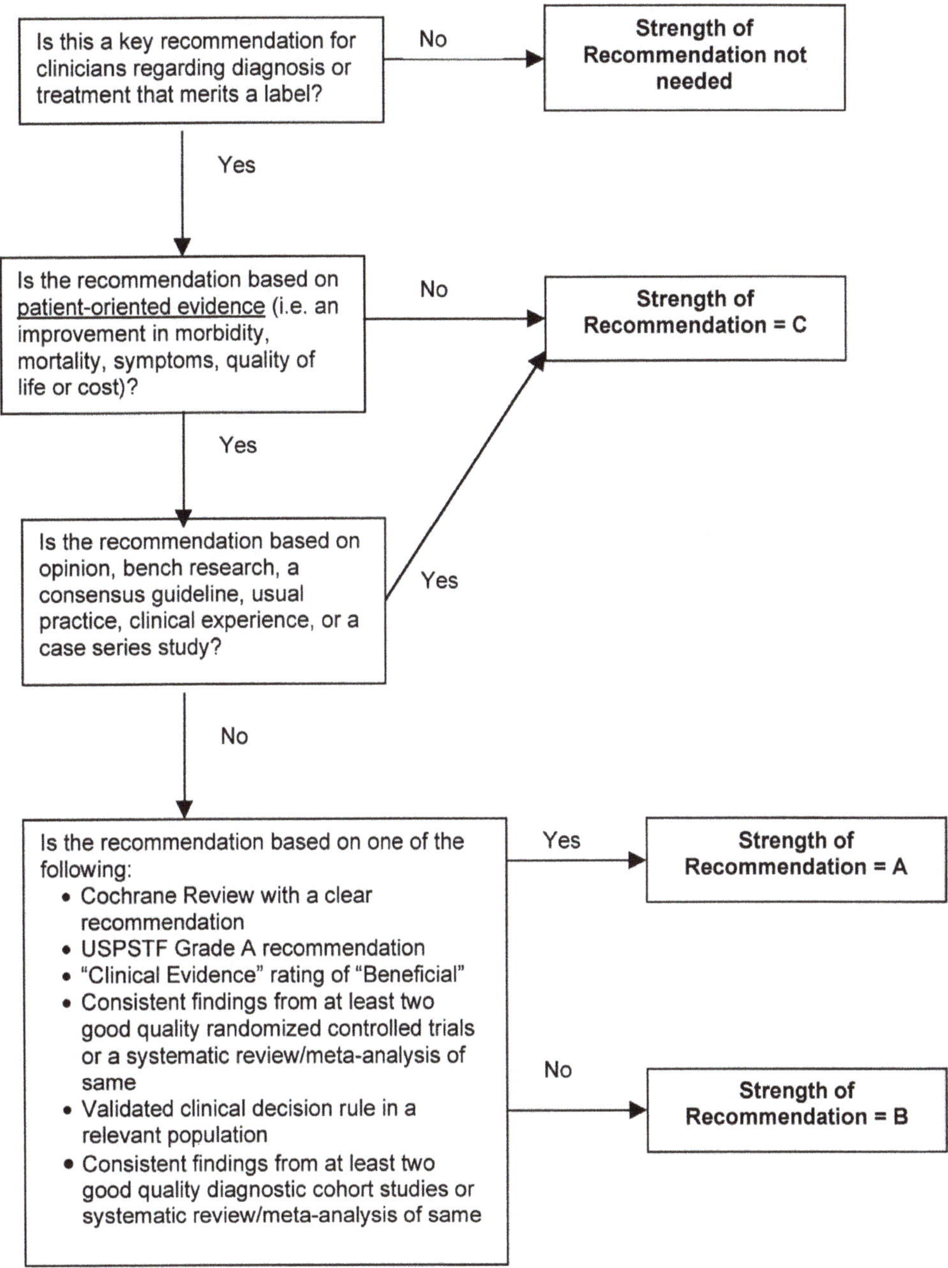

READING 9.2 "Algorithm for Determining the Strength of a Recommendation Based on a Body of Evidence." (Mark H. Ebell et al., Selection from "Strength of Recommendation Taxonomy (SORT): A Patient-Centered Approach to Grading Evidence in the Medical Literature," *The Journal of the American Board of Family Practice*, vol. 17, no. 2, p. 63. Copyright © 2004 by American Board of Family Medicine, Inc. Reprinted with permission.)

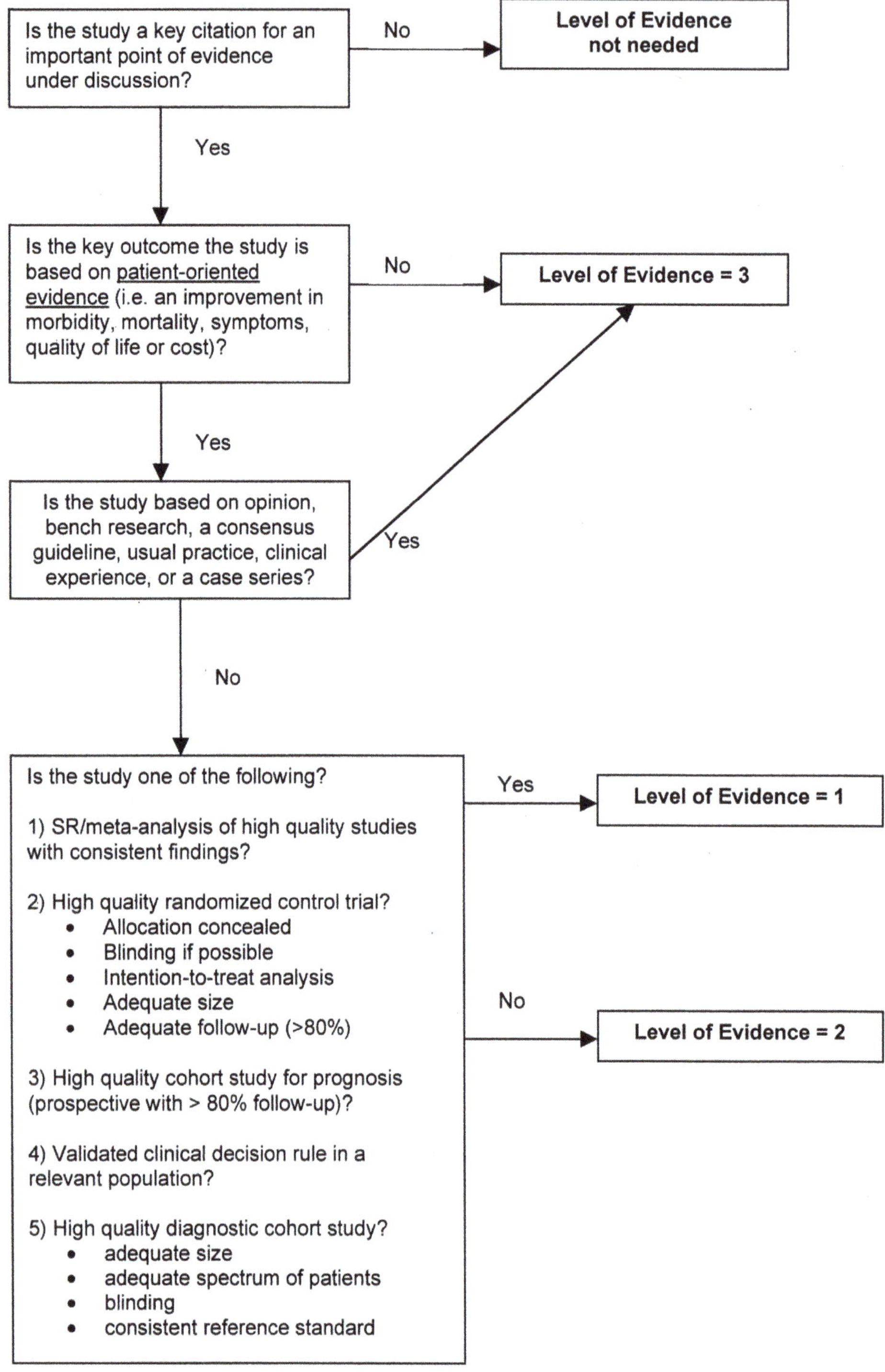

READING 9.3 "Algorithm for Determining the Level of Evidence for an Individual Study." (Mark H. Ebell et al., Selection from "Strength of Recommendation Taxonomy (SORT): A Patient-Centered Approach to Grading Evidence in the Medical Literature," *The Journal of the American Board of Family Practice*, vol. 17, no. 3, p. 64. Copyright © 2004 by American Board of Family Medicine, Inc. Reprinted with permission.)

Likewise, in Family therapy, Sexton et al. (2011) put together a framework to depict the levels of evidence in couple and family therapy research (see Figure 9.3).

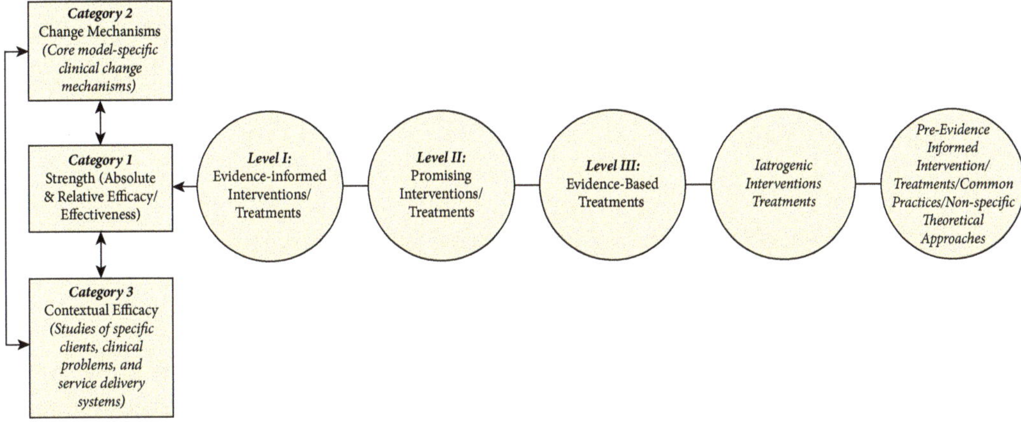

FIGURE 9.3 Level of evidence in couple and family therapy.

Efficacy and Effectiveness in FHI

The different approaches discussed in the previous section help *family health* professionals understand quality evidence that is generated from efficacy and effectiveness studies in person-centered care. Efficacy is as "the performance of an intervention under ideal and controlled circumstances, whereas effectiveness refers to intervention performance under 'real-world' conditions" (Singal et al., 2014, p. 1; see Table 9.6).

TABLE 9.6 **Differences Between Efficacy and Effectiveness Studies**

	Efficacy Study	**Effectiveness Study**
Question	Does the intervention work under ideal circumstances?	Does the intervention work in real-world practice?
Setting	Resource-intensive "ideal setting"	Real-world everyday clinical setting
Study Population	Highly selected, homogenous population Several exclusion criteria	Heterogeneous population Few to no exclusion criteria
Providers	Highly experienced and trained	Representative usual providers
Intervention	Strictly enforced and standardized No concurrent interventions	Applied with flexibility Concurrent interventions and cross-over permitted

In addition to evidence-based practice, practice-based evidence should be integrated for effective implementation in real-life settings beyond controlled environments.

Practice-based evidence refers to relevant, more actionable, and tailored evidence that is generated from clinical expertise and experience through participatory methods (Green, 2008). This approach can provide solutions to complex problems in person-centered care, especially for people living with comorbidities (Reeve et al., 2013). To be able to contribute practice-based knowledge for clinical reasoning in *family health* care, clinicians and providers must develop a culture of reflective practice (Stange et al., 2001).

Implementation FHI Challenges and Opportunities in Person-Centered Care Within 4HEALTH

Despite an increase in studies that show FHI efficacy in improving individual and *family health*, family functioning, and family process outcomes, implementation of in family-centered care presents unique challenges and opportunities across the 4HEALTH context and warrant more effectiveness studies. For example, at the *individual health* and *family health* levels, efficacious PFCC studies demonstrate that physical support, patient empowerment, and family involvement are key FHIs (Park et al., 2018; Xyrichis et al., 2021). Similarly, the Agency for Healthcare Research and Quality (2018) reports that engaging with patients and families is one of the key drivers for evidence-based care and quality improvement. Such claims of evidence are good news; however, in reality, translation to practice efforts to meet the needs of many families have slowed. The limitation is compounded by a lack of consideration of implementation evidence that captures barriers and facilitating factors from the most vulnerable families that usually contact health care systems when they are critically ill and may be less likely to be active participants in their own care. In general, these families are characterized as low-income families who are often unemployed, have unstable housing or experience homelessness, and have low levels of literacy or language fluency. While making evidence-informed care plans, *family health* professionals should avoid generalization. They should acknowledge the fact that families and individual family members have different needs and preferences regarding the FHI structure (e.g., timing, length, intensity, content of the intervention, and qualification of the care provider) and one-size-fits-all interventions will not work (Jukes et al., 2024; Selick et al., 2017). Tailoring FHIs to families is important to promote health equity in person-centered care (National Academies of Sciences, Engineering, and Medicine, 2019). Tailoring should include assessing for familial religious beliefs that can impend family-centered care (Phiri et al., 2020; Wong et al., 2023).

At the *population health* level, organizational barriers are key drivers for evidence-based FHI implementation. A culture of *family health* and a health care organization shift toward working with families to promote *population health* and health care quality is a necessity in person-centered care. For example, efficacy studies have demonstrated positive outcomes with interprofessional teams in family-centered care, but implementation is slow due to lack of reimbursable integrated health care. Reimbursement challenges are only for acute care, even in community-based family-focused programming (Leslie et al., 2016). Such uncertainties in funding do not sustain FHIs. They limit opportunities for collaborative referral agreements to meet patient and family needs. Likewise, lack of integration of family-centered goals in health care systems is a barrier for FHI implementation, especially with increased opportunities for innovation in technology (Lin et al., 2022). It is understandable that it is difficult for health care systems to change rapidly from the biomedical model. The shift to *family health* will require clinical teams to reestablish new working routines that facilitate family involvement approaches (Eassom et al., 2014). Organizations should reconfigure who should be in teams and what new roles should be established. For example, some organizations that implement FHIs have established the role of rounding coordinators in acute care settings. This approach has proved to be beneficial in the implementation of family-centered care by increasing team engagement and patient satisfactions (Bekmezian et al., 2019).

At the level of public health, evidence-based policies and practices that ensure a diverse and skilled workforce to implement evidence-based FHIs are needed. Providers still need training in family-centered care and FHI strategies (Hansson et al., 2022). Health education institutions and health care organizations should incorporate basic training policies in *family health* care to counteract professionals' negative attitudes and lack of competencies and self-confidence in working with families. How providers learn should be evaluated to make sure they both are equipped with evidence-based practice and practice-based knowledge for effective family involvement. FHIs that promote effective communication and interaction to ensure positive patient experiences are needed, especially post-COVID-19 with diminished public trust and security in health care delivery. Trusting relationships can take different forms, including innovative communication strategies such as inpatient texting (Bruce et al., 2023).

Evidence-based public health work policies that promote FHIs should also be reinforced to enable equitable access to care. For example, evidence-based barriers related to staff workloads and task shifting and task sharing should be translated to practice. This approach can only happen if public health puts *family health* first, before individual and *population health*. In addition, policies that build and maintain evidence-based infrastructures for coordination of care across settings (Council on Children with Disabilities and Medical Home Implementation Project Advisory Committee, 2014; Turchi et al., 2014) and those that support efficient and accessible financing and record-keeping are needed to permit FHI integration (Mitchell, 2020).

Overall, assuring the best evidence is available to the public is a challenge for FHI implementation. Thus, there needs to be investment in person-centered and whole-health initiatives to improve and innovate *family health* through evaluation, research, and quality improvement measures. This process needs consumers to work together to be able to evaluate the quality of FHI studies for any flaws and limitations before use and further evidence creation (Park et al., 2018).

Conclusion

In this chapter, basic knowledge of evidence-based practice in *family health* care was introduced. *Family health* professionals need to understand how to utilize the evidence related to the different *family health* interventions that fit their context. This can happen by understanding the steps of the evidence-based process. Likewise, collaborating with family is essential for advancing FHI implementation. Effective communication is discussed in the next chapter as one of the key factors in FHI implementation.

Suggested Websites

Agency for Healthcare Research and Quality: https://www.ahrq.gov/patient-safety/patients-families/index.html

American Psychological Association, Family Interventions: https://www.apa.org/pi/about/publications/caregivers/practice-settings/intervention/family

National Cancer Institute, Transforming Research into Community and Clinical Practice: https://ebccp.cancercontrol.cancer.gov/index.do

International Family Nursing Association, Family Measures Project: https://internationalfamilynursing.org/resources-for-family-nursing/research/measurement-resources/

The Substance Abuse and Mental Health Services Administration: https://www.samhsa.gov/resource-search/ebp

National Institute of Health, Evidence-Based Practices: https://prevention.nih.gov/research-priorities/dissemination-implementation/evidence-based-practices-programs

World Health Organization, Guidelines: https://www.who.int/publications/who-guidelines

Suggested Readings

Knafl, K. A., Havill, N. L., Leeman, J., Fleming, L., Crandell, J. L., & Sandelowski, M. (2017). The nature of family engagement in interventions for children with chronic conditions. *Western Journal of Nursing Research*, *39*(5), 690–723.

Martire, L., Lustig, A., Schulz, R., Miller, G., & Helgeson, V. (2004). Is it beneficial to involve a family member? A meta-analysis of psychoeducational interventions for chronic illness. *Health Psychology*, *23*, 599–611. https://doi.org/10.1037/0278- 6133.23.6.599

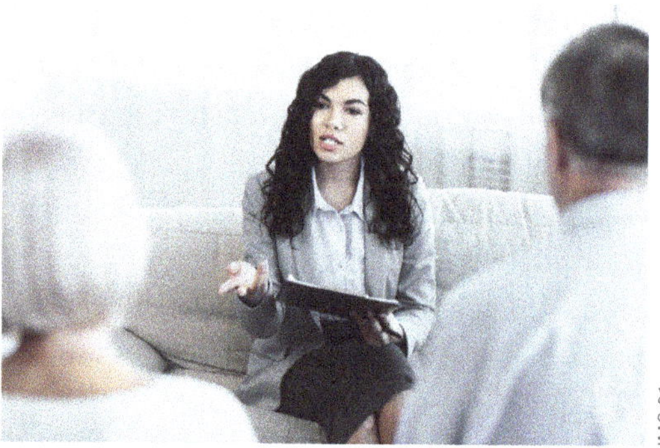

IMG 9.1

Nur, A. B. S. S., Chua, J. Y. X., & Shorey, S. (2023). Effectiveness of community-based family-focused interventions on family functioning among families of children with chronic health conditions: A systematic review and meta-analysis. *Family process*, *62*(4), 1408–1422.

Park, M., Giap, T., Lee, M., Jeong, H., Jeong, M., & Go, Y. (2018). Patient- and family-centered care interventions for improving the quality of health care: A review of systematic reviews. *International Journal of Nursing Studies*, *87*, 69–83. https://doi.org/10.1016/J.IJNURSTU.2018.07.006

Reflection Questions

1. What *family health* interventions have you encountered in health care?
2. Did the *family health* interventions work for you? Why?
3. If the *family health* interventions did not work, what do you think could have been done to make them work better for you?
4. What skills do you think are the most important in delivering a *family health* intervention?

References

Agency for Healthcare Research and Quality. (2018). *Key Driver 5: Engage with Patients and Families in Evidence-Based Care and Quality Improvement.* https://www.ahrq.gov/evidencenow/tools/key-drivers/engage-patients-families.html

Agency for Healthcare Research and Quality (2023, September). *What Is Patient Experience?* https://www.ahrq.gov/cahps/about-cahps/patient-experience/index.html

Alfheim, H. B., Hofsø, K., Småstuen, M. C., Tøien, K., Rosseland, L. A., & Rustøen, T. (2019). Post-traumatic stress symptoms in family caregivers of intensive care unit patients: A longitudinal study. *Intensive and Critical Care Nursing, 50*, 5–10.

Allen, S. R., Pascual, J., Martin, N., Reilly, P., Luckianow, G., Datner, E., ... & Kaplan, L. J. (2017). A novel method of optimizing patient-and family-centered care in the ICU. *Journal of Trauma and Acute Care Surgery, 82*(3), 582–586.

American Psychological Association. (2024, March 27. *Family Interventions.* https://www.apa.org/pi/about/publications/caregivers/practice-settings/intervention/family

Arnason, A., Langarica, N., Dugas, L. R., Mora, N., Luke, A., & Markossian, T. (2020). Family-based lifestyle interventions: What makes them successful? A systematic literature review. Preventive medicine reports, 21, 101299. https://doi.org/10.1016/j.pmedr.2020.101299

August-Brady, M. (2000). Prevention as intervention. *Journal of Advanced Nursing, 31*(6), 1304–1308.

Barnes, M. D., Hanson, C. L., Novilla, L. B., Magnusson, B. M., Crandall, A. C., & Bradford, G. (2020). Family-Centered Health Promotion: Perspectives for Engaging Families and Achieving Better Health Outcomes. Inquiry : a journal of medical care organization, provision and financing, 57, 46958020923537. https://doi.org/10.1177/0046958020923537

Bekmezian, A., Fiore, D. M., Long, M., Monash, B. J., Padrez, R., Rosenbluth, G., & Sun, K. I. (2019). Keeping Time: Implementing Appointment-based Family-centered Rounds. *Pediatric quality & safety, 4*(4), e182. https://doi.org/10.1097/pq9.0000000000000182

Bell, J. M. (2012). Making ideas "stick": The 15-minute family interview. *Journal of Family Nursing, 18*(2), 171–174.

Binumon, K. V., Ezhumalai, S., Janardhana, N., & Chand, P. K. (2024). Development and Validation of Brief Family Intervention for Young Adults with Substance Use Disorder: A Qualitative Study. *Journal of psychiatry spectrum, 3*(1), 28–35.

Bodenheimer, T., & Sinsky, C. (2014). From triple to quadruple aim: Care of the patient requires care of the provider. *The Annals of Family Medicine, 12*(6), 573–576.

Bruce, C. R., Kamencik-Wright, A., Zuniga-Georgy, N., Vinh, T. M., Shah, H., Shallcross, J., Giammattei, C., O'Rourke, C., Smith, M., Bruchhaus, L., Bowens, Y., Goode, K., Arabie, L. A., Sauceda, K., Pacha, M., Martinez, S., Chisum, J., Benjamin Saldaña, R., Nicholas Desai, S., Awar, M., ... Vernon, T. R. (2023). Design and Integration of a Texting Tool to Keep Patients' Family Members Updated During

Hospitalization: Clinicians' Perspectives. Journal of patient experience, 10, 23743735231160423. https://doi.org/10.1177/23743735231160423

Campbell, T. L. (2003). The effectiveness of family interventions for physical disorders. *Journal of Marital and family Therapy, 29*(2), 263–281.

Chesla, C. A. (2010). Do family interventions improve health? *Journal of family nursing, 16*(4), 355–377.

Claxton, M., Onwumere, J., & Fornells-Ambrojo, M. (2017). Do Family Interventions Improve Outcomes in Early Psychosis? A Systematic Review and Meta-Analysis. Frontiers in psychology, 8, 371. https://doi.org/10.3389/fpsyg.2017.00371

Council on Children with Disabilities and Medical Home Implementation Project Advisory Committee (2014). Patient- and family-centered care coordination: a framework for integrating care for children and youth across multiple systems. Pediatrics, 133(5), e1451–e1460. https://doi.org/10.1542/peds.2014-0318

Davidson, J. E., Aslakson, R. A., Long, A. C., Puntillo, K. A., Kross, E. K., Hart, J., … & Curtis, J. R. (2017). Guidelines for family-centered care in the neonatal, pediatric, and adult ICU. *Critical care medicine, 45*(1), 103–128.

Davidson, J. E., Daly, B. J., Agan, D., Brady, N. R., & Higgins, P. A. (2010). Facilitated sensemaking: A feasibility study for the provision of a family support program in the intensive care unit. *Critical care nursing quarterly, 33*(2), 177–189.

Eassom, E., Giacco, D., Dirik, A., & Priebe, S. (2014). Implementing family involvement in the treatment of patients with psychosis: a systematic review of facilitating and hindering factors. BMJ open, 4(10), e006108. https://doi.org/10.1136/bmjopen-2014-006108

Ebell, M. H., Siwek, J., Weiss, B. D., Woolf, S. H., Susman, J., Ewigman, B., & Bowman, M. (2004). Strength of recommendation taxonomy (SORT): A patient-centered approach to grading evidence in the medical literature. *The Journal of the American Board of Family Practice, 17*(1), 59–67.

Ellenwood, A. E., & Jenkins, J. E. (2007). Unbalancing the effects of chronic illness: Non-traditional family therapy assessment and intervention approach. *The American Journal of Family Therapy, 35*(3), 265–277.

Eustace, R., & Fawcett, J. (2019). *Closing the "Secondary" Research-Theory-Practice-Application Gap: Charting a Path for Advancement of Nursology Knowledge in Implementation Science.* Nursology. https://nursology.net/2022/05/24/closing-the-secondary-research-theory-practice-gap-charting-a-path-for-advancement-of-nursology-knowledge-in-implementation-science/

Eustace, R. W., Gray, B., & Curry, D. M. (2015). The meaning of family nursing intervention: what do acute care nurses think? Research and theory for nursing practice, 29(2), 125–142. https://doi.org/10.1891/1541-6577.29.2.125

Fawcett, J. & Neuman, B. (1992). *The Neuman Systems Model* (5th ed.). Pearson.

Gervais, C., Verdon, C., deMontigny, F., Leblanc, L., & Lalande, D. (2020). Creating a space to talk about one's experience of suffering: Families' experience of a family nursing intervention. *Scandinavian journal of caring sciences, 34*(2), 446–455.

Gitlin, L. N., Corcoran, M., Martindale-Adams, J., Malone, C., Stevens, A., & Winter, L. (2000). Identifying mechanisms of action: Why and how does intervention work? In R. Schulz (Ed.), *Handbook on dementia caregiving: Evidence-based interventions for family caregivers* (pp. 225–248). Springer.

Glasgow, R. E., Lichtenstein, E., & Marcus, A. C. (2003). Why don't we see more translation of health promotion research to practice? Rethinking the efficacy-to-effectiveness transition. *American journal of public health, 93*(8), 1261–1267.

Green, L. W. (2008). Making research relevant: if it is an evidence-based practice, where's the practice-based evidence? *Family practice, 25*(1), i20–i24.

Hanson, C. L., Crandall, A., Barnes, M. D., Magnusson, B., Novilla, M. L. B., & King, J. (2019). Family-Focused Public Health: Supporting Homes and Families in Policy and Practice. Frontiers in public health, 7, 59. https://doi.org/10.3389/fpubh.2019.00059

Hansson, K. M., Romøren, M., Pedersen, R., Weimand, B., Hestmark, L., Norheim, I., Ruud, T., Hymer, I. S., & Heiervang, K. S. (2022). Barriers and facilitators when implementing family involvement for persons with psychotic disorders in community mental health centres - a nested qualitative study. BMC health services research, 22(1), 1153. https://doi.org/10.1186/s12913-022-08489-y

Hawe, P., & Potvin, L. (2009). What is *population health* intervention research? *Canadian journal of public health, 100,* I8–I14.

Ho, Y. L., Mahirah, D., Ho, C. Z., & Thumboo, J. (2022). The role of the family in health promotion: a scoping review of models and mechanisms. Health promotion international, 37(6), daac119. https://doi.org/10.1093/heapro/daac119

Hsiao, P. R., Redley, B., Hsiao, Y. C., Lin, C. C., Han, C. Y., & Lin, H. R. (2017). Family needs of critically ill patients in the emergency department. *International emergency nursing, 30,* 3–8.

Jacob, M., Horton, C., Rance-Ashley, S., Field, T., Patterson, R., Johnson, C., ... & Frobos, C. (2016). Needs of patients' family members in an intensive care unit with continuous visitation. *American Journal of Critical Care, 25*(2), 118–125.

Jensen, C. B. (2015). The continuum of health professions. *Integrative Medicine: A Clinician's Journal, 14*(3), 48–53.

Jukes, L. M., Di Folco, S., Kearney, L., & Sawrikar, V. (2024). Barriers and facilitators to engaging mothers and fathers in family-based interventions: A qualitative systematic review. *Child Psychiatry & Human Development, 55*(1), 137–151.

Keitner, G. I. (2012). Family assessment in the medical setting. *The Psychosomatic Assessment, 32,* 203–222.

Knafl, K. A., Havill, N. L., Leeman, J., Fleming, L., Crandell, J. L., & Sandelowski, M. (2017). The nature of family engagement in interventions for children with chronic conditions. *Western Journal of Nursing Research, 39*(5), 690–723.

Leahey, M., & Wright, L. M. (2016). Application of the Calgary family assessment and intervention models: Reflections on the reciprocity between the personal and the professional. *Journal of family nursing, 22*(4), 450–459.

Leahey, M., & Svavarsdottir, E. K. (2009). Implementing family nursing: How do we translate knowledge into clinical practice? *Journal of Family Nursing, 15*(4), 445–460.

Leslie, L. K., Mehus, C. J., Hawkins, J. D., Boat, T., McCabe, M. A., Barkin, S., ... & Beardslee, W. (2016). Primary health care: Potential home for family-focused preventive interventions. *American journal of preventive medicine, 51*(4), S106–S118.

Lin, J. L., Huber, B., Amir, O., Gehrmann, S., Ramirez, K. S., Ochoa, K. M., Asch, S. M., Gajos, K. Z., Grosz, B. J., & Sanders, L. M. (2022). Barriers and Facilitators to the Implementation of Family-Centered Technology in Complex Care: Feasibility Study. Journal of medical Internet research, 24(8), e30902. https://doi.org/10.2196/30902

Martire, L., Lustig, A., Schulz, R., Miller, G., & Helgeson, V. (2004). Is it beneficial to involve a family member? A meta-analysis of psychoeducational interventions for chronic illness. *Health Psychology, 23,* 599–611. https://doi.org/10.1037/0278- 6133.23.6.599

Melnyk, B. M., Fineout-Overholt, E., Stillwell, S. B., & Williamson, K. M. (2010). Evidence-based practice: Step by step: the seven steps of evidence-based practice. *AJN The American Journal of Nursing, 110*(1), 51–53.

Melnyk, B., & Morrison-Beedy, D. (2012). *Intervention research: Designing, conducting, analyzing, and funding.* Springer.

Mileski, M., McClay, R., Heinemann, K., & Dray, G. (2022). Efficacy of the Use of the Calgary Family Intervention Model in Bedside Nursing Education: A Systematic Review. Journal of multidisciplinary healthcare, 15, 1323–1347. https://doi.org/10.2147/JMDH.S370053

Mitchell, E. (2020, February, 24). What is the Continuum of Care? *EOScu.* https://blog.eoscu.com/blog/what-is-the-continuum-of-care

Naef, R., Filipovic, M., Jeitziner, M. M., von Felten, S., Safford, J., Riguzzi, M., & Rufer, M. (2022). A multicomponent family support intervention in intensive care units: study protocol for a multicenter cluster-randomized trial (FICUS Trial). Trials, 23(1), 533. https://doi.org/10.1186/s13063-022-06454-y

National Cancer Institute. (2024, April 29). Mechanism of Action. NCI's Dictionary of Cancer Terms. https://www.cancer.gov/publications/dictionaries/cancer-terms/def/mechanism-of-action

National Institute of Health. (2019). *Risk and Protective Factors of Family Health and Family Level Interventions.* https://grants.nih.gov/grants/guide/pa-files/PAR-21-358.html

Nur, A. B. S. S., Chua, J. Y. X., & Shorey, S. (2023). Effectiveness of community-based family-focused interventions on family functioning among families of children with chronic health conditions: A systematic review and meta-analysis. *Family process, 62*(4), 1408–1422.

Östlund, U., & Persson, C. (2014). Examining family responses to family systems nursing interventions: An integrative review. *Journal of Family Nursing, 20*(3), 259–286.

Park, M., Giap, T., Lee, M., Jeong, H., Jeong, M., & Go, Y. (2018). Patient- and family-centered care interventions for improving the quality of health care: A review of systematic reviews. *International Journal of Nursing Studies, 87,* 69–83. https://doi.org/10.1016/J.IJNURSTU.2018.07.006

Persson, C., & Benzein, E. (2014). *Family health* conversations: how do they support health?. Nursing research and practice, 2014, 547160. https://doi.org/10.1155/2014/547160

Pineros-Leano, M., Parchment, T. M., & Calvo, R. (2023). Family interventions to improve mental, emotional, and behavioral health outcomes among Latinx youth: A systematic review. *Children and Youth Services Review, 145,* 106756. https://doi.org/10.1016/j.childyouth.2022.106756

Phiri, P. G., Chan, C. W., & Wong, C. L. (2020). The scope of family-centred care practices, and the facilitators and barriers to implementation of family-centred care for hospitalised children and their families in developing countries: An integrative review. *Journal of Pediatric Nursing, 55,* 10–28.

Reeve, J., Blakeman, T., Freeman, G. K., Green, L. A., James, P. A., Lucassen, P., ... & Van Weel, C. (2013). Generalist solutions to complex problems: Generating practice-based evidence-the example of managing multi-morbidity. *BMC family practice, 14,* 1–8.

Selick, A., Durbin, J., Vu, N., O'Connor, K., Volpe, T., & Lin, E. (2017). Barriers and facilitators to implementing family support and education in early psychosis intervention programmes: A systematic review. *Early intervention in psychiatry, 11*(5), 365–374.

Sexton, T., Gordon, K. C., Gurman, A., Lebow, J., Holtzworth-Munroe, A. M. Y., & Johnson, S. (2011). Guidelines for classifying evidence-based treatments in couple and family therapy. *Family process, 50*(3), 377–392.

Sigurdson, K., Profit, J., Dhurjati, R., Morton, C., Scala, M., Vernon, L., Randolph, A., Phan, J. T., & Franck, L. S. (2020). Former NICU Families Describe Gaps in Family-Centered Care. Qualitative health research, 30(12), 1861–1875. https://doi.org/10.1177/1049732320932897

Singal, A. G., Higgins, P. D., & Waljee, A. K. (2014). A primer on effectiveness and efficacy trials. *Clinical and translational gastroenterology, 5*(1), e45. https://doi.org/10.1038/ctg.2013.13

Sittner, B. J., Hudson, D. B., & Defrain, J. (2007). Using the concept of family strengths to enhance nursing care. *MCN: The American Journal of Maternal/Child Nursing, 32*(6), 353–357.

Smith, R. C., Fortin, A. H., Dwamena, F., & Frankel, R. M. (2013). An evidence-based patient-centered method makes the biopsychosocial model scientific. *Patient education and counseling, 91*(3), 265–270.

Stange, K. C., Miller, W. L., & McWhinney, I. (2001). Developing the knowledge base of family practice. *Family Medicine, 33*(4), 286–297.

Tharinger, D. J., Finn, S. E., Wilkinson, A. D., & Schaber, P. M. (2007). Therapeutic assessment with a child as a family intervention: A clinical and research case study. *Psychology in the Schools, 44*(3), 293–309.

Turner-Cobb, J. M., Smith, P. C., Ramchandani, P., Begen, F. M., & Padkin, A. (2016). The acute psychobiological impact of the intensive care experience on relatives. *Psychology, health & medicine, 21*(1), 20–26.

Utz, R. L., Terrill, A. L., & Thompson, A. (2023). Online interventions to support family caregivers: The value of community-engaged research practices. *Journal of prevention & intervention in the community, 51*(3), 238–253.

Wacharasin, C. (2010). Families suffering with HIV/AIDS: What family nursing interventions are useful to promote healing? *Journal of Family Nursing, 16*(3), 302–321.

Wäsche, H., Niermann, C., Bezold, J., & Woll, A. (2021). *Family health* climate: a qualitative exploration of everyday family life and health. BMC public health, 21(1), 1261. https://doi.org/10.1186/s12889-021-11297-4

Weihs, K., Fisher, L., & Baird, M. (2002). Families, health, and behavior: A section of the commissioned report by the Committee on Health and Behavior: Research, Practice, and Policy Division of Neuroscience and Behavioral Health and Division of Health Promotion and Disease Prevention Institute of Medicine, National Academy of Sciences. *Families, Systems, & Health, 20*(1), 7–46. https://doi.org/10.1037/h0089481

Weiss-Laxer, N. S., Crandall, A., Hughes, M. E., & Riley, A. W. (2020). Families as a Cornerstone in 21st Century Public Health: Recommendations for Research, Education, Policy, and Practice. Frontiers in public health, 8, 503. https://doi.org/10.3389/fpubh.2020.00503

Wolffbrandt, M. M., Soendergaard, P. L., Biering-Sørensen, F., Sundekilde, L., Kjeldgaard, A., Schow, T., Arango-Lasprilla, J. C., & Norup, A. (2024). A manual-based family intervention for families living with acquired brain or spinal cord injury: a qualitative study of families' experiences. Disability and rehabilitation, 46(19), 4503–4513. https://doi.org/10.1080/09638288.2023.2280063

Wong, C. L., Phiri, P. G., Chan, C. W., & Tse, M. (2023). Nurse' and families' perceptions and practices and factors influencing the implementation of family-centred care for hospitalised children and their families. *Journal of Clinical Nursing, 32*(17–18), 6662–6676.

Wright, L. M., & Leahey, M. (1994). Calgary family intervention model: One way to think about change. *Journal of Marital and Family Therapy, 20*(4), 381–395.

Xyrichis, A., Fletcher, S., Philippou, J., Brearley, S., Terblanche, M., & Rafferty, A. M. (2021). Interventions to promote family member involvement in adult critical care settings: a systematic review. BMJ open, 11(4), e042556. https://doi.org/10.1136/bmjopen-2020-042556

Yu, C., Xian, Y., Jing, T., Bai, M., Li, X., Li, J., Liang, H., Yu, G., & Zhang, Z. (2023). More patient-centered care, better healthcare: the association between patient-centered care and healthcare outcomes in inpatients. Frontiers in public health, 11, 1148277. https://doi.org/10.3389/fpubh.2023.1148277

Figure credits

Fig. 9.1: R. Eustace and J. Fawcett, "Closing the "Secondary" Gap," https://nursology.net/2022/05/24/closing-the-secondary-research-theory-practice-gap-charting-a-path-for-advancement-of-nursology-knowledge-in-implementation-science/. Copyright © 2019 by Nursology.net.

Fig. 9.2a: B. Melnyk and D. Morrison-Beedy, "Intervention Research and Evidence-Based Quality Improvement: Designing, Conducting, Analyzing, and Funding," *Intervention Research and Evidence-Based Quality Improvement: Designing, Conducting, Analyzing, and Funding*, p. 2. Copyright © 2012 by Springer Publishing Company.

Fig. 9.3: Thomas Sexton et al., "Guidelines for Classifying Evidence-Based Treatments in Couple and Family Therapy," *Family Process*, vol. 50, no. 3. Copyright © 2011 by John Wiley & Sons, Inc.

IMG 9.1: Copyright © 2020 Depositphotos/Milkos.

CHAPTER 10

Advocating for Evidence-Based Person- and Family-Centered Health Policies, Programs and Practices

Advocacy is empathy, compassion and community at work.

—Janna Cachola

Learning Objectives

By the end of this chapter, learners will do the following:

- Examine the basic concepts related health policy issues in *family health* care.
- Discuss the importance of a family perspective in evidence-based health policy decision-making processes.
- Describe the phases of the health policy process.
- Explore the roles of *family health* care professionals in building health and public health policies that support person and family-centered care across the life cycle.
- Analyze the factors influencing the uptake of family-focused evidence-based health policies within the 4HEALTH contexts.

Before you read on, consider the following questions:

- Are individuals or families the basic unit of the society?
- Does the family as a unit contribute or communicate any value to the society?
- Should *family health* be in all policies?
- Does an evidence-based perspective matter to stakeholders, including health policymakers, during the health policy decision-making process?

It is well known that in many countries worldwide, health policies are usually designed with either an individual or population focus in mind. The concept of family as a unit of analysis or policy development and implementation is seldom considered among policymakers (Bogenschneider et al., 2011; Ortiz et al., 2017). This chapter provides an overview of the importance of advocating for family-focused evidence-based health policy decision-making on matters of health and public health care delivery systems.

The questions provide an initial opportunity to contextualize the importance of *family* and *family health* in family-centered care as complex matters but important concepts in health policy decision-making processes for effective and equitable health systems that intend to achieve better health status for diverse individuals, families, communities, and populations across the life span. For instance, decisions on matters of health have been increasingly influenced by the concept, scope, and evolution of the family (Kumar et al., 2023). Topics and concepts discussed earlier in the book—the theoretical underpinnings of family and *family health*, whole-health care, patient and family-centered care (PFCC), social determinants of health (SDOH), patient and family engagement, multisectoral approach (MSA) and interprofessional family-focused care, family assessment, and evidence-based family intervention approaches—provide a foundational and philosophical basis for advocating for inclusion of families in policymaking in the health and illness continuum. The goal of this chapter is to provide information to expand *family health* professionals' policy stewardship to address health and public challenges.

Definition of Policy and Health Policy

Policy development is one of the core functions of public health functions that aims to protect the health of the population (CDC, Office of Policy, Performance, and Evaluation 2015; Pan American Health Organization, 2020). A *policy* is defined as a "law, regulation, procedure, administrative action, incentive or voluntary practice in the public sector (e.g., government, judiciary) or the private sector (e.g., employers, nonprofit organizations)" (CDC, Office of Policy, Performance and Evaluation, 2015, para. 1). A *health policy* is an "agreement or consensus on the health issues, goals and objectives to be addressed, the priorities among those objectives, and the main directions for achieving them" (Zahidie, Asif, & Iqbal , 2023, p. 1). Health policies include formal and informal rules that guide individual and collective behaviors to improve population-based outcomes, often with limited resources (Jilcott et al., 2007). Policies can be conceptualized in three levels: formal written agreements such as codes or regulations, written standards that guide choices made, and unwritten social norms that influence values, beliefs, and behavior (Jilcott et al., 2007). These policies vary and range from local, state, territorial, and federal to international policies, including organizational policies (e.g., employment; Jilcott et al., 2007). The policies can be health sector specific or multisectoral. Sectorial and multisectoral health policies are essential in the policymaking process because they foster collaboration to influence individual, interpersonal, and organization/systems behavior change to promote public health.

The Importance of a Family Perspective in Evidence-Based Policymaking

As discussed in previous chapters, ecological models provide an excellent framework for examining the interconnections among the family, the individual, and broader contexts (Haehnel et al., 2022; Trzcinski, 1995). Communities and populations are comprised of individuals and families who together affect the health of the community, and vice versa. The family system is considered the core social context for health development (Bogenschneider, 2014; Weiss-Laxer et al., 2020; WHO, 2013). It provides the context, care, continuity, and connections for health (Hanson et al., 2019; Weiss-Laxer et al., 2020). Table 10.1 provides information on the unique influences of families on health. Preliminary research in health promotion practice confirms the importance of the family unit as the primary player for keeping family members healthy through health-promotion behaviors and disease prevention strategies across the life course (Barnes et al., 2020). In addition, the family system provides initial disease management for sick family members, access to medical care for those who need outpatient care, and support during hospitalization and after discharge (Kumar et al., 2023). See Table 10.2 for a summary of the role of family in health and illness.

TABLE 10.1 **Unique Influence of Families on Health**

Nature of Influence	Examples of Influence	Examples of Effects
Context: An early, proximal, persistent, encompassing, and long-term environment is created by each family.	Adults' skills capacities, needs, and resources create physical and social living environments that vary in terms of safety, predictable caring access to resources, and health care when sick	The myriad family environments individually and collectively support or hinder health-related actions.
Care: Individuals depend on families to provide for basic needs, including a sense of security and belonging.	Nurturance early in life, support throughout life, sharing of nutritional health care, and other tangible resources are ways families provide the foundation for health and coping.	Family members, especially adults, communicate their caring through verbal and nonverbal communication, shared time, food preparation, and the sharing of meals.
Continuity: Family ties persist, enduring even across generations	Positive, long-term relationships are health promoting through the dependability and predictability they provide.	One's experience that others are accessible provides security and meaning and helps prevent isolation and loneliness. Family celebrations support continuity.
Connections: Families provide social capital connecting members with the communities and the larger world.	Health is shaped by opportunities for learning and growing, and also by the inter-relationships that give meaning. Families can and often do assist in both.	Family members understand members' needs and often help to identify others outside the family who can help create opportunities and/or enrich relationships.

TABLE 10.2 **Summary of the Role of Family in Health and Illness**

Health Care Components	Role of Family in ...	
	Health	**Disease**
Health Promotion	Diet: Food type, quantity, quality, frequency, cooking, and storage; physical activity; exercise, how frequently; alcohol, tobacco, and drug use Primordial prevention of risk factors	Maintaining the desirable behaviors as a nonpharmaceutical intervention in illness Compliance to treatment Prevention and early detection of complications
Life Course and Inter-generational Care	Desirable behavior and practices during prepregnancy, pregnancy, childhood, adolescence, youth, middle age, and healthy aging Prevention of conditions such as LBW, risk factors	Managing risk factors in those with disease
Traditional and Sociocultural Early Detection	Diseases and seeking prompt treatment	Complications and prompt, appropriate referral in various diseases such as diabetes, hypertension, and infections
Compliance	Desirable health behaviors	Treatment, including non-pharmaceutical interventions
Support to Care Givers	Care from caregivers and other family members	Engaging in hospital and posthospital care, including palliative care

Sanjiv Kumar, Pankaj Bhardwaj, and Neeta Kumar, Selection from "Need to Bring Family to the Heart of Healthcare as It Is Home, Not a Hospital, Where Healthcare Begins and Ends," *Indian Journal of Community Medicine*, vol. 48, no. 2, p. 211.

Advocating for Evidence-Based Family-Focused Public Health Policies, Programs, and Practices

Advocacy is a common word with multiple meanings in the political and policy world. In health care, the word could be described as one's involvement in the process of doing for or taking action on behalf of a person or recommending a health policy or arrangement to meet the needs of a person (i.e., individual, group, community) (Kalaitzidis & Jewell, 2015). It is an essential part of the *family health* professional's role in promoting collaborative PFCC models (Kokorelias et al., 2019; MacKean et al., 2005). To advocate for evidence-based, family-focused health policies, professionals, policymakers, and public and other key stakeholders must endorse the importance of *family health* and family functioning using an ecological lens because policy decisions in one sector interact with those of other sectors. For example, a family that is low income cannot provide sufficient economic resources and appropriate allocations to meet the family's needs. As a result, the family is at increased risk of not meeting health care function needs

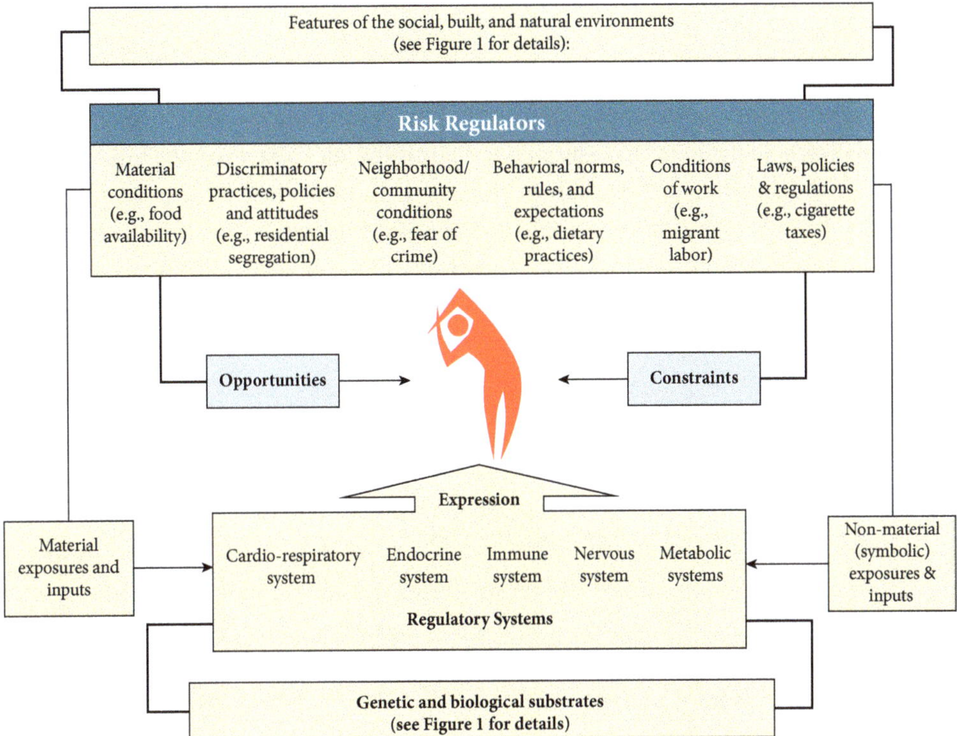

FIGURE 10.1 An illustration of risk regulators from an ecological (i.e., social and biological) context (Glass & McAtee, 2006, p. 1661).

on things such as healthy foods, health care, and housing. In this case, laws, policies, and regulations associated with family poverty can act as "risk regulators" that influence the family's exposure to risk factors such as behaviors and environmental risks, increasing the risk for poverty and poor health and well-being outcomes (AAFP, 2022). Figure 10.1 illustrates how the ecological risk regulators such as material conditions, neighborhood and community conditions, work conditions, behavioral norms, rules and expectations, and laws, policies, and regulations affect *individual health*. Thus, it is obvious that understanding the root causes of health problems and the problems' impact on *individual health* and *population health* without including family and *family health* as upstream factors is quite limiting. The family unit should be valued as the primary community stakeholder because their living, working, playing, worshiping, learning, and aging environments are constantly affected by proposed health policies. Efforts have been underway to support *family health* spillovers in economic evaluation in the health care sector (Al-Janabi ete al., 2016).

Likewise, advocating for evidence-based, family-focused care requires a good grasp of how family, *family health*, heath equity, health disparity, and evidence-based informed decision-making (EIDM) are conceptualized in health policy development and implementation.

Family and Family Health

Health policy decisions are influenced by the broadness or narrowness of the definitions and scopes of *family* or *family health* in health care delivery systems. For example, a narrow definition related to the health policy, family medical leave, can be limiting if the statutory law of a given context defines "family" using a traditional lens versus a non-traditional lens (Weiss-Laxer et al., 2020). The following textbox provides information on consensus definitions of family and *family health* in the context of family-centered health promotion. Table 10.3 provides a summary of family definitions used in primary care and their clinical significance.

DEFINITION OF FAMILY AND FAMILY HEALTH

Family is: two or more persons related by blood adoption, marriage or choice and whose relationship is characterized by at least one of the following:

Social and/or legal rights and obligations

Affective and emotional ties, and Endurance or intended endurance of the relationships

Relations by choice be characterized by an emotional connection strong enough to be perceived by individuals as a kingship tie

Family health is: a resource at the level of the family unit that develops from the intersection of the health of each family member, their interactions and capacities, as well as the family's physical, social, emotional, economic, and medical resources. *Family health* is greater than the sum of its parts. Positive *family health* promotes family members' sense of belonging and capacity to develop and adapt, to care for one another, and to meet responsibilities. (Riley et al., 2018, p. XX)

Michael D. Barnes et al., Selection from "Family-Centered Health Promotion: Perspectives for Engaging Families and Achieving Better Health Outcomes," *INQUIRY: The Journal of Health Care Organization, Provision, and Financing*, vol. 57.

TABLE 10.3 Summary of Clinical Significance of Family Definitions

Family Definition	Major Family Situation	Clinical Significance
Primary		
Census Definition (Blood, Marriage, Adoption)	Routine contact with all new patients	Inventory of family morbidity, mortality, and biologic relationships
Biologic	Genetic and/or familial disorder	Diagnosis of family/genetic transmission; identification of high-risk members and their early treatment or prevention
Household	Infectious diseases	Determine the origin of infection; prevent, ameliorate, or treat contacts

Functional	Chronic disease or illness	Identify caregiver and support system of patient and caregiver to help with care at that particular time
Secondary		
Crisis	Sudden death, illness, or accident	Identify key members to participate with physician in dealing with situation
Bereaved	Terminal phase of disease and following death of patient	Prepare patient and family for death and continue follow-up, especially of spouse, after death of patient
Cultural	Cultural beliefs of patient impact on medical decisions and care	Determine beliefs and reasons for behavior to negotiate treatment and care
Relationship	Conflicted relationships leading to violence, abuse, psychosomatic problems, depression, and unclear results of treatment	Evaluate relationships within family to directly treat or make appropriate referral

Health Equity and Health Disparity

The terms *health equity* and *health disparity* have been widely used in public health and health literature to describe the actions put in place that reflect justice for the sick and well (Braveman, 2022). They are rooted in social values, norms, and ethical and human rights, including the right to value all individuals equally, the right to health and adequate standard of living for health, and nondiscriminatory acts, especially among social disadvantaged groups (Braveman et al., 2011). In the health policy process, they are considered issues related to social justice and distributive justice. Social justice entails the righteous and sustainable acts of balancing benefits and burdens in a society that results in equitable living for all and a just order with fairness and equity in the distribution of power, resources, and processes in just institutions, systems, structures, policies, and processes (Buettner-Schmidt & Lobo, 2012). Distributive justice refers to acts of fairness, equitable and appropriate distribution of resources that are allocated by justifiable collaborative norms, and standards to reflect fair opportunities for all involved (Baumrucker et al., 2012). In public health, the terms have the benefit of promoting shared understanding in prioritization of needs in collaborative relationships to improve health for all (U.S. Department of Health and Human Services (USDHHS), 2022):

Health equity means that everyone has a fair and just opportunity to be as healthy as possible. This requires removing obstacles to health such as poverty, discrimination, and their consequences, including powerlessness and lack of access to good jobs with fair pay, quality education and housing, safe environments, and health care (USDHHS, 2022).

Broadly, health disparities are referred to as "health differences that adversely affect socially disadvantaged groups" (USDHHS, 2022, p. 13.).

Definition of Evidence-Informed Policy Decision-Making

As mentioned in Chapter 9, evidence-based practice demonstrates promising results related to quality care, improved patient outcomes, reduced costs, and greater provider satisfaction compared to usual/traditional care (Melnyk et al., 2010). In policymaking, evidence-informed policy decision-making (EIDM) processes reassure viable policy options and actionable health intervention for better health outcomes. According to the WHO (2021), an EIDM process is "a systematic and transparent approach that applies structured and replicable methods to identify, appraise, and make use of evidence across decision-making processes, including for implementation" (p. 6). The process emphasizes the use of the best-available evidence from research, as well as other factors such as context, public opinion, equity, and implementation outcomes (acceptability, adoption, appropriateness, cost, feasibility, fidelity, penetration, and sustainability) to make policy decisions for improved *population health*. Evidence-based policies derived from EIDM processes are considered "informed, more effective and less expensive" (Strydom et al., 2010, p. 1). Additionally, evidence-based health policies that have a family focus provide an important criterion for assessing health policy impact and means of achieving other policy goals (Bogenschneider, 2011). As an explicit goal, family-focused healthy policies "protect, promote and strengthen families" by supporting family functioning (Bogenschneider, 2014, p. 43). Effective health policies that support *family health* and functioning contribute to improved health, health equity, and thriving communities (i.e., stable, resilient and durable communities; Weiss-Laxer et al., 2020). Table 10.4 provides examples of different health policy priority areas across the five family functions: affective, socialization and social placement, health care, reproductive function, and economic function. The examples in the health policy priority areas cut across the family functions and SDOH. This observation supports the need of multisectoral collaborative approaches in health policy decision-making for successful policy development and implementation (Regional Office for Europe, European Observatory on Health Systems and Policies et al., 2019).

TABLE 10.4 **Health Policy Issues Across the Friedman's Five Family Functions**

Family Function	Definition	Health Policy Family-Related Priority Issues
Affective Function	Healthy families provide affection and understanding to meet the socioemotional needs of all their members. This includes providing healthy communication, intimacy, cooperation, and conflict management.	Social support (family and community) to address social isolation
Socialization and Social Placement Function	Healthy families raise and nurture the next generation to be productive members of the society. This function is important for societal survival and transmittal of cultural heritage, values, and privileges. The function is shared with other institutions such as schools and recreational and childcare facilities.	Adolescent crime and violence, parenting (childrearing patterns), childcare, early childhood education, school, breastfeeding, children's rights, parental rights, duties and responsibilities, guardianship, welfare, language, motherhood, fatherhood

Health Care Function	Healthy families provide protective family care across the life span, which includes food, clothing, shelter, health care, and safety measures.	Family care giving (e.g., caring for older family members or family members who are disabled), patient and family engagement, access to care (physical, mental, social, etc.), safe water (insurance), environmental health, maternal, infant, and child health, women and men's health, communicable and noncommunicable disease prevention, screening and management, disability and health, nutrition and weight status, wellness policies, family access to safe neighborhoods (leisure and recreation), patient-centered care and teams
Reproductive Function	Families ensure continuity of the intergenerational family and bringing new individuals into the society.	Childbirth, marriage (traditional, same-sex marriages), divorce, adoption, foster care, inheritance, abortions, sex education (abstinence and HPV), contraception (family planning), infertility
Economic Function	Families provide sufficient economic resources (financial, space, and material) and appropriate allocation to meet their dependents' basic needs for shelter, food, and clothing.	Income, welfare, food, housing, job counseling and training, maternal employment, financial assistance (e.g., tax subsidies/credits), financial counseling, equitable/subsidized housing, employment programs, childcare programs, zoning, workplace policies

Defining the Health Policymaking Process

Advocacy also involves a better understanding of the health policymaking processes in one's context of practice to better grasp the prescriptive (how policies occur in the controlled environment) versus the descriptive (how they are actually occurring in real settings) nature of policies. The health policymaking process resembles Ida Jean Orlando's (1990) deliberate nursing process that is nonlinear, cyclical, and made of stages (assessment, diagnosis, planning, implementation, and evaluation) that are influenced by an individual's characteristics and needs as well as their environment.

There are several conceptual approaches for policymaking in the literature (Rawat & Morris, 2016). The most commonly cited models have been the Walt and Gilson's (1994) policy triangle conceptual framework, Kingdon's (1995) policy streams model, and Longest's (2010) policy cycle model. Walt and Gilson's policy triangle conceptual framework helps identify the contextual factors related to policies, such as the people (policymakers, groups, and communities) who influence policy formulation, policy content (components, implementation plans, and gaps), and processes (problem formulation, strategy, implementation, and related challenges). Figure 10.2 shows how these three policy contextual factors are interrelated.

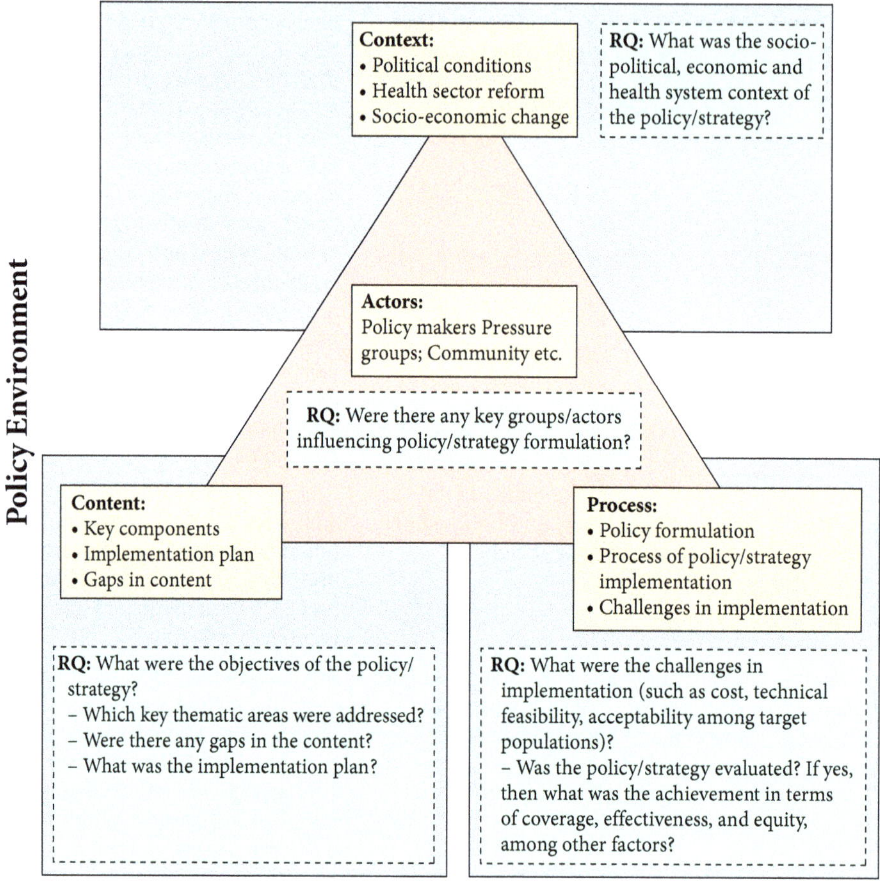

FIGURE 10.2 Policy triangle framework (adapted from Walt & Gilson 1994).

John Kingdon's model proposes multiple streams of policy activity that are used to explain policy formulation process: problem, policy, and political streams. The model sheds light on the key players in each stream who can influence policymaking and how they are central in bringing the three streams together by creating what is called the window of opportunity for policy development or modification (Rawat & Morris, 2016). Longest's (2010) model (2010) focuses on the interrelationships of the actors in three phases of the policy process: policy formulation, policy implementation, and policy modification. The policy formulation includes finding the window of opportunity, defining the problem, and analyzing the political context. The implementation phase refers to the monitoring of the legislative and rule-making process. Lastly, the policy modification phase is when regulations or rules proposed are revised and evaluated. All three models emphasize the involvement of key stakeholders in the policy process and consideration of the contextual influences that include political, ideological, and economic factors (Lilly et al., 2023; Strydom et al., 2010).

In public health practice, the CDC (2013) proposed a systematic health process to guide the development of health policies, which has four major domains (problem identification, policy analysis, strategy and policy development, policy enactment, and policy implementation) and two overachieving domains (stakeholder engagement and evaluation). Table 10.5 provides a summary of each domain, activities involved, and potential *family health* professional roles.

TABLE 10.5 **The Domains of the CDC's Health Policy Process**

Policymaking Stage	**Definition**	**Activities**	**Examples of *Family Health* Professional Roles**
Problem Identification	Clarify and frame the problem or issue in terms of the effect on *population health*.	• Collect, summarize, and interpret information relevant to a problem or issue (e.g., nature of the problem, cause of the problem). • Define the characteristics (e.g., frequency, severity, scope, economic and budgetary impacts) of the problem or issue. • Identify gaps in the data. • Frame the problem or issue in a way that lends itself to potential policy solutions.	Collect and analyze family-focused data from various sources using a biosocialecological perspective beyond the biomedical perspective.
Policy Analysis	Identify different policy options to address the problem/issue and use quantitative and qualitative methods to evaluate the policy options to determine the most effective, efficient, and feasible option.	• Research and identify policy options. • Describe (a) how the policy will impact morbidity and mortality (health impact); (b) the costs to implement the policy and how the costs compare with the benefits (economic and budgetary impacts); and (c) the political and operational factors associated with adoption and implementation (feasibility). • Assess and prioritize policy options.	Review family-related literature for policy options and assess policy options according to health and economic impact to support family-focused health interventions within the context of *population health*.
Strategy and Policy Development	Identify the strategy for getting the policy adopted and how the policy will operate.	• Identify how the policy will operate and what is needed for policy enactment and implementation (e.g., understand jurisdictional context and identify information and capacity needs). • Define strategy for engaging stakeholders and policy actors. • Possibly draft the policy (law, regulation, procedures, actions, etc.).	Participate in providing evidence-based information to inform the *family health* policy development process and drafting guidelines, standards, and organizational policies that support *family health* and functioning.

Policy Enactment	Follow internal or external procedures for getting policy enacted or passed.	• Enact law, regulation, procedure, administrative action, incentive, or voluntary practice.	Monitor policy enactment by serving as the knowledge expert to policymakers/legislators, public officials and administrators, and state and local board members.
Policy Implementation	Translate the enacted policy into action, monitor uptake, and ensure full implementation.	• Translate policy into operational practice and define implementation standards. • Implement regulations, guidelines, recommendations, directives, and organizational policies. • Identify indicators and metrics to evaluate implementation and impact of the policy. • Coordinate resources and build capacity of personnel to implement policy. • Assess implementation and ensure compliance with policy. • Support postimplementation sustainability of policy.	Participate in implementation of the policy at respective levels.
Stakeholder Engagement and Education (Overachieving Domain)	Identify and connect with decision-makers, partners, those affected by the policy, and the general public.	• Identify key stakeholders, including supporters and opponents (e.g., community members, decision-makers, nonprofit, and for-profit agencies). • Assess relevant characteristics (e.g., knowledge, attitudes, needs). • Implement communication strategies and deliver relevant messages and materials. • Solicit input and gather feedback.	Identify and engage relevant stakeholders/actors (e.g., individuals and organizations) throughout the policy process.
Evaluation (Overachieving Domain)	Formally assess the appropriate steps of the policy cycle, including the impact and outcomes of the policy.	• Define evaluation needs, purpose, and intended uses and users. • Conduct evaluation of prioritized evaluation questions (e.g., Was the problem defined in a way that prioritized action? How were stakeholders engaged? Is the policy being implemented as intended? What is the impact of the policy?). • Disseminate evaluation results and facilitate use.	Evaluate the policy process, impact, and outcomes of the policy impact and outcomes to foster EIDM.

Adapted from Centers for Disease Control and Prevention, "CDC Policy Process," CDC.gov, Centers for Disease Control and Prevention, 2022.

Expanding stewardship for evidence-based policy practices by engaging diverse stakeholders from the problem identification process is vital for addressing public health challenges, eliminating health disparities, and improving *population health* outcomes (Bowen & Zwi, 2005; Chhetri & Zacarias, 2021). The following is a list of potential stakeholders who can be considered across the CDC (2019) policy process:

- those who are affected by the policy (directly or indirectly)
- those directly involved with or responsible for the policy
- people whose jobs or lives are affected by the policy or any part of the policy process
- community members and leaders
- neighborhood associations and networks
- those with strong influence in the community (e.g., doctors, media, clergy, health system CEOs)
- state and local health departments
- interest groups (e.g., business, activities, academics)
- funders and other resources providers
- schools and educational groups
- evaluators
- legislators, government officials, and other policymakers

Overall, the health policy process is a complex and multifaceted process that involves incremental decisions and gains. During the evidence-based policymaking process, it is important that *family health* professionals cultivate a culture of curiosity as part of finding the best solutions for complex health topics. Some of the essential questions posed from the policy triangle framework and the multiple streams model include these:

- What was the sociopolitical, economic, and health system context of the policy/strategy?
- Were there any key groups/actors influencing policy/strategy formulation?
- What was the process of policy formulation?
- What were the objectives of the policy/strategy? Which key thematic areas were addressed? Were there any gaps in the content?
- What was the implementation plan?
- What were the challenges in implementation (e.g., cost, technical feasibility, acceptability among target populations)?
- Was the policy/strategy evaluated? If yes, what was the achievement in terms of coverage, effectiveness, and equity, among other factors (Jilcott et al., 2007)?

Likewise, in the emerging field of evidence-based public health, assessing the impact of policies on public health is highly needed to find answers to the most interesting questions to policymakers:

- What are the main priority issues/problems for decision-making?
- What are the potential effective and safe policy options?
- Are the policy options cost-effective and affordable?
- Are the policy options feasible to implement and sustainable?

Although different models of have been proposed to guide planning and evaluation of evidence-based public health, focusing on behavior change, few models have been used in policy evaluation (Jilcott et al., 2007). The conceptual model of nursing and health policy (Russell & Fawcett, 2005) is an evaluation models to guide the assessment of nursing and health policy outcomes such as efficacy and effectiveness of nursing care, equity of access to nursing practice, efficiency, and cost-effective nursing practice delivery systems in a research environment. The model conceptualizes issues of social and economic justice. One other proposed model to assess policy planning and evaluation is the RE-AIM (reach, effectiveness, adoption, implementation, and maintenance) framework (Jilcott et al., 2007). Table 10.6 provides information on how the RE-AIM model can be applied in health policy. Questions that can be addressed in health policy activity using the RE-AIM include these:

- Whose health is to be improved as a result of the policy (e.g., children younger than 8 years old, all residents of a community, smokers)?
- What organization or governing body is responsible for passing, or adopting, the policy?
- Who is responsible for adhering to or complying with the policy?
- What organization, institution, or governing body is responsible for enforcing the policy (Jilcott et al., 2007)?

TABLE 10.6 **RE-AIM Perspective of Policy Translation Issues**

Dimension	Key Issues	Policy Issues, Questions, and Examples
Reach	How many people are impacted, and are they representative or those most at risk?	Extent that populations most exposed to environmental risks are reached
Effectiveness	Impact/risk reduction results Robustness and impact on quality of life. Unanticipated consequences.	How robust or consistent are outcomes? Impact on other prevention activities or environmental risks
Adoption	What percent of the target setting will participate, especially if it is voluntary?	How many and which coal-burning power plants will decrease emissions under Policy A?
Implementation	Cost (and different types of cost) Level of enforcement or delivery variability	What happens to adherence over time? Are some parts of a policy implemented and enforced more consistently that others? What are the economic implications of Policy A in terms of both development and outcomes?
Maintenance	Long-term effects and sustainability Re-invention and variation in policy interpretation	Policy may lose impact over time; policy may be rescinded in difficult economic times New scientific findings may require policy revisions over time

A new evaluation tool known as the public health family impact (PHFI) checklist was designed to facilitate the evaluation of the impact of a health policy or program from a family-focused lens (Crandall et al., 2019). The PHFI checklist is a revised version of the family impact checklist (Bogenschneider et al., 2012). The checklist includes 14 items across four major thinking family principles: family engagement, family responsibility, family stability, and family diversity. Table 10.7 provides the principles and their definitions.

TABLE 10.7 **Principles of the PHFI Checklist**

Family Impact Principle	A "think family"
Family Engagement	Public health practitioners who "think family" ensure that families are actively involved in all programming phases.
Family Responsibility	Public health practitioners who "think family" plan and deliver programs that support and empower family members to perform their responsibilities. The program also supports the family's choices in performing these responsibilities. Examples of such functions include family formation, partner relationships, economic and financial support, childrearing, and caregiving.
Family Stability	Public health practitioners who "think family" strive to plan and deliver programs that encourage stability within the family and recognize the importance of family relationships to individual and *family health*.
Family Diversity	Public health practitioners who "think family" understand that programs can have varied effects on families from different cultures and ethnic backgrounds. Through the program, practitioners acknowledge and respect the diversity of families and do not discriminate against or penalize families based on economic situation, educational attainment, family structure, geographic locale, disability, religious affiliation, or gender and sexual minority status of individual family members.

Factors Influencing the Uptake of Evidence-Based Health Policy-Making Processes Within the 4HEALTHS Context

A call to action is needed to advance family-focused policy development and implementation among *family health* professionals. Prioritizing family capacity during health and illness with the aim of reducing health care spending, improving health systems and *population health* outcomes, improving care and patient experience, and improving provider satisfaction and well-being post-COVID-19 is a timely matter (Kumar et al., 2023). This means that the role of family should be considered in every health policy, standard treatment protocol, and guideline. Most important is the need to acknowledge the role of value judgments in the uptake of evidence-based policy decision-making in health and public health (Strydom et al., 2010). Value discussions can provide a better understanding of how health and access are viewed by key stakeholders (a right of privilege; Jones, 2022; Verulava, 2021).

According to the Merriam-Webster online dictionary, *value judgment* is a judgment of assigning a value to something, such as good or bad. Understanding value judgments that influence decision-making processes at the individual, family, societal, health system, and policy process levels can create windows of opportunities for new health policies or policy modifications/reforms (Shams et al., 2021). In addition, sharing values in the policy decision-making process promotes shared policy options for better individual, family, community, and *population health*. Shared policy strategies promote "objectivity, transparency, public trust and good policy" in the policy-making process (Pelley, 2014, p. A192).

At the individual and *family health* level, possible evidence on value determinants include health beliefs and social norms related to health care–seeking behaviors and access to health care. Policy and politics is an intergenerational family affair (Jennings et al., 2009). Thus, value assessment of individuals' and families' understanding, interpretation, perceptions, and meanings of family, *family health*, cure, and prevention in the policymaking would be appropriate in this case. In addition to understanding disease burdens (the norm in policymaking), *family health* professionals should include evidence that demonstrates how individuals and families conceptualize health and illness from multiple sources by family type, culture, socioeconomic status, region, and country across time.

At the *population health* level, the same is true for community organizations and other interest groups. At the organizational level, the evidence on value assessment should be on how *family health* care in patient and family engagement and clinician–patient partnerships and relationships in curative, promotive, preventive, rehabilitative, and palliative and end-of-life aspects inform health outcomes and health equity. The role of the family as a key decision-maker and partner at the organizational level should also be appraised (Slowther, 2006). Organizational values, vision, and mission are sources of evidence for value determinants for policy formulation or modification related to health care service delivery, financing (reimbursement and incentives), innovative technologies, and health care work force models to promote *population health*. For example, health systems that value family involvement may support organizational policy change to try new family communication strategies (Jazieh et al., 2018).

At the public health level, assuring a well-rounded workforce that is not only competent in conducting and translating basic and intervention research studies but is also informed of policy implementation and dissemination studies and methods is crucial for generating evidence to influence policymaking and uptake in real settings (Chriqui et al., 2023; Innvaer et al., 2002). A competent health workforce and other key stakeholders are instrumental in narrowing the science–policy divide in evidence-based policymaking (Strydom et al., 2010). Emancipatory methods that are integral to empirical, ethical, personal, and aesthetic knowing (Lindell & Chinn, 2024) are highly needed because of their benefits in promoting health equity and fostering necessary value reflexivity among policy implementation scientists (Snell-Rood et al., 2021). Rational decision-making models such as the health belief model and other family and public health promotions models are instrumental in generating value data that can be of use in shared value-driven goal settings and prioritizations to inform evidence-based health policy (Friedman et al., 2003).

Data from participatory family workshops can be utilized to understand the family's value on health and illness for health promotion (Grabowski et al., 2022). Moreover, value-determinant metrics for health equity should be in place to account for both economic and social cost (National Academies of Sciences, Engineering, and Medicine, 2016). Lastly, it is important to acknowledge the need for building capacity to strengthen evidence-based policymaking processes in communities and institutions/organizations to help priority setting for better *population health* (Niessen et al., 2000; WHO, 2021).

Conclusion

This chapter provided an overview of the importance of the role of family in policymaking processes and the role that *family health* care professionals can take to advocate for value recognition in evidence-based policymaking. The information presented provides *family health* professionals and other public health professionals with information that can broaden their horizon on the need for including the family, key stakeholders, and value assessments in health and public health matters.

Suggested Websites

CDC, Policy Process: https://www.cdc.gov/policy/polaris/policyprocess/index.html

Healthy People 2020, Health Equity in Health People 2030: https://health.gov/healthypeople/priority-areas/health-equity-healthy-people-2030

Nursology: https://nursology.net/category/emancipatory-nursing/

WHO, Health Equity: https://www.who.int/health-topics/health-equity#tab=tab_1

WHO Checklist: https://www.who.int/publications/i/item/9789240056145

Suggested Readings

Braveman, P. (2022). Defining health equity. *Journal of the National Medical Association, 114*(6), 593–600.

Chriqui, J. F., Asada, Y., Smith, N. R., Kroll-Desrosiers, A., & Lemon, S. C. (2023). Advancing the science of policy implementation: A call to action for the implementation science field. *Translational Behavioral Medicine, 13*(11), 820–825.

Crandall, A., Novilla, L. K. B., Hanson, C. L., Barnes, M. D., & Novilla, M. L. B. (2019). The public health family impact checklist: A tool to help practitioners think family. *Frontiers in Public Health, 7*, 458526.

Harris, M., & Haines, A. (2010). Brazil's *family health* programme. *BMJ, 341.*

Kumar, S., Bhardwaj, P., & Kumar, N. (2023). Need to bring family to the heart of healthcare as it is home, not a hospital, where healthcare begins and ends. *Indian Journal of Community Medicine, 48*(2), 209–213.

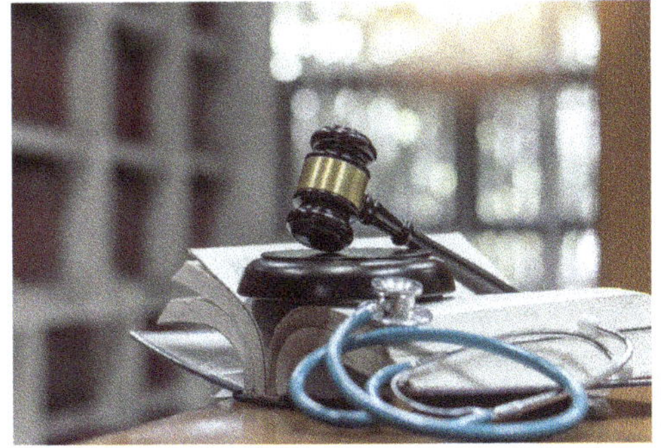
IMG 10.1

Medalie, J. H., & Cole-Kelly, K. (2002). The clinical importance of defining family. *American Family Physician, 65*(7), 1277–1280.

Snell-Rood, C., Jaramillo, E. T., Hamilton, A. B., Raskin, S. E., Nicosia, F. M., & Willging, C. (2021). Advancing health equity through a theoretically critical implementation science. *Translational Behavioral Medicine, 11*(8), 1617–1625.

Reflection Questions

1. What *family health* policy do you want to see changed in health care?
2. What problem did the *family health* policy try to solve?
3. What other policy options do you have in mind to help address the problem?
4. Who do you want to include as a key stakeholder in your policy decision-making team?
5. Is there evidence to bolster your policy option? What is the best available evidence?
6. What values are you bringing with you to the policy decision table to address the problem?
7. How might your values conflict with the other key stakeholders around the policy decision-making table?

References

Al-Janabi, H., Van Exel, J., Brouwer, W., & Coast, J. (2016). A framework for including *family health* spillovers in economic evaluation. *Medical Decision Making, 36*(2), 176–186.

American Academy of Family Physicians. (2022, January). *Poverty and Health.* https://www.aafp.org/about/policies/all/poverty-health.html#:~:text=SDoH%2C%20especially%20poverty%2C%20structural%20racism,primary%20drivers%20of%20health%20inequities.&text=Economic%20prosperity%20can%20provide%20individuals,buffer%20exposure%20to%20health%20risks

Barnes, M. D., Hanson, C. L., Novilla, L. B., Magnusson, B. M., Crandall, A. C., & Bradford, G. (2020). Family-Centered Health Promotion: Perspectives for Engaging Families and Achieving Better Health Outcomes. *Inquiry: A journal of medical care organization, provision and financing, 57.* https://doi.org/10.1177/0046958020923537

Baumrucker, S. J., Stolick, M., Mingle, P., Oertli, K. A., Morris, G. M., & VandeKieft, G. (2012). The principle of distributive justice. *American Journal of Hospice and Palliative Medicine, 29*(2), 151–156.

Bogenschneider, K. (2011, June). Family policy: Why we need it and how to communicate its value. In *United Nations Expert Group Meeting Assessing Family Policies: Confronting family poverty and social exclusion & ensuring work family balance.* https://www.un.org/esa/socdev/family/docs/egm11/Bogenschneider-paper.pdf

Bogenschneider, K. (2014). *Family Policy Matters: How Policy Making affects families and What Professionals Can Do* (3rd ed.). Routledge.

Bogenschneider, K., Little, O. M., Ooms, T., Benning, S., Cadigan, K., & Corbett, T. (2012). The family impact lens: A family-focused, evidence-informed approach to policy and practice. *Family Relations, 61*(3), 514–531.

Bowen, S., & Zwi, A. B. (2005). Pathways to "evidence-informed" policy and practice: a framework for action. *PLoS medicine, 2*(7), e166. https://doi.org/10.1371/journal.pmed.0020166

Buettner-Schmidt, K., & Lobo, M. L. (2012). Social justice: A concept analysis. *Journal of advanced nursing, 68*(4), 948–958.

Braveman, P. (2022). Defining health equity. *Journal of the National Medical Association, 114*(6), 593–600.

Braveman, P. A., Kumanyika, S., Fielding, J., LaVeist, T., Borrell, L. N., Manderscheid, R., & Troutman, A. (2011). Health disparities and health equity: The issue is justice. *American journal of public health, 101*(S1), S149–S155.

Centers for Disease Control and Prevention. (2013). *CDC policy process.* https://www.cdc.gov/policy/polaris/policyprocess/index.html

Centers for Disease Control and Prevention. (2019). *Problem identification: Stakeholders on your policy journey.* https://www.cdc.gov/policy/polaris/policyprocess/problem-identification/index.html

Centers for Disease Control and Prevention, Office of Policy, Performance and Evaluation. (2015). *Policy definition.* https://www.cdc.gov/policy/paeo/process/definition.html

Chhetri, D., & Zacarias, F. (2021). Advocacy for evidence-based policy-making in public health: Experiences and the way forward. *Journal of Health Management, 23*(1), 85–94.

Chriqui, J. F., Asada, Y., Smith, N. R., Kroll-Desrosiers, A., & Lemon, S. C. (2023). Advancing the science of policy implementation: A call to action for the implementation science field. *Translational Behavioral Medicine, 13*(11), 820–825.

Crandall, A., Novilla, L. K. B., Hanson, C. L., Barnes, M. D., & Novilla, M. L. B. (2019). The Public Health Family Impact Checklist: A Tool to Help Practitioners *Think Family*. *Frontiers in public health, 7,* 331. https://doi.org/10.3389/fpubh.2019.00331

Friedman. M. M, R., Bowden, V. R., & Jones, E., G. (2003). *Family nursing: Research, theory, and practice* (5th ed.). Prentice Hall.

Glass, T. A., & McAtee, M. J. (2006). Behavioral science at the crossroads in public health: Extending horizons, envisioning the future. *Social science & medicine, 62*(7), 1650–1671.

Grabowski, D., Pals, R. A. S., Hoeeg, D., Ingersgaard, M. V., DeCosta, P., & Jespersen, L. N. (2022). Participatory family workshops in psychosocial health and illness research: experiences from Danish health promotion projects. *Health promotion international, 37*(Supplement_2), ii73–ii82. https://doi.org/10.1093/heapro/daac014

Haehnel, Q., Whitehead, C., Broadbent, E., Hanson, C. L., & Crandall, A. (2022). What Makes Families Healthy? Examining Correlates of *Family Health* in a Nationally Representative Sample of Adults in the United States. *Journal of Family Issues, 43*(12), 3103–3126. https://doi.org/10.1177/0192513X211042841

Hanson, C. L., Crandall, A., Barnes, M. D., Magnusson, B., Novilla, M. L. B., & King, J. (2019). Family-Focused Public Health: Supporting Homes and Families in Policy and Practice. *Frontiers in public health, 7,* 59. https://doi.org/10.3389/fpubh.2019.00059

Innvaer, S., Vist, G., Trommald, M., & Oxman, A. (2002). Health policy-makers' perceptions of their use of evidence: A systematic review. *Journal of health services research & policy, 7*(4), 239–244.

Jazieh, A. R., Volker, S., & Taher, S. (2018). Involving the family in patient care: A culturally tailored communication model. *Global Journal on Quality and Safety in Healthcare, 1*(2), 33–37.

Jennings, M. K., Stoker, L., & Bowers, J. (2009). Politics across generations: Family transmission reexamined. *The Journal of Politics, 71*(3), 782–799.

Jilcott, S., Ammerman, A., Sommers, J., & Glasgow, R. E. (2007). Applying the RE-AIM framework to assess the public health impact of policy change. *Annals of Behavioral Medicine, 34*(2), 105–114.

Jones L. (2022). Including a wider range of values in healthcare policy: how can public value evaluation help?. *Future healthcare journal, 9*(3), 222–225. https://doi.org/10.7861/fhj.2022-0109

Kalaitzidis, E., & Jewell, P. (2015). The concept of advocacy in nursing: A critical analysis. *The health care manager, 34*(4), 308–315.

Kingdon, J. W. (1995). *Agendas, Alternatives, and Public Policies.* Longman.

Kokorelias, K. M., Gignac, M. A., Naglie, G., & Cameron, J. I. (2019). Towards a universal model of family centered care: A scoping review. *BMC health services research, 19,* 1–11.

Kumar, S., Bhardwaj, P., & Kumar, N. (2023). Need to Bring Family to the Heart of Healthcare as it is Home, not a Hospital, Where Healthcare Begins and Ends. *Indian Journal of Community Medicine, 48*(2), 209–213.

Lilly, K., Kean, B., Hallett, J., Robinson, S., & Selvey, L. A. (2023). Factors of the policy process influencing health in all policies in local government: A scoping review. *Frontiers in Public Health, 11*, 1010335.

Lindell, D., & Chinn, P. (January, 19, 2024). *Emancipatory and Sociopolitical Knowing.* Nursology. https://nursology.net/patterns-of-knowing-in-nursing/emancipatory-knowing/#:~:text=Emancipatory%20knowing%20is%20integral%20to,practices%20that%20influence%20nursing%20practice

Longest B. (2010). *Health policymaking in the United States* (5th ed.). Health Administration Press.

MacKean, G. L., Thurston, W. E., & Scott, C. M. (2005). Bridging the divide between families and health professionals' perspectives on family-centred care. *Health expectations, 8*(1), 74–85.

Medalie, J. H., & Cole-Kelly, K. (2002). The clinical importance of defining family. *American Family Physician, 65*(7), 1277–1280.

Melnyk, B. M., Fineout-Overholt, E., Stillwell, S. B., & Williamson, K. M. (2010). Evidence-based practice: Step by step: the seven steps of evidence-based practice. *The American Journal of Nursing, 110*(1), 51–53.

National Academies of Sciences, Engineering, and Medicine. (2016). *Metrics That Matter for Population Health Action: Workshop Summary.* Washington, DC: The National Academies Press. https://doi.org/10.17226/21899.

Niessen, L. W., Grijseels, E. W., & Rutten, F. F. (2000). The evidence-based approach in health policy and health care delivery. *Social science & medicine, 51*(6), 859–869.

Orlando I. J. (1990). The dynamic nurse-patient relationship. Function, process, and principles. 1960. *NLN publications*, (15-2341), v, 1–97.

Ortiz, Y., Suárez-Villa, M., & Expósito, M. (2017). Importance and recognition of the family in health care: A reflection for nursing. *Nurse Care Open Acces J, 3*(5).

Pan American Health Organization. (2020). *The Essential Public Health Functions in the Americas: A Renewal for the 21st Century.*

Pelley, J. L. (2014). Science and policy: Understanding the role of value judgments. *Environmental health perspectives, 122*(7), A192. https://doi.org/10.1289/ehp.122-A192

Rawat, P., & Morris, J. C. (2016). Kingdon's "streams" model at thirty: Still relevant in the 21st century? *Politics & Policy, 44*(4), 608–638.

Regional Office for Europe, European Observatory on Health Systems and Policies, Rechel, B., Williams, G., & Wismar, M. (2019). What are the conditions for successful health policy implementation? Lessons learnt from WHO's regional health policy health 2020: Policy brief. https://iris.who.int/handle/10665/340360

Russell, G. E., & Fawcett, J. (2005). The conceptual model for nursing and health policy revisited. *Policy, Politics, & Nursing Practice, 6*(4), 319–326.

Shams, L., Sari, A. A., Yazdani, S., & Nasiri, T. (2021). Model for value-based policy-making in health systems. *International Journal of Preventive Medicine, 12.*

Slowther, A. M. (2006). The role of the family in patient care. *Clinical Ethics, 1*(4), 191–193.

Snell-Rood, C., Jaramillo, E. T., Hamilton, A. B., Raskin, S. E., Nicosia, F. M., & Willging, C. (2021). Advancing health equity through a theoretically critical implementation science. *Translational behavioral medicine, 11*(8), 1617–1625.

Strydom, W. F., Funke, N., Nienaber, S., Nortje, K., & Steyn, M. (2010). Evidence-based policymaking: A review. *South African Journal of Science, 106*(5), 1–8.

Trzcinski, E. (1995). An ecological perspective on family policy: A conceptual and philosophical framework. *J Fam Econ Iss, 16*, 7–33. https://doi.org/10.1007/BF02353665

U.S. Department of Health and Human Services. (2022). *Health Equity and Health Disparities Environmental Scan.* Office of the Assistant Secretary for Health, Office of Disease Prevention and Health Promotion.

Verulava, T. (2021). Access to Healthcare as a Fundamental Right or Privilege? *Siriraj Medical Journal, 73*(10). 721–726. https://doi.org/10.33192/Smj.2021.92

Walt, G., & Gilson, L. (1994). Reforming the health sector in developing countries: The central role of policy analysis. *Health policy and planning, 9*(4), 353–370. https://doi.org/10.1093/heapol/9.4.353

Weiss-Laxer, N. S., Crandall, A., Hughes, M. E., & Riley, A. W. (2020). Families as a Cornerstone in 21st Century Public Health: Recommendations for Research, Education, Policy, and Practice. *Frontiers in public health, 8*, 503. https://doi.org/10.3389/fpubh.2020.00503

World Health Organization. (2013). *Family as centre of health development: Report of the regional meeting, Bangkok, Thailand, 18–20 March 2013* (No. SEA-HSD-363). WHO Regional Office for South-East Asia.

World Health Organization. (2021). *Evidence, policy, impact: WHO guide for evidence-informed decision-making.* Geneva: World Health Organization. Licence: CC BY-NC-SA 3.0 IGO. https://iris.who.int/bitstream/handle/10665/350994/9789240039872-eng.pdf?sequence=1

Zahidie, A., Asif, S., & Iqbal, M. (2023). Building on the Health Policy Analysis Triangle: Elucidation of the Elements. *Pakistan journal of medical sciences, 39*(6), 1865–1868. https://doi.org/10.12669/pjms.39.6.7056

Figure credits

Fig. 10.1: Thomas A. Glass and Matthew J. McAfee, "An Illustration of Risk Regulators from an Ecological (i.e. Social and Biological) Context," *Social Science & Medicine*, vol. 62, no. 7, p. 1661. Copyright © 2006 by Elsevier B.V.

Fig. 10.1a: Copyright © 2015 Depositphotos/cteconsulting.

Fig. 10.2: Gill Walt and Lucy Gilson, "Policy Triangle Framework," *Health Policy and Planning*, vol. 9, no. 4. Copyright © 1994 by Oxford University Press.

IMG 10.1: Copyright © 2021 Depositphotos/Chinnapong.

PART III

FAMILY HEATH PRACTICE OPPORTUNITIES

CHAPTER 11

Experiential Learning for 21st-Century Family Health Professionals

Education must not simply teach work, it must teach life.

—W. E. B. Du Bois

Learning Objectives

By the end of this chapter, learners will do the following:

- Describe the meaning of experiential learning, internship, volunteerism, and service-learning.
- Describe the importance of service-learning opportunities in higher education.
- Describe the benefits of family-focused service-learning opportunities in *family health* care.
- Identify the core principles in developing service-learning pedagogy.

Before you read on, consider the following questions:

- What is the difference among clinical, volunteering, and service-learning experiences?
- What are the benefits of service-learning in *family health* and family science?
- How can you effectively engage with families through service-learning?

Importance of Experiential Learning in Higher Education

Experiential learning is a common terminology in the literature that has evolved from various schools of thoughts, including the classic work of John Dewey and David. A. Kolb (Kraft, 1990). It is described as the process of learning from experience also known as "learning by doing," "experienced-based learning," "applied experiential learning," and "real-world learning" while promoting student participation and self-evaluation/reflection (Gentry, 1990, p. 10). During experiential learning, learners observe, review, and reflect on what they have practiced and consciously link the knowledge/content to practice (Bartle,

2015). The process reflects the stages in Kolb's (1984) experiential learning cycle known as concrete experience (feeling or experiencing), reflective observation (watching), abstract conceptualization (thinking), and active experimentation (doing). Experiential learning can take different forms and structure (Austin & Rust, 2015). These include internships, cooperative education, simulation (Underberg, 2003), study abroad (Strange & Gibson, 2017) and service-learning (Moore, 2010). Educational programs that offer experiential learning opportunities positively influence student recruitment, retention, completion rate, and future enrollment in postgraduate studies (Bartle, 2015).

Importance of Service-Learning Programs

Simulation and service-learning (SL) pedagogy have benefitted students in health and health-related education programs in many different ways (Siefer, 1998; Stewart & Wubbena, 2015; Zhu et al., 2022). For example, simulation learning experiences promote students acquisition of interprofessional competencies and standards (Fewster-Thuente & Batteson, 2018), facilitate nursing students' family assessment clinical skills in a home environment (see examples in suggested website for the *family health* promotion scenarios at the end of the chapter), and foster patient-centered communication and empathy skills (Bauchat et al., 2016). Service-learning opportunities have also contributed to health care professionals' acquisitions of clinical reasoning skills and interprofessional competencies (Seif et al., 2014). In addition, SL has helped medical and nursing students engage with vulnerable populations to address SDOH, thus building health equity and eliminating health disparities (Bickerton et al., 2020; Fredrick, 2011; Gillis & Mac Lellan, 2010; Sabo et al., 2015). Patient-centered SL opportunities reinforce skills in communication and building partnership (Lévesque et al., 2013; Parent, Jones, Phillips et al., 2016). In global settings, SL enhances globalization (García & Longo, 2013) and global health competencies (Evert et al., 2007).

Overall, SL programs provide students with experiential opportunities that go beyond career development competencies to include preparations of generations of responsible citizens (Bringle & Hatcher, 1996). Thus, most instructors help students achieve outcomes in general categories of academic enhancement, personal growth, and civic learning (Ash & Clayton, 2009). To achieve mutual benefits, quality SL programs need well-articulated goals that are explicitly student and community focused (Clayton et al., 2013). For example, community partners, not just students, should benefit from the SL initiatives (Hamner et al., 2002).

Components in SL programs include a "community service, preparation/reflection, an activity in response to community needs, learning about service context, roles in the community, and the connection between academics and service-learning activities" (Douglas, 2009, p. 1). According to Barbara Holland, a U.S. based service-learning expert, SL primarily focuses on all key players (students, faculty, community, and institution; Kenworthy-U'Ren et al., 2006). Enhancement of students' depth of learning and critical thinking skills through guided reflections is an essential component of SL programs (Elverson & Klawiter, 2019, Hatcher et al., 2011; Nierenberg et al., 2018). Reflection activities embedded in a course with clear guidelines and directions positively promote personal growth and community self-efficacy (Sanders et al., 2016). However, it is important to note that SL differs from internships and volunteerism. Internships primarily focus on students who are expected to meet professional-led learning goals for career and professional development, while volunteerism mostly benefits communities and is largely self-directed with or without assessed learning goals (Kenworthy-U'Ren et al., 2006). Internships and volunteerism may or may not include reflections. Figure 11.1 shows the differences among internship, SL, and volunteerism per Holland's experimental pedagogy continuum.

Experiential Pedagogy	Internships	Service-learning	Volunteerism
Primary Beneficiary	Student	Mutual benefits	Community
Inclusion of Reflection	Sometimes	Always	Rarely

FIGURE 11.1 Experiential pedagogy continuum (Kenworthy-U'Ren et al., 2006, p. 122).

Benefits of Family-Focused SL Programs

In family science, family-focused experiential learning programs facilitate concepts of family through students' reflections of their own family experience and experiences working with or for families in societies (Eby, 2001; Jacobson et al., 2011; Wiersma-Mosley & Garrison, 2022). The programs provide *family health* professional trainees with learning opportunities to assess and address health-related individual, family, and societal risk and protective factors in places where families live (Finello et al., 2016; Peacock et al., 2013). For example, home visiting programs promote assessment of social determinants of health (SDOH) in family medical (Clair et al., 2019; Cline et al., 2020; Essel et al., 2016; Nothelle et al., 2018; Pereles, 2000) and family nursing (Kearney et al., 2000; Kemp et al., 2011). SL has also been used in family life education to engage students in human development content through integrated intergenerational projects (Hamon & Way, 2001; Lamson et al., 2006) and in family volunteering as a tool for strengthening relationships and family functioning whereby families learn together while giving back to their community (Lewton & Nievar, 2012).

Core Principle of SL Programs

The quality of any SL program depends on how the faculty and community work together to design culturally appropriate activities that match the learning goals for the students (Alexander-Ruff & Kinion, 2019). In other words, instructor and community interests must align (Kenworthy-U'Ren et al., 2006). To help facilitate this process, McKinnon and Fealy (2011) propose seven global core principles for faculty to consider when developing service culturally effective and sustainable SL programs that foster ethical and compassionate learning experiences: compassion, curiosity, courage, collaboration, creativity, capacity building, and competence (see Table 11.1).

TABLE 11.1 **Global Core Principles for Developing Service**

Core Principle	Description	Faculty Considerations
Compassion	This is the impetus or driver for change and key motivator for establishing the service program.	• Do you have passion to teach new professionals? • Do you have passion for the clients and communities you plan to serve? • Do you aspire for social responsibility?
Curiosity	Exploring ways to create opportunities for students can lead to innovative approaches to program development.	• Are you curious about other cultures and issues? • Are you interested in the learning needs of students? • Are you curious about the learning site?
Courage	Have the commitment, trust, willingness, and ability to lead by example.	• Are you ready to embark on uncertain, unfair, sometimes risk territories with the confidence of gaining personal and professional rewards?
Collaboration	Create dynamic partnerships between educational institutions and communities, whereby the needs of program participants and the communities they serve are of equal importance.	• Are you ready and capable to negotiate key program structures and processes, such as who controls access to resources, the relative contributions of staff, and the pattern and flow of relationships in a reciprocal exchange manner?
Creativity	Create effective program development both at the macro level, when partnerships are sought and formed, and at the micro level of service provision and in the conduct of pedagogical activities associated with the service.	• Can you provide opportunities for innovation that are especially appropriate for helping to link education and a commitment to community service either locally or globally? • Do you work effectively with individuals and communities?
Capacity building	Empower the host community to develop the necessary capacity to create its own resources for health care and community development.	• Do you avoid service interventions that cultivate a dependent relationship? • Do you make sure institutional-community partnerships are based not only on the host community's needs for health improvement, but that they build on identified strengths and assets? • Is the program ethical? • Is the program demonstrating components of capacity building within communities that include synergy, sustainability, and evaluation research, in which a mutually beneficial relationship is the ultimate outcome?
Competence	This is the means of measuring the behaviors/competencies of all three partners: students, faculty, and community	• Does the program include evaluation processes of cultural competence, civic engagement, and student leadership skills?

Source: McKinnon and Fealy (2011)

Conclusion

In this chapter, experiential learning options in health care education courses and programs in higher education were introduced. Specifically, SL was highlighted with key considerations for developing, implementing, and evaluating quality future family-focused programs.

Suggested Websites

American Red Cross: https://www.redcross.org/about-us/who-we-are/nursing-health/academic-service-learning.html

Association of Community Health Nursing Educators (ACHNE): https://www.achne.org/aws/ACHNE/pt/sp/innovative-teaching-strategies

National medical fellowships: https://nmfonline.org/

National Youth Leadership Council: https://nylc.org/

Sigma Theta Tau International Honor Society of Nursing: https://www.sigmanursing.org/advance-elevate/research/international-collaborative-research-guidelines

Suggested Readings

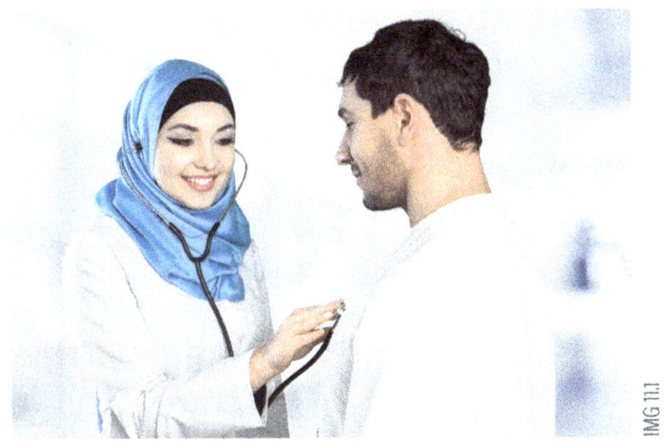
IMG 11.1

Ash, S. L., & Clayton, P. H. (2009). Generating, deepening, and documenting learning: The power of critical reflection in applied learning. *Journal of Applied Learning in Higher Education*, *1*, 25–48.

Eustace et al., Geriatric *Family Health* Promotion Simulation Strategy: https://www.achne.org/aws/ACHNE/asset_manager/get_file/641038?ver=1

Eustace et al., Teenager *Family Health* Promotion Simulation Strategy: https://www.achne.org/aws/ACHNE/asset_manager/get_file/641037?ver=1

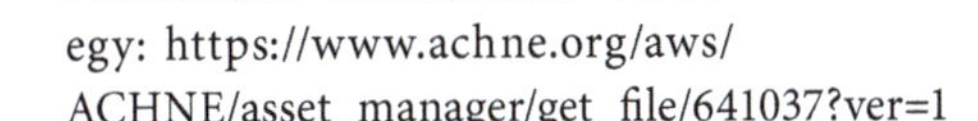
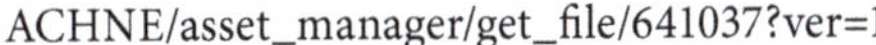

Essel, K. D., Yalamanchi, S., Hysom, E., & Lichtenstein, C. (2016). Healthy homes, healthy futures: A home visitation curriculum for pediatric residents. *MedEdPORTAL*, *12*, 10480.

Fredrick, N. (2011). Teaching social determinants of health through mini-service learning experiences. *MedEdPORTAL*, *7*, 9056.

Kenworthy-U'Ren, A., Petri, A., & Taylor, M. L. (2006). Components of successful service-learning programs: Notes from Barbara Holland, director of the US National Service-Learning Clearinghouse. *International Journal of Case Method Research and Application*, *18*(2), 120–129.

McKinnon, T. H., & Fealy, G. (2011). Core principles for developing global service-learning programs in nursing. *Nursing Education Perspectives*, *32*(2), 95–101.

Reflection Questions

1. Describe experiential learning.
2. Why did you participate in the experience?
3. What did you learn about yourself in the experience?
4. What knowledge did you apply?
5. How did the experience help you become a good citizen?
6. Did the experience involve working with or for families? Briefly explain.
7. What did you do after the experiential learning?

References

Ash, S. L., & Clayton, P. H. (2009). Generating, deepening, and documenting learning: The power of critical reflection in applied learning. *Journal of Applied Learning in Higher Education, 1*, 25–48.

Austin, M. J., & Rust, D. Z. (2015). Developing an Experiential Learning Program: Milestones and Challenges. *International Journal of Teaching and Learning in Higher Education, 27*(1), 143–153.

Bartle, E. (2015, March). Experiential learning: An overview. *Institute for teaching and learning innovation. Australia: The University of Queensland.* https://itali.uq.edu.au/files/1264/Discussion-paper-Experiential_learning%20_an_overview.pdf

Bauchat, J. R., Seropian, M., & Jeffries, P. R. (2016). Communication and empathy in the patient-centered care model—why simulation-based training is not optional. *Clinical Simulation in Nursing, 12*(8), 356–359.

Bickerton, L., Siegart, N., & Marquez, C. (2020). Medical Students Screen for Social Determinants of Health: A Service Learning Model to Improve Health Equity. *PRiMER, 4*, 27. https://doi.org/10.22454/PRiMER.2020.225894

Bringle, R. G., Clayton, P. H., & Hatcher, J. A. (2013). Research on service learning: An introduction. In R. G. Bringle, B. J. Hatcher & P. H. Clayton *Research on service learning* (1st Ed., pp. 335–358). Routledge.

Bringle, R. G., & Hatcher, J. A. (1996). Implementing service learning in higher education. *The Journal of Higher Education, 67*(2), 221–239.

Clair, M. C. S., Sundberg, G., & Kram, J. J. F. (2019). Incorporating Home Visits in a Primary Care Residency Clinic: The Patient and Physician Experience. Journal of patient-centered research and reviews, 6(3), 203–209. https://doi.org/10.17294/2330-0698.1701

Cline, M., Pagels, P., Gimpel, N., & Day, P. G. (2020). Utilizing Home Visits to Assess Social Determinants of Health During Family Medicine Residency. *PRiMER, 4*, 31. https://doi.org/10.22454/PRiMER.2020.448665

Eby, J. W. (2001). The promise of service-learning for family science: An overview. *Journal of Teaching in Marriage & Family, 1*(3), 1–13.

Elverson, C. A., & Klawiter, R. (2019). Using guided reflection to link cultural and service learning in a study abroad course. *Journal of professional nursing, 35*(3), 181–186.

Essel, K. D., Yalamanchi, S., Hysom, E., & Lichtenstein, C. (2016). Healthy homes, healthy futures: A home visitation curriculum for pediatric residents. *MedEdPORTAL, 12*, 10480.

Evert, J., Bazemore, A., Hixon, A., & Withy, K. (2007). Going global: considerations for introducing global health into family medicine training programs. *Family medicine, 39*(9), 659–665.

Fewster-Thuente, L., & Batteson, T. J. (2018). Kolb's experiential learning theory as a theoretical underpinning for interprofessional education. *Journal of allied health, 47*(1), 3–8.

Finello, K. M., Terteryan, A., & Riewerts, R. J. (2016). Home visiting programs: What the primary care clinician should know. *Current problems in pediatric and adolescent health care, 46*(4), 101–125.

Fredrick, N. (2011). Teaching social determinants of health through mini-service learning experiences. *MedEdPORTAL, 7,* 9056.

García, N. A., & Longo, N. V. (2013). Going global: Re-framing service-learning in an interconnected world. *Journal of higher education outreach and engagement, 17*(2), 111–136.

Gentry, J. W. (1990). What is experiential learning. *Guide to business gaming and experiential learning, 9*(1), 20–32.

Gillis, A., & Mac Lellan, M. (2010). Service learning with vulnerable populations: review of the literature. International journal of nursing education scholarship, 7, Article41. https://doi.org/10.2202/1548-923X.2041

Hamner, J. B., Wilder, B., & Byrd, L. (2007). Lessons learned: Integrating a service learning community-based partnership into the curriculum. *Nursing outlook, 55*(2), 106–110.

Hamon, R. R., & Way, C. E. (2001). Integrating intergenerational service-learning into the family science curriculum. *Journal of Teaching in Marriage & Family, 1*(3), 65–83.

Hatcher, J. A., Bringle, R. G., & Muthiah, R. (2004). Designing Effective Reflection: What Matters to Service-Learning? *Michigan Journal of Community Service Learning, 11*(1), 38–46.

Jacobson, J., Oravecz, L., Falk, A., & Osteen, P. (2011). Proximate outcomes of service-learning among family studies undergraduates. *Family Science Review, 16*(1), 22–33.

Kearney, M. H., York, R., & Deatrick, J. A. (2000). Effects of home visits to vulnerable young families. *Journal of nursing scholarship, 32*(4), 369–375.

Kenworthy-U'Ren, A., Petri, A., & Taylor, M. L. (2006). Components of successful service-learning programs: Notes from Barbara Holland, director of the US National Service-Learning Clearinghouse. *International Journal of Case Method Research and Application, 18*(2), 120–129.

Kemp, L., Harris, E., McMahon, C., Matthey, S., Vimpani, G., Anderson, T., ... & Zapart, S. (2011). Child and family outcomes of a long-term nurse home visitation programme: A randomised controlled trial. *Archives of disease in childhood, 96*(6), 533–540.

Kolb, D. A. (1984). *Experiential learning: Experience as the source of learning and development.* Prentice Hall.

Kraft, R. J. (1990). Experiential learning. In J.C. Miles. & S. Priest (Eds.) *Adventure education,* (pp.175–183. State College, PA

Lamson, A., Ballard, S. M., & LaClaire, S. (2006). Creating an effective intergenerational service-learning experience: Components of the UGIVE Program. *Journal of Teaching in Marriage and Family, 6,* 186–205.

Lévesque, M. C., Hovey, R. B., & Bedos, C. (2013). Advancing patient-centered care through transformative educational leadership: A critical review of health care professional preparation for patient-centered care. *Journal of Healthcare Leadership,* 5, 35–46. https://doi.org/10.2147/JHL.S30889

Lewton, A. R., & Nievar, M. A. (2012). Strengthening families through volunteerism: Integrating family volunteerism and family life education. *Marriage & Family Review, 48*(7), 689–710

McKinnon, T. H., & Fealy, G. (2011). Core principles for developing global service-learning programs in nursing. *Nursing Education Perspectives, 32*(2), 95–101.

Molee, L. M., Henry, M. E., Sessa, V. I., & McKinney-Prupis, E. R. (2011). Assessing learning in service-learning courses through critical reflection. *Journal of Experiential Education, 33*(3), 239–257.

Moore, D. T. (2010, May, 4). Forms and issues in experiential learning. In D. A. Qualters & C. Wehlburg Experiential Education: Making the Most of Learning Outside the Classroom. *New Directions for Teaching and Learning, 124* (pp. 3–13).

Nierenberg, S., Hughes, L. P., Warunek, M., Gambacorta, J. E., Dickerson, S. S., & Campbell-Heider, N. (2018). Nursing and Dental Students' Reflections on Interprofessional Practice After a Service-Learning Experience in Appalachia. *Journal of Dental Education, 82*(5), 454–461.

Nothelle, S. K., Christmas, C., & Hanyok, L. A. (2018). First-year internal medicine residents' reflections on nonmedical home visits to high-risk patients. *Teaching and learning in medicine, 30*(1), 95–102.

Parent, K., Jones, K., Phillips, L., Stojan, J. N., & House, J. B. (2016). Teaching patient-and family-centered care: integrating shared humanity into medical education curricula. *AMA Journal of Ethics, 18*(1), 24–32.

Peacock, S., Konrad, S., Watson, E., Nickel, D., & Muhajarine, N. (2013). Effectiveness of home visiting programs on child outcomes: a systematic review. *BMC public health, 13*, 1–14.

Pereles, L. (2000). Home visits: An access to care issue for the 21st century. *Canadian Family Physician, 46*(10), 2044–2048.

Sabo, S., De Zapien, J., Teufel-Shone, N., Rosales, C., Bergsma, L., & Taren, D. (2015). Service learning: A vehicle for building health equity and eliminating health disparities. *American Journal of Public Health, 105*(S1), S38–S43.

Sanders, M. J., Van Oss, T., & McGeary, S. (2016). Analyzing reflections in service learning to promote personal growth and community self-efficacy. *Journal of Experiential Education, 39*(1), 73–88.

Seif, G., Coker-Bolt, P., Kraft, S., Gonsalves, W., Simpson, K., & Johnson, E. (2014). The development of clinical reasoning and interprofessional behaviors: service-learning at a student-run free clinic. *Journal of interprofessional care, 28*(6), 559–564.

Seifer, S. D. (1998). Service-learning: Community-campus partnerships for health professions education. *Academic medicine, 73*(3), 273–277.

Stewart, T., & Wubbena, Z. C. (2015). A systematic review of service-learning in medical education: 1998–2012. *Teaching and Learning in Medicine, 27*(2), 115–122.

Strange, H., & Gibson, H. J. (2017). An investigation of experiential and transformative learning in study abroad programs. *Frontiers: The Interdisciplinary Journal of Study Abroad, 29*(1), 85–100.

Underberg, K. E. (2003, August). Experiential learning and simulation in health care education. *SSM, 9*(4), 31–34, 36.

Wiersma-Mosley, J. D., & Garrison, M. B. (2022). Developing intercultural competence among students in family science: The importance of service learning experiences. *Family Relations, 71*(5), 2070–2083.

Zhu, Z., Xing, W., Liang, Y., Hong, L., & Hu, Y. (2022). Nursing students' experiences with service learning: A qualitative systematic review and meta-synthesis. *Nurse Education Today, 108*, 105206. https://doi.org/10.1016/j.nedt.2021.105206

Figure credits

Fig. 11.1: Amy Kenworthy-U"Ren, Alexis Petri, and Marilyn L. Taylor, "Experiential Pedagogy Continuum," *International Journal of Case Method Research and Application*, vol. 18, p. 122. Copyright © 2006 by Amy Kenworthy-U"Ren, Alexis Petri, and Marilyn L. Taylor.

IMG 11.1: Copyright © 2017 Depositphotos/billiondigital.

CHAPTER 12

Career in Family Health Teams

A Connecting Bridge Between Individual and Population Health in 21st-Century Person-Centered Health Care and Public Health Systems

Bridges symbolize change and flexibility.

—Mehmet Murat ildan

Learning Objectives

By the end of this chapter, learners will do the following:

- Examine the following key terminologies: *family health* teams, scope of practice, licensure, and credentials.
- Describe the importance of *family health* teams for the 21st-century person-centered health care and public health systems.
- Identify health care settings for 21st-century *family health* teams in person-centered health care and public health systems.
- Describe the essential knowledge, skills, and attitudes for 21st-century *family health* teams in person-centered health care and public health systems.

Before you read on, consider the following questions:

- Why do you think *family health* professional teams are vital for improving individual and *population health* within the 4HEALTH context?
- How can someone become a competent *family health* team member in 21st-century person-centered health care and public health systems?

The Importance of Culturally Competent Family Health Professional Teams

As reflected in the previous chapters, the need for family science in health care is evident. The overall evidence related to health care delivery systems clearly supports the need to intervene with family systems to bridge the gaps between individual-focused and *population health* outcomes (Anderson & Tomlison, 1992; Barnes et al., 2020; Doherty & McCubbin, 1985). Innovative multidisciplinary and interdisciplinary family interventions that encompass the prevention, screening, treatment, management, and rehabilitation of biopsychosocial problems are essential services in health care (Doherty, 1985). These essential services rely on a qualified and competent workforce that is ready to deal with complex health care needs in diverse settings utilizing solutions beyond biomedical strategies. As mentioned in previous chapters, behavioral, psychological and social solutions are needed to meet SDOH within the contexts of the individual, family, population, and public health (4HEALTH).

Diverse Health Care Settings for Family Health Teams in the 21st Century

The diverse health care settings suitable for delivery of essential health and public health services in the 21st century include traditional and nontraditional places where individuals and families live (home), pray (faith based), work (employment sites), learn (schools), and play (community centers). For example, potential traditional and nontraditional settings for direct care or indirect care family science professional include these (National Council on Family Relations (NCFR), 2023):

- Hospitals, health clinics, or agencies:
  - Disability services organizations
  - Funeral services
  - Holistic health centers
  - Hospice programs
  - Nutrition education programs
  - Prenatal and maternity services
  - Public health programs and services
- Community education organizations
- Courts and corrections systems
- Development or support organizations for children, youth, or seniors
- Family or human services agencies (nonprofit, faith based, secular)
- Government agencies (administrative or human services)
- Military-related organizations
- Policy analysis, advocacy, or research organizations
- Private practice or consulting
- Schools (K–12, early childhood)
- Universities and colleges (academic units and/or cooperative extension)
- Workplace education programs

The ultimate goal for establishing these diverse settings in the delivery of essential health and public health service delivery is to achieve health for all and improve *population health* outcomes. Efforts to adopt value-based approaches and strengthen integrated services and systems of care (i.e., hospital, primary, public health) are also part of the process (Zieff et al., 2020). In addition, initiatives that promote health for all across the life span through integrated family- and community-oriented primary health care have been on the rise. Examples include the HEALTH21 framework by the WHO's Regional Office for Europe (1998) and the U.S. healthcare for all framework proposed by the American Academy of Family Physicians (AAFP, 2009). Both frameworks establish the need to increase access to comprehensive care, improve coordination and continuity of care, care management, and patient and family engagement through a well-rounded interdisciplinary workforce.

Specifically, there is a strong need to develop and implement health care teams using a *family health* team approach (Gocan et al., 2014; Soklaridis, Oandasan & Kimpton, 2007; Somé et al., 2020). *Family health* teams (FHTs) are instrumental in ensuring the delivery of essential service, including continuum of care among family/home, the community, social support systems, and health care systems. FHT members are made up of health care workers with career backgrounds such as family and community / public health nursing, family medicine, medical family therapy, medical/clinical social work, and clinical family psychology / mental health and family life education. Most FHTs include physicians and nurses, but there are efforts to integrate pharmacists (Gillespie et al., 2017), physical therapists (Cott et al., 2011), social workers (Ashcroft et al., 2018), and mental health providers (Gryschek & Pinto, 2015) and to collaborate with public health teams (Green et al. 2013). These efforts facilitate the integration of essential behavioral, social, psychological, and spiritual (clerical) services.

The FHT can be formed in private or public health care settings. Private settings can be for profit or nonprofit. The roles and responsibilities of FHT members vary depending on credentials (licenses, certificates, and educational backgrounds) and level of involvement with families as per each member's scope of practice as either a generalist or specialist with advanced practice. FHT members' scopes of practice include legal standards of practice. Educational background includes medical or nonmedical and a family science background or a family science degree. Licenses, which are legally binding documents, show a FHT member has met the requirements and competencies of a specific professional program to perform a related job.

FHT members may demonstrate professional certifications to verify advanced skills in a given area. For example, licensed registered nurses (RNs) can be certified as generalists to work with well-functioning families, whereas advanced nurse practitioners can be licensed and certified to work with families experiencing interpersonal challenges (Hassan et al., 2022). Likewise, physicians and nurses are usually academically prepared, as well as licensed and certified to perform certain biomedical tasks (direct care or indirect care activities) within their full scopes of practice (Coutinho et al., 2015; Eagar et al., 2010; Heale et al., 2018).

Essential Competencies for FHTs in Primary Care and Community-Oriented Care

It is important to note that the major goal of the FHT in primary care and community-oriented care is to change families' experiences within family processes. For example, changing targets include family processes such as interactive (e.g., communication, support); developmental (e.g., transitions, tasks); coping (e.g., problem solving, adaptation); integrity (e.g., shared meanings, values); and health (e.g., *family health* beliefs, *family health* practices) processes (Anderson, 2000; Anderson & Tomlinson, 1992). Thus, to achieve this goal, there needs to be a competent FHT member workforce.

As the largest health care profession, nursing has been an integral part of FHTs in primary and community care (Lopes-Júnior, 2021; Norful et al., 2017; WHO Regional Office for Europe, 2000). Nurses practicing to the full extent of their professional scope of practice are capable of providing quality, cost-effective, and efficient services such as episodic and preventive care, chronic disease management, and practice operations, including telephone triage, assessment and documentation, hospital transition management, delegated care, health coaching, medication reconciliation, staff supervision, and improvement in leadership (Smolowitz et al., 2015). In addition to clinical skills within one's scope of practice, competencies in building relationships with individuals, families, and communities; assessment of a family system's response to health and illness; and the application of evidence-based informed family interventions and application of family strengths are unique to *family health* professionals. The 21st-century competencies include new sets of foundational, disciplinary (generalists or specialists), and integrative competencies (Frenk et al., 2022). These competencies reflect basic knowledge on theories, facts, and concepts within a practice discipline, specialized knowledge and skills of the discipline or a specialty, and emerging capabilities that meet the complexities of health and social needs and of health care systems innovations such as information technology, leadership, systems thinking, relationship-based care, collaboration, and partnership. These capabilities help families develop abilities in critical thinking skills, numeracy, creativity, emotional intelligence, ethical considerations, effective communication, and teamwork. See the framework of the professional competencies in Figure 12.1.

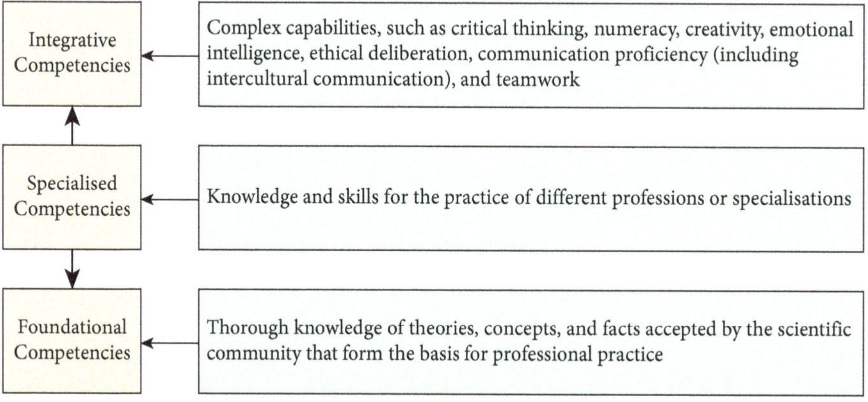

FIGURE 12.1 Framework of health care professional competencies (Frenk et al., 2022).

Nurses as well as other FHT members must be capable of empowering diverse and complex persons presenting or dealing with transitional, acute, and chronic health problems. Empowerment skills include curing, caring, and coaching strategies to promote health and resilience and prevent disease. Likewise, skills in communication and promotion of health behavior change are essential (Baker, 2001; Sibille et al., 2010) in providing effective chronic condition preventions and self-care management interventions (Lawn et al., 2009).

In addition, systems thinking is a high priority as it offers an understanding the interconnections between the components of health (physical, social, psychological, and spiritual) and family-level dynamics and relationships. Systems thinking captures the multilayered aspects of illness within the social context in which people live (Tramonti et al., 2021). Culturally competent FHTs apply knowledge of power dynamics in human functioning to understand clients, the intervention process, and themselves at multiple levels of the ecological influences as well as within the 4HEALTH context. Knowledge in community assessment and *population health* is also necessary to meet the complex health care needs of the target individual/family, community, and population. Likewise, a good understanding of the complexity and adaptive nature of the individual/person system, family system, and health care system is also essential (Waldman, 2007). Systems thinking promotes patient safety and teamwork (Aboumatar et al., 2012; Batt et al., 2021; Dolansky & Moore, 2013; Swanson & Widmer, 2018; Will & Essary, 2021; Vetere, 2007) and behavioral interventions across family systems (May et al., 2017). Likewise, competencies in leadership, delegation, and information technology are important to ensure coordination, continuity of care, and a sustainable health care system as part of achieving the triple and quadruple aims via interprofessional *family health* teams. Applications of artificial intelligence (AI) is increasingly considered in health care to lower costs and improve standardizations such as in diagnostic algorithm applications (Frenk et al., 2022). Although health care workers have voiced concerns regarding AI applications such as ethics and morals dilemmas, job security issues, redefined workforce roles, regulations, and quality of care issues (Rony et al., 2024), there is a positive outlook of AI use in enhancing humane and compassionate care and improved provider–patient interactions (Frenk et al., 2022). These competencies are highly needed for the 21st-century *family health* care workforce.

Professional organization have identified disciplinary FHT competencies that capture the knowledge, attitudes and skills needed to work with families in the contexts of the 4HEALTH. Likewise, the WHO has proposed 10 self-care competencies for health care workers to support self-care in their clinical practice, focusing on key family-focused areas that include people centeredness, decision-making, effective communication, collaboration, evidence-informed practice, and personal conduct. Effective implementation of the competencies across disciplines requires investment in reforming the academic preparation and licensing of the health care and public health workforce to fit the needs of individuals, families, and populations at different levels of practice. With the increased shortage of health care providers after the COVID-19 pandemic, designing effective task delegations, task shifting, and sharing strategies is inevitable. This includes eliminating role confusion and dynamics in health care decision-making processes and reimbursement barriers for effective *family health* professional teams.

Examples of Professional Family Health Competencies

The WHO European Region Initiative of HEALTH21

The WHO European Region initiative of HEALTH21 is a health policy framework developed for the *family health* nurse role within *family health* teams, focusing on primary care. The *family health* nurse was expected to have certain competencies to make key contributions in a multidisciplinary team of health care professionals to attainment targets for the 21st century. These skills include the following:

- Identify and assess the health status and health needs of individuals and families within the context of their cultures and communities.
- Make decisions based on ethical principles.
- Plan, initiate, and provide care for families within their defined caseload.
- Promote health in individuals, families and communities.
- Apply knowledge of a variety of teaching and learning strategies with individuals, families, and communities.
- Use and evaluate different methods of communication.
- Participate in disease prevention.
- Coordinate and manage care, including what has been delegated to other people and personnel.
- Systematically document their practice.
- Generate, manage, and use clinical, research-based and statistical information (data) for planning care and prioritizing health- and illness-related activities.
- Support and empower individuals and families to influence and participate in decisions concerning their health.
- Set standards and evaluate the effectiveness of *family health* nursing activities.
- Work independently and as members of a team.
- Participate in the prioritization of health- and illness-related activities.
- Manage change and act as agents for change.
- Maintain professional relationships and a supportive collegiate role with colleagues.
- Display evidence of a commitment to lifelong learning and continuing professional development.

The International Family Nursing Association (IFNA)

The International Family Nursing Association (IFNA) has developed the prelicensure family nursing education and generalist practice and advanced practice (IFNA, 2018).

Generalist Competencies for Family Nursing Practice

The following are competencies for family nursing practice at the generalist level:

- Enhance and promote *family health*.
- Focus nursing practice on families' strengths, the support of family and individual growth, the improvement of family self-management abilities, the facilitation of successful life transitions, the improvement and management of health, and the mobilization of family resources.
- Demonstrate leadership and systems thinking skills to ensure the quality of nursing care with families in everyday practice and across every context.
- Commit to self-reflective practice based on examination of nurse actions with families and family responses.
- Practice using an evidence-based approach. (IFNA, 2015)

Advanced Practice Competencies for Family Nursing

- Establish a relationship with the family for health promotion, disease prevention, health restoration, and symptom management during complex health transitions.
- Collect comprehensive data pertinent to the family's health status.
- Continually assess and process with the family the family's response to health and disease conditions during complex health transitions.
- Systematically use evidence- and practice-informed clinical reasoning to develop family nursing judgments.
- Consistently intervene with the family in preventing, maintaining, and restoring well-being during complex health transitions.
- Facilitate the resolution of family responses to complex health transitions.
- Actively engage in deliberate family nursing practice.
- Draw on a formal approach to monitor and evaluate family responses to interventions.
- Collaborate with interprofessional health teams to mobilize resources to support family care provision.
- Champion *family health* care at the larger systems level.
- Integrate practice-based research and evidence-based practice into family nursing advanced practice (FN-AP) care provided to families.
- Provide leadership in ethical conduct in the care of families at the systems level.
- Engage in reflective practice with families. (IFNA, 2017)

National Council on Family Relations: Family Life Education

Certified family life educators are expected to demonstrate competencies in the following 10 family life education content areas (NCFR, 2020):

- Families and individuals in societal contexts
- Internal dynamics of families
- Human growth and development across the life span
- Human sexuality across the life span
- Interpersonal relationships
- Family resource management
- Parenting education and guidance
- Family law and public policy
- Professional ethics and practice
- Family life education methodology

The Erasmus+ Project: European Curriculum for Family and Community Nurses

Proposed competencies for the family and community nurses' role in the field of primary care according to the European Curriculum for Family and Community Nurses (ENhANCE) include the following:

- Use the best scientific evidence available.
- Systematically document and evaluate their own practice.
- Plan, implement, and assess nursing care to meet the needs of individuals, families, and the community within their scope of competence.
- Identify and assess the health status and health needs of individuals and families within the context of their cultures and communities.
- Provide patient education and build a therapeutic relationship with patients, informal carers, and their families.
- Work together with the multidisciplinary team to prevent disease and promote and maintain health.
- Apply educational strategies to promote the health and safety of individuals and families.
- Involve individuals and families in decisions concerning their own health and well-being.
- Monitor and provide long-term care to people affected by chronic and rare illnesses in one community in collaboration with other members of the multidisciplinary team.
- Communication competencies should be based on evidence in relation to a specific context.

- Promote health in individuals, families, and communities
- Mentor students to promote the health and well-being of the community.
- Make decisions based on professional ethical standards.
- Maintain professional and interprofessional relationships and a supportive role with colleagues to ensure that professional standards are met.
- Engage in multidimensional community health needs assessments to implement appropriate clinical interventions and care management
- Demonstrate an ability to negotiate health care with patients and their families, the multidisciplinary team, and health care centers.
- Assess the social, cultural, and economic context in which the nurse's patient lives.
- Coordinate and be accountable for attributing community health care activities to support workers.
- Demonstrate accountability for the outcomes of nursing care in individuals, families, and communities.
- Develop nurse leadership and decision-making skills to ensure clinical and health care effectiveness and appropriateness.
- Alleviate patient suffering.
- Participate in the prioritization of activities of the multidisciplinary team to address problems related to health and illness.
- Set standards and evaluate the outcomes related to nursing activities in people's homes and in the community.
- Manage diversity and foster inclusiveness.
- Engage in analytic assessment, cultural competence, program planning, and community dimensions of practice to pursue community health promotion goals with the community multidisciplinary team.
- Manage change and act as agents for change to improve family and community nursing practice.
- Show leadership and development and participate in the implementation and evaluation of policies for the family and the community for purposes of health promotion
- Manage health promotion, education, treatment ,and monitoring supported by information and communication technologies (ICTs) (e-health). (Bagnasco et al., 2022)

Medical Family Therapy

Six Competency Domains for Family Therapists Working in Healthcare Settings include:

- Systems
- Biopsychosocial-spiritual
- Collaboration
- Leadership
- Ethics
- Diversity (AAMFT, n.d.)

WHO Self-Care Competencies

The WHO (2023) designed the following competencies to serve as standards for how health and care workers can support self-care among individuals, families, and communities. *Self-care* is defined as the ability of individuals, families, and communities to promote health, prevent disease, maintain health, and cope with illness and disability with or without the support of a health worker.

Domain I: People-Centeredness

- Competency 1: Promotes self-care by individuals, caregivers, families, and their communities
- Competency 2: Provides people-centered support for self-care by individuals, caregivers, and families

Domain II: Decision-Making

- Competency 3: Takes an adaptive and collaborative approach to decision-making about self-care by individuals

Domain III: Communication

- Competency 4: Communicates effectively with individuals, caregivers, and families

Domain IV: Collaboration

- Competency 5: Collaborates with other health and care and community workers to support self-care

Domain V: Evidence-Based Practice

- Competency 7: Supports evidence-informed self-care practice by individuals, caregivers, and families

Domain VI: Personal Conduct

- Competency 8: Demonstrates high standards of ethical conduct
- Competency 9: Undertakes reflective learning and practice about self-care
- Competency 10: Manages own health and well-being

Conclusion

This chapter sheds light on the importance of creating *family health* teams for the 21st-century health care and public health systems. The emphasis on FHTs is to build a competent health workforce capable of delivering comprehensive and equitable health care services that protect and promote health for all across the family life span and in all community settings by bridging individual and *population health* outcomes.

Suggested Readings

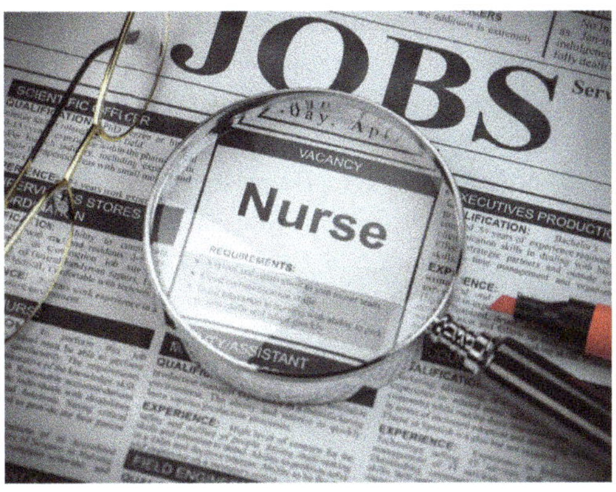

IMG 12.1

Breton, M., Lévesque, J. F., Pineault, R., & Hogg, W. (2011). Primary care reform: Can Quebec's family medicine group model benefit from the experience of Ontario's *family health* teams? *Healthcare Policy, 7*(2), e122.

Fardousi, N., Nunes da Silva, E., Kovacs, R., Borghi, J., Barreto, J. O., Kristensen, S. R., ... & Powell-Jackson, T. (2022). Performance bonuses and the quality of primary health care delivered by *family health* teams in Brazil: A difference-in-differences analysis. *PLoS Medicine, 19*(7), e1004033.

Silva, I. S., & Arantes, C. I. S. (2017). Power relations in the *family health* team: Focus on nursing. *Revista Brasileira de Enfermagem, 70*(3), 580–587.

Reflection Questions

Look for any health care job announcement or advertisement in primary care or in a community setting. Read the announcement and answer the following questions:

1. What skills do they need?
2. What skills do they prefer?
3. What kind of license is required?
4. What kind of credentials are required or preferred?
5. What is the work experience requirement?
6. Is the job a *family health* job?

References

Aboumatar, H. J., Thompson, D., Wu, A., Dawson, P., Colbert, J., Marsteller, J., ... & Pronovost, P. (2012). Development and evaluation of a 3-day patient safety curriculum to advance knowledge, self-efficacy and system thinking among medical students. *BMJ quality & safety, 21*(5), 416–422.

Anderson, K. H. (2000). The *family health* system approach to family systems nursing. *Journal of family nursing, 6*(2), 103–119.

Anderson, K. H., & Tomlinson, P. S. (1992). The *family health* system as an emerging paradigmatic view for nursing. *Image: The Journal of Nursing Scholarship, 24*(1), 57–63.

Ashcroft, R., McMillan, C., Ambrose-Miller, W., McKee, R., & Brown, J. B. (2018). The emerging role of social work in primary health care: A survey of social workers in Ontario *family health* teams. *Health & Social Work, 43*(2), 109–111.

Bagnasco, A., Catania, G., Zanini, M., Pozzi, F., Aleo, G., Watson, R., ... & Stavropoulos, K. (2022). Core competencies for family and community nurses: A European e-Delphi study. *Nurse Education in Practice, 60*, 103296.

Baker, A. (2001). Crossing the quality chasm: a new health system for the 21st century. *British Medical Journal, 323*(7322), 1192.

Barnes, M. D., Hanson, C. L., Novilla, L. B., Magnusson, B. M., Crandall, A. C., & Bradford, G. (2020). Family-centered health promotion: Perspectives for engaging families and achieving better health outcomes. *INQUIRY: The Journal of Health Care Organization, Provision, and Financing, 57.*

Batt, A. M., Williams, B., Brydges, M., Leyenaar, M., & Tavares, W. (2021). New ways of seeing: Supplementing existing competency framework development guidelines with systems thinking. *Advances in Health Sciences Education, 26*(4), 1355–1371.

Cott, C. A., Mandoda, S., & Landry, M. D. (2011). Models of integrating physical therapists into *family health* teams in Ontario, Canada: challenges and opportunities. *Physiotherapy Canada, 63*(3), 265–275.

Coutinho, A. J., Cochrane, A., Stelter, K., Phillips, R. L., & Peterson, L. E. (2015). Comparison of intended scope of practice for family medicine residents with reported scope of practice among practicing family physicians. *JAMA, 314*(22), 2364–2372.

Doherty, W. J. (1985). Family interventions in health care. *Family Relations, 34*(1),129–137.

Doherty, W. J., & McCubbin, H. I. (1985). Families and health care: An emerging arena of theory, research, and clinical intervention. *Family Relations: An Interdisciplinary Journal of Applied Family Studies, 34*(1), 5–11. https://doi.org/10.2307/583751

Dolansky, M. A., & Moore, S. M. (2013). Quality and Safety Education for Nurses (QSEN): The Key is Systems Thinking. *Online Journal of Issues in Nursing, 18*(3). Manuscript 1. https://doi.org/10.3912/OJIN.Vol18No03Man01

Eagar, S. C., Cowin, L. S., Gregory, L., & Firtko, A. (2010). Scope of practice conflict in nursing: A new war or just the same battle? *Contemporary Nurse, 36*(1–2), 86–95.

Frenk, J., Chen, L. C., Chandran, L., Groff, E. O. H., King, R., Meleis, A., & Fineberg, H. V. (2022). Challenges and opportunities for educating health professionals after the COVID-19 pandemic. *Lancet, 400*(10362), 1539–1556. https://doi.org/10.1016/S0140-6736(22)02092-X

Gillespie, U., Dolovich, L., & Dahrouge, S. (2017). Activities performed by pharmacists integrated in *family health* teams: Results from a web-based survey. *Canadian Pharmacists Journal, 150*(6), 407–416.

Gocan, S., Laplante, M. A., & Woodend, K. (2014). Interprofessional collaboration in Ontario's *family health* teams: A review of the literature. *Journal of Research in Interprofessional Practice and Education, 3*(3). 1–19. https://doi.org/10.22230/jripe.2014v3n3a131

Green, M. E., Weir, E., Hogg, W., Etches, V., Moore, K., Hunter, D., & Birtwhistle, R. (2013). Improving collaboration between public health and *family health* teams in Ontario. *Healthcare Policy, 8*(3), e93.

Gryschek, G., & Pinto, A. A. M. (2015). Mental health care: How can *family health* teams integrate it into primary healthcare? *Ciência & Saúde Coletiva, 20*, 3255–3262.

Hassan, I. S., AbdulKareem, A. K., Alrabee, N. H. K., Mansour, S. F., Fadlelmoula, S. A., Elhassan, E. A., Abdelgadir, M. M., Mohamed, M. A., Adam, S. A., Bedawi, F. O., Yousif, M. A., Ahmed, R. A., & Kashif, T. A. (2022). A Systems Thinking approach for the creation of effective competency-based medical education programs. The Pan African medical journal, 41 (203), 1–9. https://doi.org/10.11604/pamj.2022.41.203.28896

Heale, R., Dahrouge, S., Johnston, S., & Tranmer, J. E. (2018). Characteristics of nurse practitioner practice in *family health* teams in Ontario, Canada. *Policy, Politics, & Nursing Practice, 19*(3–4), 72–81.

International Family Nursing Association (IFNA) (2018). *IFNA position statements.* https://internationalfamilynursing.org/association-information/position-statements/

Lawn, S., Battersby, M., Lindner, H., Mathews, R., Morris, S., Wells, L., … & Reed, R. (2009). What skills do primary health care professionals need to provide effective self-management support? Seeking consumer perspectives. *Australian Journal of Primary Health, 15*(1), 37–44.

Lopes-Júnior, L. C. (2021). Advanced practice nursing and the expansion of the role of nurses in primary health care in the Americas. *SAGE Open Nursing, 7.*

May, C., Chai, L. K., & Burrows, T. (2017). Parent, partner, co-parent or partnership? The need for clarity as family systems thinking takes hold in the quest to motivate behavioural change. *Children (Basel, Switzerland), 4*(4), 29. https://doi.org/10.3390/children4040029

Murray, I. (2008). *Family health* nurse project—an education program of the world health organization: The University of Stirling experience. *Journal of Family Nursing, 14*(4), 469–485.

National Council for Family Relations (2020). Family Life Education Content Areas: Content and Practice Guidelines. https://www.ncfr.org/sites/default/files/2021-03/FLE%20Content%20and%20Practice%20Guidelines%202020.pdf

National Council for Family Relations (2023). *Where are Family Life Educators Employed?* https://www.ncfr.org/cfle-certification/what-family-life-education/where-are-family-life-educators-employed

Norful, A., Martsolf, G., de Jacq, K., & Poghosyan, L. (2017). Utilization of registered nurses in primary care teams: A systematic review. *International journal of nursing studies, 74*, 15–23.

Pinderhughes, E. (1995). Empowering diverse populations: Family practice in the 21st century. *Families in Society, 76*(3), 131–140.

Rony, M. K. K., Parvin, M. R., Wahiduzzaman, M., Debnath, M., Bala, S. D., & Kayesh, I. (2024). "I Wonder if my Years of Training and Expertise Will be Devalued by Machines": Concerns About the Replacement of Medical Professionals by Artificial Intelligence. *SAGE open nursing, 10*. https://doi.org/10.1177/23779608241245220

Sibille, K., Greene, A., & Bush, J. P. (2010). Preparing Physicians for the 21 Century: Targeting Communication Skills and the Promotion of Health Behavior Change. *Annals of behavioral science and medical education : journal of the Association for the Behavioral Sciences and Medical Education, 16*(1), 7–13. https://doi.org/10.1007/BF03355111

Smolowitz, J., Speakman, E., Wojnar, D., Whelan, E. M., Ulrich, S., Hayes, C., & Wood, L. (2015). Role of the registered nurse in primary health care: Meeting health care needs in the 21st century. *Nursing Outlook, 63*(2), 130–136.

Soklaridis, S., Oandasan, I., & Kimpton, S. (2007). *Family health* teams: Can health professionals learn to work together? *Canadian Family Physician, 53*(7), 1198–1199.

Somé, N. H., Devlin, R. A., Mehta, N., Zaric, G. S., & Sarma, S. (2020). Team-based primary care practice and physician's services: Evidence from *Family Health* Teams in Ontario, Canada. *Social science & medicine, 264*, 113310.

Swanson, C., & Widmer, M. (2018). Transforming health education to catalyze a global paradigm shift: Systems thinking, complexity, and design thinking. In S. P. Sturmberg Putting systems and complexity sciences into practice: Sharing the experience (1st Ed. pp. 119–131). 10.1007/978-3-319-73636-5_9

Tramonti, F., Giorgi, F., & Fanali, A. (2021). Systems thinking and the biopsychosocial approach: A multilevel framework for patient-centred care. *Systems Research and Behavioral Science, 38*(2), 215–230.

Vetere, A. (2007). Bio/Psycho/Social Models and Multidisciplinary Team Working: Can Systemic Thinking Help? *Clinical child psychology and psychiatry, 12*(1), 5–12.

Will, K. K., & Essary, A. (2021). Competency-based interprofessional continuing education focusing on systems thinking and health care delivery for health care professionals. *Journal of Continuing Education in the Health Professions, 41*(2), 153–156.

World Health Organization, Regional Office for Europe. (1998). *HEALTH21—Health for all in the 21st century: An introduction.* https://iris.who.int/handle/10665/107327

World Health Organization, Regional Office for Europe. (2000). *The family health nurse: Context, conceptual framework and curriculum.* https://iris.who.int/handle/10665/107930

Zieff, G., Kerr, Z. Y., Moore, J. B., & Stoner, L. (2020). Universal Healthcare in the United States of America: A Healthy Debate. Medicina (Kaunas, Lithuania), 56(11), 580. https://doi.org/10.3390/medicina56110580

Figure credits

Fig. 12.1: Julio Frenk et al., "Framework of Health-Care Professional Competencies," *The Lancet*, vol. 400, no, 10362. Copyright © 2022 by Elsevier B.V.

IMG 12.1: Copyright © 2019 Depositphotos/maxxyustas.

CHAPTER 13

The Future of Family Research in 21st-Century Health Care and Public Health System(s)

Complex questions take complex methods.

—Wendy Nilsen

Learning Objectives

By the end of this chapter, learners will do the following:

- Examine the following key terminologies: family research and family-related research.
- Describe the importance of family research in health care and public health.
- Identify Feethman's criteria for quality family research in health care and public health.
- Describe the steps of building a program of family research.

Before you read on, consider the following questions:

- What is family research?
- What makes a research study a family research study?

Importance of Family Research in Health Care and Public Health in the 21st Century

The study of families has been a contemporary evolution and change in health care and public health efforts to respond to the growing complexities in societies' needs and opportunities to improve individual and *population health* outcomes worldwide. Family scholars are faced with the need to evolve to contribute to advancements in knowledge development in biomedical, biopsychosocial, economic, and behavioral family research in the health care space. Previous chapters provided the premise for the following discussion that explores the importance of including a family lens or "think family" in health care and public health research efforts. Specifically, the chapter provides a discussion that identifies opportunities for health research to think family across the individual and family life spans and the continuum of heath care, especially in the areas of health promotion, disease prevention, disease control and management, and end-of-life and palliative care.

The discussion here indicates an emphasis on the proposed rules for the 21st-century healthcare system, outlined in Table 13.1, that stress the need for research that will contribute to health equity by addressing medical issues as well as social determinants of health (SDOH) through evidence-based, cost-effective, collaborative, quality, and safe humanistic and caring relationships. In addition, the chapter introduces future family scientists to the steps of building a program of family research.

TABLE 13.1 **Simple Rules for the 21st-Century Healthcare System**

Current Approach	New Rule
Care is based primarily on visits.	Care is based on continuous healing relationships.
Professional autonomy drives variability.	Care is customized according to patient needs and values.
Professionals control care.	The patient is the source of control.
Information is a record.	Knowledge is shared and information flows freely.
Decision-making is based on training and experience.	Decision-making is evidence based.
Do no harm is an individual responsibility.	Safety is a system property.
Secrecy is necessary.	Transparency is necessary.
The system reacts to needs.	Needs are anticipated.
Cost reduction is sought.	Waste is continuously decreased.
Preference is given to professional roles rather that the system.	Cooperation among clinicians is a priority.

By definition, *family research* is the study of the family structure, function, transitions, and processes evolving among diverse families across the life span and across contextual aspects of relationships (Coontz, 2000). In health care, the focus of family research/studies has been on the role of family in influencing health outcomes. The emphasis of family studies is on the "conditions, for which outcomes, for whom, and through which pathways do family structure, context, and process affect health" (Carr & Springer, 2010, p. 743). *Health outcomes* in this aspect are broadly defined as the physical, social, psychological, and spiritual well-being of the individual family members, the family as a unit, populations, and overall communities. The main purposes of family research on health include the need to (a) build basic foundational research to advance the knowledge of family to improve care and outcomes for families; (b) conduct intervention research (i.e., efficacy and feasibility studies) to determine sustainable interventions to improve health outcomes; and (c) utilize policy integration strategies to sustain change that advance the health and well-being of families (Danford et al., 2024;

Feethman, 2018). Research on families can be divided into two categories: (a) family research that examines how the family system as a whole or its subsystems functions and makes health care decisions and (b) family-related research that examines how the process constructs or how variables within the family, such as roles, communication, and relationships, influence health (Feethman, 2018). Explanatory models of *family health* and illness, described as "culturally determined beliefs that individuals hold about misfortune, suffering, illness and health" and shaped by "societal expectations of the sick role, individual illness behavior and help-seeking," are essential in describing family research phenomena (Dinos et al., 2017, p. 106). For example, the family illness beliefs model has been used to show the importance of health beliefs in relation to health outcomes within family systems (Bell & Wright, 2015). Family research and family-related research studies use both single and multilayered full explanatory and partial explanatory models (the predominant model in family research) to describe, explain, or predict the interdependence within and between families and the ecological context.

Diverse family researchers or scientists continue to make great strides in advancing family science knowledge in the many ways family life health, illness, and death intersect. Family research efforts facilitate knowledge development in understanding health disparities and health inequities, especially among vulnerable populations (Deatrick, 2017). Biomedical family scientists shed light on the epigenetics of precision medicine through *family health* history and clinical decision support systems in health care settings (Ginsburg & Willard, 2009). Likewise, biomedical family professionals use biomarkers to integrate social processes to advance the science of symptom management (Dodd et al., 2001). Family research scientists have also utilized neuro-education with families (i.e., couples) to help families adapt to stress (Walsh, 2012).

Biopsychosocial, behavioral, and environmental family scientists have also contributed to the advancement of family science on the growing topic on SDOH that affects *family health*, functioning, and quality of life and contributes to health disparities and inequities (Gray et al., 2023). For example, understanding where families live and work sheds light on evidence-based health policy initiatives that eliminate disparities to meet the actual needs of the person in health care. Family scholarship related to family-work balance, men involvement, parenting practices advances the science of the intersection of SDOH and *family health* (Bianchi & Milkie, 2010). Family studies on the social environment in which children live have also been instrumental in the study of SDOH with the hope to achieve health equity for vulnerable families (Institute of Medicine and National Research Council of the National Academies, 2011; McNeill, 2010). Moreover, family studies on the relationship between poverty and family financial challenges have contributed important information on how families can adapt and adjust when caring for children with medical complexities (Mooney-Doyle & Lindley, 2019). Family research also contributes a robust body of scientific evidence to demonstrate the psychology of human social relationships and health risk markers in public health priorities (Holt-Lunstad et al., 2017), especially among the elderly (National Academies of Sciences, Engineering and Medicine, 2019; Ryff & Singer, 2005). It is also important to mention that family studies shed light on the conceptualizing family structure as a socially stratified grouping within an SDOH framework (Russell et al., 2018). This conceptualization enhances family science scholarship in understanding living arrangements and family stability (Institute of Medicine and National Research Council of the National Academies, 2011). Such data assists family professionals in putting forth effective strategies that serve vulnerable families.

It is important to delineate the settings for family research as the concept and scope of family-focused practice is recommended across diverse health care settings (e.g., mental health care settings; Foster et al., 2016). Family research contributions in acute care settings have been on the rise with the introduction and institutionalization of the philosophy of patient and family-centered care (PFCC), especially in pediatric settings (Lankin, 2020). However, in 21st century, more efforts should be put to advance family knowledge development in the area of family practice and family primary care settings. Primary care family scholars are well suited to address social aspects of health care (Pinto & Bloch, 2017). Studies reveal that primary care is linked to better *population health* outcomes at lower costs compared to acute care (Future of Family Medicine Project Leadership Committee, 2004). A family research area that needs attention in primary care is the science of family and health promotion and its contribution to *population health* (Ho et al., 2022) across generations (Christensen, 2004).

These examples demonstrate the need to support the advancement of the family research and science in public health and health care systems. In addition, the studies highlight the need to acknowledge the role of culture in person-conceptualized health, illness, health, and health care practices, as well as in leveraging opportunities for cultural competency care within health care systems (Levesque & Li, 2014).

Criteria for Family Research

Many tips for how to write for family research have been proposed in the literature. The tips provide *family health* professional with valuable information that can aid *thinking family* while writing for publication or funding in family research. Specific criteria for addressing conceptual and methodological considerations include the adoption of methods that capture the complexities of *family health* units of focus, family definitions, and family ecological contexts to facilitate the development of family intervention. Methodological considerations are crucial for advancing the science of health equity (Gray et al., 2023).

Methods recommended for family research include mixed-method approaches and designs (qualitative and quantitative) that contribute to the development of family knowledge and to health. Qualitative research builds contextualized evidence-based family-focused practice (Chironda et al., 2023). Case study methods offer an approach that overcomes some of the sampling and analysis obstacles researchers face when studying families (Schulz et al., 2021). New methods, like participatory methods, that engage researchers and stakeholders throughout the research process are also critical for family research (Turnbull et al., 1998). In addition, consideration of a family-focused recruitment and consenting approach is important in enhancing research participation that impacts the health of individuals, families, and communities (Polfuss et al., 2023). *Family health* theories and family theories also play a critical role in guiding methods used in family research. For example, symbolic interaction theory is used in qualitative family research to delineate family roles and identities (Luxford et al., 2011).

Moreover, it is important to pay attention to the process of constructing family interventions through the advancement of foundational work through efficacy testing and policy integration (Danford et al. 2024). In this process, qualitative methods are instrumental in determining the barriers and facilitating factors to implementation of evidence-informed family programs and understanding health beliefs and practices across diverse groups. The methods bring patient and provider experiences into practice. Moreover, since family research is interdisciplinary, developing a common language in methods and theories facilitates common knowledge development in *family health* (Institute of Medicine and National Research Council of the National Academies, 2011). Family research that reflects cross-disciplinary perspectives addresses the complex health issues encountered by patients, families, and communities (Loeb et al., 2008). Interdisciplinary teams are also instrumental in ensuring study aims and designs are in sync in family synthesis research—meaning research that draws conclusion from multiple studies using multiple methodological approaches (Knafl, 2015). Interdisciplinary teams should also demonstrate education and training in family research to facilitate translation of family knowledge into clinical practice (Svavarsdottir et al., 2015). The criteria proposed by Feetham's (2018) is a useful resource to help interdisciplinary *family health* professionals address the complexity of families and further *family health* and well-being through family research (see Table 13.2).

TABLE 13.2 **Feetham's (2018) Criteria for Family Research**

Criterion	Definition	Examples of Guiding Questions
Conceptualization of Family	The investigator's conceptualization of family as informed by the specific discipline, theoretical underpinnings, contextual factors such as culture, and the social and public policy of the specific setting	What is family? How is family conceptualized from other groups (e.g., family as an environment, a mediator; family as strengths, resilience, and resource)? Is the study family research or family-related research?
Family Is Defined	The investigator's conceptualization of family, which may be based on biological, structural, functional, or subjective criteria	Who is the family addressed in the study? Who is meeting the functions of the family under study?
Advance Knowledge of Family Functioning and Structure	Describes the different family functions that are generic across all family forms; also includes the difference descriptions of family structures	What family function or family structure is addressed? How is the family function or family structure defined? Are the family functions culturally relevant?

Design, Instruments, Analysis, and Interpretation Have Consistent Application in the Study and Alignment With Family Constructs	The family research methodology demonstrates consistent alignment of family throughout all aspects of a study	How are the methods (design, research questions, theories, recruitment, measures, analysis, and interpretation) conceptualized to think family?
Relevancy to Practice	Description of value of collaborating with clinicians to inform the direction of family research and scholarship	How does the study demonstrate successful partnerships to facilitate clinical expectation? What is the nature of the researchers–clinician relationship?
Family Research That Informs Health and Social Policy	Demonstration of an understanding of the policy context and the impact of policy on the issues influencing family well-being	How are families affected by the policy? In what ways, if any, do families contribute to the policy issue? Would providing data on families result in more effective policies and programs?
Evidence of Clear Program of Family Research	Description of the what and where of the research	How does the study fit in the program of research? How does the study address gaps in the science and moves toward the goals of the program to advance the health and well-being of family and inform family policy?

How to Build a Program of Family Research

Building a program of research is important in family research and scholarship. Holzemier (2009) defines a *program of research* as a "iterative coherent expression of a researcher's area of interest that has public health significance, builds from published research literature in the field, has relevance for clinical practice and captures the passion and commitment of the researcher" (p. 1). A program of family research can be conceptualized using Holzemeir's (2009) outcome model for health care research, which incorporates horizontal dimensions, namely *inputs*, *processes*, and *outcomes* that represent time and the vertical dimensions of care that represent the client (i.e., patients, families, populations, and communities), provider, and health care system/setting (see Figure 13.1).

	Inputs ⇨	⇨ Processes	Outcomes
Client			
Provider			
Setting			

FIGURE 13.1 Outcomes model for health care research (Holzeimer, 2009).

From a family research perspective, inputs would be considered background information of the family unit of analysis, *family health* professionals' characteristics, and health systems characteristics (family-centered care philosophy, availability and functioning of *family health* professional teams, and family focused information technology, collaboration, and partnerships, etc.). Family-related processes would be family self-care interventions (disease prevention and management, health promotion, screening, etc.), family communication, family decision-making, family support and coping, family routines and rituals, family roles and relationships, family disease management, and so forth. *Family health* professional processes may include family–provider relational practices such as ability to communicate effectively, using strength-based approaches, intervening with families using strategies that are culturally responsive to family needs, and so on. Health care systems processes include family-centered practice, availability of *family health* teams, family-focused referral, and coordinated care. A good program of family research that is well organized with targeted inputs and processed is likely to be impactful on related health and health care service delivery outcomes for clients, providers, and health care systems. For example, outcomes related to the client would be improvement in *family health*, patient and family satisfaction with care and family engagement, enhanced family relationships, and family functioning. *Family health* professional outcomes would be provider satisfaction with work environment, improved provider–family relationships, and improved professional development help-giving practices. Health care systems family-focused outcomes include family spillover cost analysis, family quality of life, and morbidity and mortality rates. Table 13.3 presents steps for building a successful program of research (Holzemier, 2009, p. 5) that can help *family health* scholars conceptualize their plans to contribute to family research.

TABLE 13.3 **Steps for Building a Program of Family Research**

	Steps	**Examples of questions to consider in a program of family research**
1	Know your passion.	Why are you passionate about family or *family health*? Are you interested in family research or family-related research?
2	Ensure high public health significance.	What are you observing in your clinical practice when working with patients and families? What is working well? What areas might work better?
3	Know the literature in your field.	Consider overall status and theoretical and methodological implications: What level of evidence does the family research represent? Is the research basic family research or applied family research? What is the design? What are the sample criteria? Who is included and excluded? What family measures are you using?

		What family theoretical framework, constructs, or variables are you using? Is the family study cross-sectional or longitudinal? What is hypothesized about the phenomenon of interest? Who is the family (biological, structural, functional, subjective)? What *family health* need are addressed (physical, social, psychological, spiritual, family functions and health, family processes and health)? What good research question on family phenomena of interest are you deriving from the literature? Is your research question feasible, interesting, novel, and relevant (FINER)?
4	Understand clinical practice in your area.	What are the practice guidelines, nursing standards, and procedural manuals indicating (innovative) about the state of the knowledge or evidence about family-focused care in your area of interest?
5	Use the outcomes model to think about the program of research.	What variables are you interested about the phenomena, who is the client (inputs), what is the intervention (processes), and what outcomes do you want to measure (outcomes)? What relationships are you interested in? What research designs would answer your questions?
6	Nurture interdisciplinary colleagues and multisectorial approaches.	Who is in your research team? Does the team include all the members you need to be able to accomplish the study on the phenomenon of interest? Is the study intersectoral or multisectorial?
7	Publish/build from one study to another study.	Have you published evidence related to understanding the phenomenon of interest (literature review, concepts analysis)? Have you published any studies on measuring the phenomenon of interest? Have you published a correctional and causal study (study relating the phenomenon to another concept)? Have you conducted and published an intervention trial to test the efficacy of causing a change in an outcome?
8	Have fun along the journey.	Are you sustaining your program of research with passion and dedication? Are you constantly building your program of research through writing small local grants and larger external grants to support your work? Do you have a grant idea in our mind, are you writing another one, do you have another in review, or do you have one that is funded and supporting your ongoing work?

Conclusion

Family research is needed in health care and public health. To effectively advance the science of family and health, there must be efforts to understand the conceptual, methodological, and ethical underpinnings considerations as an integral part of conducting family research. Doing so will facilitate the closing of gaps among clinical practice, policy development, and future research.

Suggested Websites

American Psychology Association, Caregiver Research: https://www.apa.org/pi/about/publications/caregivers/research

International Family Nursing Association, Family Nursing Research Resources: https://international-familynursing.org/resources-for-family-nursing/research/

National Cancer Institute, Dyadic Processes: https://cancercontrol.cancer.gov/brp/hbrb/dyadic-processes

National Institute on Minority Health and Health Disparities (NIMHD), Family Level Research, *Family Health*, Well-Being, and Resilience: https://www.nimhd.nih.gov/funding/approved-concepts/2019/family-health/index.html

National Cancer Institute (NCI) Division of Cancer Control and Population Sciences (DCCPS), Multilevel Intervention Training Institute (MLTI) Course Modules: https://healthcaredelivery.cancer.gov/mlti/

Suggested Readings

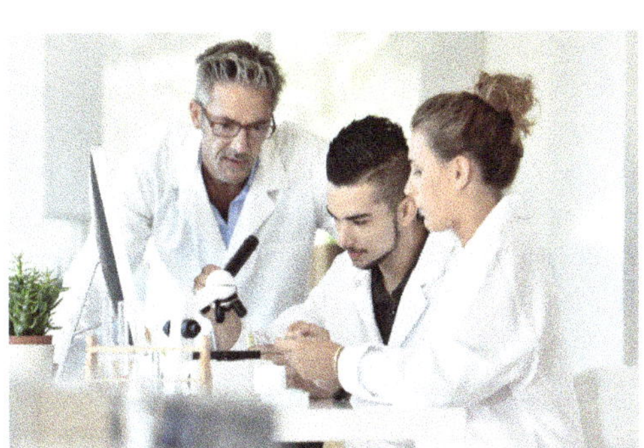
IMG 13.1

Danford, C. A., Mooney-Doyle, K., Deatrick, J. A., Feetham, S., Gross, D., Knafl, K. A., … & Swallow, V. (2024). Building family interventions for scalability and impact. *Journal of Family Nursing, 30*(2), 94–113.

Feetham, S. (2018). Guest editorial: Revisiting Feetham's criteria for research of families to advance science and inform policy for the health and well-being of families. *Journal of Family Nursing, 24*(2), 115–127.

Gray, T. F., Henderson, M. D., Barakat, L. P., Knafl, K. A., & Deatrick, J. A. (2023). Advancing family science and health equity through the 2022–2026 National Institute of Nursing Research strategic plan. *Nursing Outlook, 71*(5), 102030.

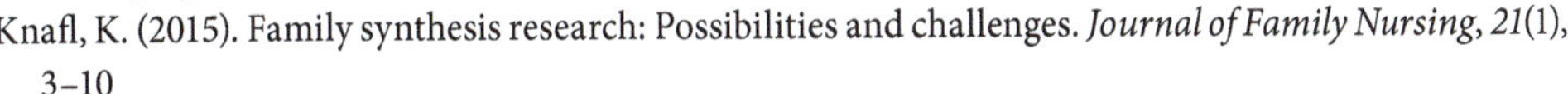

Knafl, K. (2015). Family synthesis research: Possibilities and challenges. *Journal of Family Nursing, 21*(1), 3–10

Wilson, S. J., Novak, J. R., Yorgason, J. B., Martire, L. M., & Lyons, K. S. (2024). New opportunities for advancing dyadic health science in gerontology. *The Gerontologist, 64*(1), gnac187. https://doi.org/10.1093/geront/gnac187

Reflection Questions

Read an article of your choice about a *family health* topic of your interest and answer the following questions:

1. How did the researchers conceptualize family?
2. How did the researcher define family?
3. What are the possible methodological, ethical, and theoretical limitations?
4. Was the team appropriate for the family research? Why?
5. Was there any implication for policymaking? Briefly explain.

References

Bell, J. M., & Wright, L. M. (2015). The Illness Beliefs Model: Advancing practice knowledge about illness beliefs, family healing, and family interventions. *Journal of Family Nursing, 21*(2), 179–185.

Bianchi, S. M., & Milkie, M. A. (2010). Work and family research in the first decade of the 21st century. *Journal of marriage and family, 72*(3), 705–725.

Carr, D., & Springer, K. W. (2010). Advances in families and health research in the 21st century. *Journal of marriage and family, 72*(3), 743–761.

Coontz, S. (2000). Historical perspectives on family studies. *Journal of marriage and family, 62*(2), 283–297.

Chironda, G., Jarvis, M. A., & Brysiewicz, P. (2023). Family-focused nursing research in WHO Afro-Region Member states: A scoping review. *Journal of Family Nursing, 29*(2), 136–154.

Christensen, P. (2004). The health-promoting family: a conceptual framework for future research. *Social science & medicine, 59*(2), 377–387.

Danford, C. A., Mooney-Doyle, K., Deatrick, J. A., Feetham, S., Gross, D., Knafl, K. A., ... & Swallow, V. (2024). Building Family Interventions for Scalability and Impact. *Journal of Family Nursing, 30*(2), 94–113.

Deatrick, J. A. (2017). Where is "family" in the social determinants of health? Implications for family nursing practice, research, education, and policy. *Journal of Family Nursing, 23*(4), 423–433.

Dinos, S., Ascoli, M., Owiti, J. A., & Bhui, K. (2017). Assessing explanatory models and health beliefs: An essential but overlooked competency for clinicians. *BJPsych Advances, 23*(2), 106–114.

Dodd, M., Janson, S., Facione, N., Faucett, J., Froelicher, E. S., Humphreys, J., ... & Taylor, D. (2001). Advancing the science of symptom management. *Journal of advanced nursing, 33*(5), 668–676.

Feetham, S. (2018). Guest editorial: Revisiting Feetham's criteria for research of families to advance science and inform policy for the health and well-being of families. *Journal of Family Nursing, 24*(2), 115–127.

Foster, K., Maybery, D., Reupert, A., Gladstone, B., Grant, A., Ruud, T., ... & Kowalenko, N. (2016). Family-focused practice in mental health care: An integrative review. *Child & Youth Services, 37*(2), 129–155.

Future of Family Medicine Project Leadership Committee. (2004). The future of family medicine: A collaborative project of the family medicine community. *The Annals of Family Medicine, 2*(1), S3–S32.

Ginsburg, G. S., & Willard, H. F. (2009). Genomic and personalized medicine: Foundations and applications. *Translational research, 154*(6), 277–287.

Gray, T. F., Henderson, M. D., Barakat, L. P., Knafl, K. A., & Deatrick, J. A. (2023). Advancing family science and health equity through the 2022–2026 National Institute of Nursing Research strategic plan. *Nursing Outlook, 71*(5), 102030.

Hill-Briggs, F., Adler, N. E., Berkowitz, S. A., Chin, M. H., Gary-Webb, T. L., Navas-Acien, A., Thornton, P. L., & Haire-Joshu, D. (2020). Social Determinants of Health and Diabetes: A Scientific Review. *Diabetes care, 44*(1), 258–279. Advance online publication. https://doi.org/10.2337/dci20-0053

Ho, Y. C. L., Mahirah, D., Ho, C. Z. H., & Thumboo, J. (2022). The role of the family in health promotion: A scoping review of models and mechanisms. *Health promotion international, 37*(6), daac119.

Holt-Lunstad, J., Robles, T. F., & Sbarra, D. A. (2017). Advancing social connection as a public health priority in the United States. *American Psychologist, 72*(6), 517–530. https://doi.org/10.1037/amp0000103

Institute of Medicine and National Research Council. (2011). *Toward an Integrated Science of Research on Families: Workshop Report.* National Academies Press. https://doi.org/10.17226/13085.

Knafl, K. (2015). Family synthesis research: Possibilities and challenges. *Journal of Family Nursing, 21*(1), 3–10

Lankin, K. A. (2020). *Supporting Families Through the Acute Phase of the Pediatric HSCT Experience* [Doctoral dissertation]. University of Illinois at Chicago.

Levesque, A., & Li, H. Z. (2014). The relationship between culture, health conceptions, and health practices: A qualitative–quantitative approach. *Journal of cross-cultural psychology, 45*(4), 628–645.

Luxford, K., Safran, D. G., & Delbanco, T. (2011). Promoting patient-centered care: A qualitative study of facilitators and barriers in healthcare organizations with a reputation for improving the patient experience. *International Journal for Quality in Health Care, 23*(5), 510–515.

McNeill, T. (2010). Family as a social determinant of health. *Healthc Q, 14*, 60–67.

Mooney-Doyle, K., & Lindley, L. C. (2019). The Association between Poverty and Family Financial Challenges of Caring for Medically Complex Children. *Nursing Economic$, 37*(4). 198–208.

Pinto, A. D., & Bloch, G. (2017). Framework for building primary care capacity to address the social determinants of health. *Canadian Family Physician, 63*(11), e476–e482.

Polfuss, M., Mooney-Doyle, K., Keller, M., Gralton, K. S., Giambra, B., & Vance, A. (2023). Developing a Family Resource: Considerations for Family Member Research Participation. *Journal of Family Nursing, 29*(2), 202–222.

Russell, L. T., Coleman, M., & Ganong, L. (2018). Conceptualizing family structure in a social determinants of health framework. *Journal of Family Theory & Review, 10*(4), 735–748.

Ryff, C. D., & Singer, B. H. (2005). Social environments and the genetics of aging: Advancing knowledge of protective health mechanisms. *The Journals of Gerontology Series B: Psychological Sciences and Social Sciences, 60*(1), 12–23.

Schulz, G. L., Patterson Kelly, K., Armer, J., & Ganong, L. (2021). Uncovering family treatment decision-making processes: The value and application of case study methods to family research. *Journal of Family Nursing, 27*(3), 191–198.

Svavarsdottir, E. K., Sigurdardottir, A. O., Konradsdottir, E., Stefansdottir, A., Sveinbjarnardottir, E. K., Ketilsdottir, A., … & Guðmundsdottir, H. (2015). The process of translating family nursing knowledge into clinical practice. *Journal of Nursing Scholarship, 47*(1), 5–15.

Turnbull, A. P., Friesen, B. J., & Ramirez, C. (1998). Participatory action research as a model for conducting family research. *Journal of the Association for Persons with Severe Handicaps, 23*(3), 178–188.

Walsh, F. (Ed.). (2012). *Normal family processes* (4th ed.). Guilford Press.

Wilson, S. J., Novak, J. R., Yorgason, J. B., Martire, L. M., & Lyons, K. S. (2024). New Opportunities for Advancing Dyadic Health Science in Gerontology. *The Gerontologist, 64*(1), gnac187. https://doi.org/10.1093/geront/gnac187

Figure credit

CHAPTER 14

The Role of Professional Organizations in Promoting Family Health

It is not what we get, but who we become, what we contribute that gives meaning to our lives.

—Tony Robbins

Learning Objectives

By the end of this chapter, learners will do the following:

- Examine professional organization and community of practice.
- Describe the role and benefits of professional organizations.
- Assess one's need to join a professional organization.
- Identify examples of professional organizations in family science.

Before you read on, consider the following questions:

- Why do *family health* professionals belong to a professional association?
- Where can you find family-related professional organizations?

Role of Professional Associations in Family Science and Health

As mentioned in Chapter 1, different initiatives have been on the forefront of *family health* care. The primary purpose of any professional organizations is to advance the respective profession (Benton et al., 2017). Most professional organizations in *family health* can be considered communities of practice. Weller (2017) describes a professional community of practice as "a less formal, more organic structure that develops around people engaged in common work leveraging common language, tools, stories and other artifacts of their practice." and serving primarily four roles which include "facilitating social interaction, knowledge creation, knowledge sharing, and identity building" (p. 362). The life span of professional associations goes through a seven-step evolutionary process that has the intention of building strong connections between members to achieve shared goal(s). According to Weller (2017), the first early steps of a professional evolution include seeking a shared need (potential), building relationships (coalescing), then organizing and managing knowledge (maturation), followed by maintaining relevance and attracting new members (stewarding), and lastly changing/evolving due to internal or external factors (transforming). Figure 14.1 provides a visual presentation of these seven stages adopted from Wenger et al. (2002).

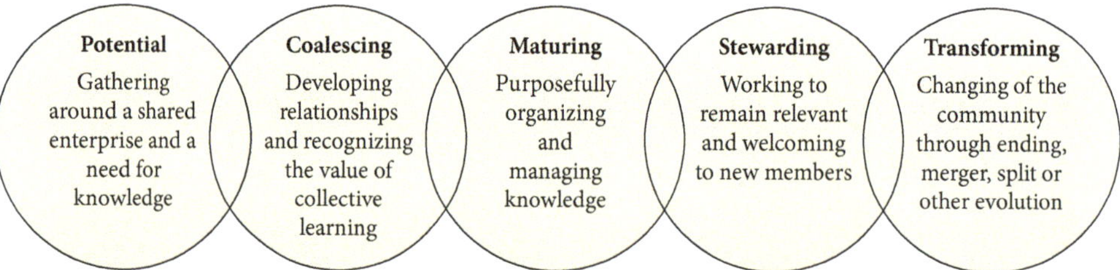

FIGURE 14.1 Five-stage evolution of a community practice.

Benefits of Professional Associations

There are many benefits of engaging in professional organizations (Escoffery et al., 2015; Markova et al., 2013; Mata et al., 2010; Thomas et al., 2013). The associations bring together individuals or members who predominantly volunteer. In *family health*-focused associations, members collectively associate to meet a common goal of advocating for families, family science, specific *family health* profession, and their contributions to health and health care systems. Membership in professional associations varies. Mostly it is through membership fees across various categories representing one's professional stage (retired/emeritus, early career/new professionals, student). The major roles of a professional association include advocating for the profession to other organizations or groups; developing professional standards such as code of ethics, certification, and accreditation and technical standards (Ernstthal & Jones, 1996); offering education and meetings that can provide employment opportunities; and providing members with access to publications and information development and utilization (Weller, 2017).

How to Assess One's Need to Join a Professional Organization

Table 14.1 presents a checklist students or professionals can use to assess personal needs to join a professional organization of their choice.

TABLE 14.1 **How to Assess Joining a Professionals Organization**

Items	Assessment Questions
Determine your career and self-development goals.	What options would you wish to pursue in your career? Do you wish to pursue practice, advocacy, research, theory, education?
Identify the gaps in your current knowledge of (a) the profession, (b) the career path you have chosen, and (c) the skills you feel will be necessary to succeed.	What professional development opportunities are you interested in? What seminar would you want to engage in, such as résumé writing, interviewing, and professional speaking and writing? Are you interested in learning about advocacy work and the role of volunteers in the success of the advocacy efforts?
Make a commitment to lifelong learning.	Do you have time to be involved? What is your commitment to the profession? What are the barriers and facilitators of your engagement? Do you want to maintain licensure to continue practicing? Do you have the moral obligation to maintain knowledge of skills and abilities beyond the minimum legal requirement for licensure?
Consider what you would lose if you were not involved.	Are you active in the association/organization? Do you feel included and involved? Do you feel served by the organization? What would you lose if you were not involved?

Source: Elliott (2004, p. 395)

Conclusion

This chapter introduced basic information on the role and benefits of professional organizations in general. *Family health* professionals can use the information to assess future interests to contribute to the field of family science in health care through active engagement in their association(s) of choice.

Suggested Websites

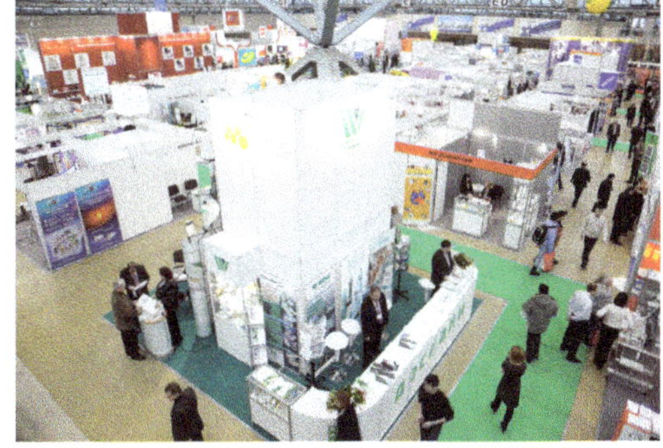
IMG 14.1

American Academy of Family Physicians Foundation: https://www.aafp.org/
American Family Therapy: https://www.afta.org/
American Association for Marriage and Family Therapy (AAMFT): https://www.aamft.org/
Association of Maternal & Child Health Programs (AMCHP): https://amchp.org/#
International Association of Marriage and Family Counselors (IAMFC): https://www.iamfconline.org/
International Family Therapy Association (IFTA): https://www.ifta-familytherapy.org/
International Family Nursing Association (IFNA): https://internationalfamilynursing.org/
Institute for Patient- and Family-Centered Care (IPFCC): https://www.ipfcc.org/about/mission.html
National Association of Social Workers (NASW) https://www.socialworkers.org/About
National Council on Family Relations (NCFR): ncfr.org

Reflection Questions

Choose a *family health* professional organization of your choice. Browse through its website and then answer the following questions:

1. What is the organization about?
2. Why did you select the association?
3. What does membership look like?
4. What educational and research opportunities does the association offer?
5. What advocacy work does the association perform?

References

Benton, D. C., Thomas, K., Damgaard, G., Masek, S. M., & Brekken, S. A. (2017). Exploring the differences between regulatory bodies, professional associations, and trade unions: An integrative review. *Journal of Nursing Regulation, 8*(3), 4–11.

Elliott, V. E. (2004). The role of professional organizations and pharmacy practices. In A. M. Peterson (Ed.), *Managing Pharmacy Practice: Principles, Strategies, and Systems* (pp. 395–425). CRC Press

Ernstthal, H. L., & Jones, B. (1996). *Principles of association management.* American Society of Association Executives.

Escoffery, C., Kenzig, M., & Hyden, C. (2015). Getting the most out of professional associations. *Health Promotion Practice, 16*(3), 309–312.

Markova, G., Ford, R. C., Dickson, D. R., & Bohn, T. M. (2013). Professional associations and members' benefits: What's in it for me?. *Nonprofit Management and Leadership, 23*(4), 491–510.

Mata, H., Latham, T. P., & Ransome, Y. (2010). Benefits of professional organization membership and participation in national conferences: Considerations for students and new professionals. *Health promotion practice, 11*(4), 450–453.

Thomas, M., Inniss-Richter, Z., Mata, H., & Cottrell, R. R. (2013). Career development through local chapter involvement: Perspectives from chapter members. *Health Promotion Practice, 14*(4), 480–484.

Weller, A. (2017). Professional associations as communities of practice: Exploring the boundaries of ethics and compliance and corporate social responsibility. *Business and Society Review, 122*(3), 359–392.

Wenger, E., McDermott, R., & Snyder, W. M. (2002). Seven principles for cultivating communities of practice. *Cultivating Communities of Practice: a guide to managing knowledge, 4*, 1–19.

Figure credits

CHAPTER 15

Building a Family Health Professional Portfolio for 21st-Century Health Care and Public Health Systems

Begin somewhere. You cannot build a reputation on what you intend to do.

—Liz Smith

Learning Objectives

By the end of this chapter, learners will do the following:

- Define the meaning of portfolio.
- Examine the benefits of building a career reputation in family-focused 21st-century health care and public health systems using *family health* portfolios.
- Explore important components in a *family health* professional portfolio.
- Create a personal portfolio for your career as a *family health* professional.

Freestone's (2020) blog highlights senior health science student Kristen Novilla's work:

> "Medical practice focuses on what can be done on the individual level to improve health, while public health focuses at the population level. Families can serve as a bridge between the two because they influence both individual and *population health*." Novilla said. "That is why I'm so eager to see public health programming be more intentional about incorporating the family and making programs more family-centered." (para. 7)

Before you read on, consider the excerpt above and following questions:

- What does the excerpt imply for 21st-century health and public health care systems?
- What should *family health* teams (FHTs) look like in the 21st-century health and public health care systems workforce?

Importance of Qualified Family Health Teams

Throughout the book, the role of family and *family health* in improving the future of health care and public health systems has been emphasized. With this emphasis comes the need for preparing a well-rounded health care workforce that is equipped to become part of future FHTs. The journey of becoming a qualified member of an FHT is multifaceted and includes schooling, training, work experience, and ongoing professional development. Licensing and accreditation requirements are also part of becoming a qualified family-focused professional in some health care disciplines. With ongoing developments and changes in the health care delivery systems, FHTs are always evolving and include diverse groups of health care workers with fewer qualifications that traditionally were not within the scope of work. Teams can be made of individuals with undergraduate and graduate education, as well as secondary education (e.g., some community health workers). This means that the FHT may include nurses in generalist and advanced roles, physicians, physician assistants, pharmacists, social workers, mental health professionals, and community health workers. The goal of the FHT is to enable each team member to practice to the full extent of their training and education while meeting the social and health needs of their targeted clients (individuals, families, populations, communities) where they live, eat, play, learn, work, worship, and heal. Working in a 21st-century FHT requires a demonstration of mastery in competencies in family science and health within one's specified professional discipline or allied program. Mastery of the competencies (i.e., knowledge, attitudes, and skills) can be achieved or accomplished and organized throughout one's academic and career trajectory in many different ways. The portfolio method is one way of demonstrating competencies in health care professional practice (Kostrzewski et al., 2008).

Components of a Family Health Professional Portfolio

A portfolio is a living document that helps individuals highlight their areas of personal and professional accomplishments and growth in knowledge in an interactive, multidimensional manner. Professional portfolios can be prepared as an online document or hard copy. *Family health* professionals can use portfolios to critically reflect on their knowledge acquisitions and application processes (Brown, 2001). This means documenting learning journeys and showing evidence of competency for employment and professional registration (Anderson et al., 2009). For instance, in the higher education settings, portfolios are useful in facilitating students' learning processes (Babaee, 2020; Buckley et al., 2009; Eskici, 2015; Lu, 2021; Marinho et al., 2021; Wright et al., 1999). Likewise, in health care organizations, portfolios help assess competency through recertification or reactivation of a credentials (Byrne et al., 2009; Hespenheide et al., 2011). Other benefits include portfolio tooling for job search, career advancement (Ciesielkiewicz, 2019) and mentorship (Mollahadi et al., 2018).

No one portfolio fits all. Thus, information in professional portfolios is usually structured and individualized to reflect disciplinary or program content and competencies. Drews (2015, p. 115) identified common portfolio components 1.

COMMON PORTFOLIO COMPONENTS

- Biographical information
- Educational background
- Professional licensure/certification
- Employment history with brief description of roles and responsibilities
- Continuing education/training
- Performance evaluations/personal development plan
- Professional development activities
- Activities to support learning and assessment of others, such as mentoring, precepting, and teaching
- Support for evidence-based practice/research publications/presentations
- Membership in professional organizations

Tracy B. Chamblee et al., Selection from "Implementation of a Professional Portfolio: A Tool to Demonstrate Professional Development for Advanced Practice," *Journal of Pediatric Health Care*, vol. 29, no. 1. Copyright © 2015 by Elsevier B.V.

An example template and guide in family science was put forth by Mitchell et al. (2014), "The Family Life Education Portfolio Template and Guide," to provide an overview of steps that are helpful in completing portfolio projects specifically for undergraduate majors in family science while integrating FLE components. The common components, together with Mitchell et al.'s (2014) guide, align well with the Carper's fundamental patterns of knowing: empirical, personal, esthetic, and ethical knowledge, used to organize professional nurses' achievement of nursing competency. See Table 15.1 for definitions of the patterns and examples.

TABLE 15.1 **Carper's Fundamental Patterns of Knowing in Nursing**

Pattern of Knowing	Definition	Example Criteria
Empirical Knowledge	Acquisition of factual knowledge	Formal education; descriptive and focused on degree; participation in nursing research; continuing education attendance and presentations
Personal Knowledge	Product of experiences occurring in work environment as a registered nurse clinical practice and interpersonal relationships; reflects unique experiences of the nurse	Work experience as a registered nurse
Esthetic Knowledge	Manual and technical skills associated	Exemplars of clinical judgment and use with delivering nursing care both of skills in patient care situations (direct); precepting, charge nurse role, competency assessment (indirect)
Ethical Knowledge	Knowledge on professional standards, codes, avalues and ethics	Membership in professional organizations; enacting the professional nursing certifications; demonstrating exemplars of ethical problem solving knowledge, attitudes and skills; engaging in community service to promote justice and equity

Lee A Schmidt, Deana Nelson and Leah Godfrey, Selection from "A Clinical Ladder Program Based on Carper's Fundamental Patterns of Knowing in Nursing," JONA: *The Journal of Nursing Administration*, vol. 33, no. 3. Copyright © 2003 by Wolters Kluwer Health.

To build on Drews's (2015), Mitchell et al.'s (2014) and Barbara Carper's work, a detailed display of family-focused components that maybe beneficial to a *family health* professional portfolio is presented in Table 15.2. These components are organized into four main areas: education, research/scholarship, service, other (e.g., theory development, policy engagement, collaboration/partnerships, technology applications and innovations, etc.). The updated components emphasize learning processes that reflect the use of emancipatory knowing—the fifth pattern of knowing in the nursing literature proposed by Peggy Chinn and Maeona Kramer (Lindell & Chinn, 2022). *Family health* professional teams are in a better position to demonstrate emancipatory knowing through building trusting relationship and engaging with multiple stakeholders to address social determinants of health (SDOH) that reduce heath disparities and eliminate health equity. Evidence on this approach of learning is exemplary in supporting patient-centered collaborative teams for the 21st century beyond personal knowing (Thorne, 2020).

TABLE 15.2 **Components for a *Family Health* Professional Portfolio**

Areas of Accomplishment	Component	Examples Reflective Knowing Patterns	Example of Supportive Materials/Evidence
Family Science Education	Educational background/ training Teaching experience	Family programs, courses, certificates, training attended Family courses taught, family presentations completed Family Seminars attended Teaching innovation in *family health* or family science	Syllabus Presentation Awards Certificates Innovative teaching strategies
Family Research	Scholarship Experience	Family studies or family research conducted Participation in family research Participation in quality improvement or appraisal family projects Research consultations Participation in family research journal clubs	Family research project reports/papers, dissertation, thesis Publications Innovative research strategies
	Theory development	Participation in family research	Publications
	Innovation in technology	Participation in developing innovative family technologies	Publications Patterns Sample projects
Family Service	Leadership	Initiative or projects Materials developed for class projects, organizations, families Mentoring in *family health*	Writing samples of projects Letters from family members Letters from faculty or supervisors

	Service (including policymaking or advocacy work)	Involvement in the community on family-focused activities Involvement in family professional organizations Involved as a *family health* consultant on a project Participate in advocacy and the political process	Presentations, projects, and initiatives
Family-Focused Collaboration and Partnerships	Collaboration and Partnerships as a component for this area of accomplishment	Participation in intraprofessional, interprofessional, and multisectoral work	Presentations, projects, and initiatives
Family Professional Development	Lifelong learning goals	Areas of interest in professional growth in *family health* (e.g., technology applications like telemedicine)	Narrative describing the ability to self-reflect and self-assess

Conclusion

This chapter introduced learners to portfolios and the benefits they can provide in demonstrating the mastery of competencies in *family health* care within the context of 4HEALTHS. Creating a portfolio is a rewarding experience that can help build confident and strong *family health* teams in the 21st-century health and public health workforce.

Suggested Website

National Institute of Health (NIH) Biosketch: https://grants.nih.gov/grants/forms/biosketch.htm

Suggested Readings

Gottlieb, M., Promes, S. B., & Coates, W. C. (2021). A guide to creating a high-quality curriculum vitae. *AEM education and training*, *5*(4), e10717. https://doi.org/10.1002/aet2.10717

Hecht, E. M., Leyendecker, J. R., Spieler, B. M., Chaturvedi, A., Fennessy, F. M., Gadde, J. A., … & Lewis, P. J. (2023). Practical tips and a template for developing your curriculum vitae. *Academic Radiology*, *30*(11), 2761–2768.

Price, B. (2014). Preparing a successful, role-specific curriculum vitae. *Nursing Standard*, *29*(5), 50–57.

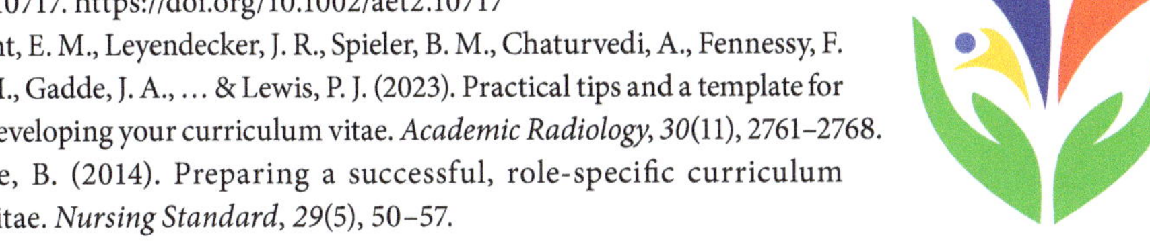

IMG 15.1

Reflection Question

Retrieve and review a sample CV on the internet for a health care job position in nursing, medicine, medical family therapy, social work, or any other health care profession. Reflect on the CV and answer the following question:

1. Is the CV family focused? Why or why not?

References

Anderson, D., Gardner, G., Ramsbotham, J., & Tones, M. (2009). E-portfolios: Developing nurse practitioner competence and capability. *Australian Journal of Advanced Nursing, 26*(4), 70–76.

Babaee, S. (2020). E-portfolio as a higher training professional tool: A comparative-descriptive study. *American Journal of Humanities and Social Sciences Research, 4*(2), 225–233.

Brown, J. O. (2001). The portfolio: A reflective bridge connecting the learner, higher education, and the workplace. *The Journal of Continuing Higher Education, 49*(2), 2–13.

Buckley, S., Coleman, J., Davison, I., Khan, K. S., Zamora, J., Malick, S., Morley, D, Pollard, D. Ashcroft, T., Popovic, C. & Sayers, J. (2009). The educational effects of portfolios on undergraduate student learning: A best evidence medical education (BEME) systematic review. *Medical teacher, 31*(4), 282–298.

Byrne, M., Schroeter, K., Carter, S., & Mower, J. (2009). The professional portfolio: An evidence-based assessment method. *The Journal of Continuing Education in Nursing, 40*(12), 545–552.

Ciesielkiewicz, M. (2019). The use of e-portfolios in higher education: From the students' perspective. *Issues in Educational Research, 29*(3), 649–667.

Drews, B. (2015). Implementation of a professional portfolio: A tool to demonstrate professional development for advanced practice. *J Pediatr Health Care, 29*, 113–117.

Eskici, M. (2015). University students' opinions on application of portfolio in higher education. *Procedia-Social and Behavioral Sciences, 174*, 2946–2955.

Hespenheide, M., Cottingham, T., & Mueller, G. (2011). Portfolio use as a tool to demonstrate professional development in advanced nursing practice. *Clinical Nurse Specialist, 25*(6), 312–320.

Lindell, D., & Chinn, P. (2022). *Overview—Patterns of Knowing in Nursing.* Nursology. https://nursology.net/patterns-of-knowing-in-nursing/

Marinho, P., Fernandes, P., & Pimentel, F. (2021). The digital portfolio as an assessment strategy for learning in higher education. *Distance Education, 42*(2), 253–267.

Mitchell, Y. T., Hartenstein, J. L., Markham, M. S., & Bernard, D. L. (2014). Portfolios in Family Science: A Template for Integrating Family Life Education. *Family Science Review,* 19 (1), 37–55.

Mollahadi, M., Khademolhoseini, S. M., Mokhtari-Nouri, J., & Khaghanizadeh, M. (2018). The portfolio as a tool for mentoring in nursing students: A scoping review. *Iranian Journal of nursing and midwifery research, 23*(4), 241–247.

Schmidt, L. A., Nelson, D., & Godfrey, L. (2003). A clinical ladder program based on Carper's fundamental patterns of knowing in nursing. *JONA: The Journal of Nursing Administration, 33*(3), 146–152.

Thorne S. (2020). Rethinking Carper's personal knowing for 21st century nursing. *Nursing philosophy: An international journal for healthcare professionals, 21*(4), e12307. https://doi.org/10.1111/nup.12307

Wright, W. A., Knight, P. T., & Pomerleau, N. (1999). Portfolio people: Teaching and learning dossiers and innovation in higher education. *Innovative higher education, 24*, 89–103.

Figure credit

Index

A

abstract conceptualization, 232
Accountable Communities of/for Health (ACH) model, 176
active experimentation, 232
active listening in health care, 154
adolescence health, 67
age-adjusted mortality rate, 65

B

belonging and love, 62, 69
biomedical perspective on *family health*, 31–33
  benefits, 32
  body and body structures, 32
  cognitions and social relations, 32
  limitations, 32–33
  organismal level, 32
  symptom experience, 32
biopsychosocial perspective on *family health*, 14, 33–39
  contexts in theorizing health and illness, 33
  levels of influence, 33, 35
  role in health promotion and risk reduction, 33
borrowed theory, 30–31
Bowen family systems theory, 35
burnout and burnout disparities among health care workforce, 112–117
  compassionate fatigue, 113
  consequences, 112–113
  during COVID-19, 113
  factors associated with, 116
  female health workers, 114
  moral distress and injury, 112–113
  rural health care workers, 114
  "whole of society" approach, 115

C

Calgary family assessment model (CFAM), 130
Calgary family intervention model (CFIM), 186
Canadian Institute for Health Information (CIHI), 66
cancer care continuum, 42, 149–150
care and caring, 10
  at family system level, 10
  at individual level, 10
  at interpersonal level, 10
care continuum, definition, 42
Carper's fundamental patterns of knowing, 271
case study, 256
CDC health impact pyramid, 59–60
Census, 66
child health, 61, 67, 126, 190
chronic diseases and disabilities, 58, 61, 65, 96, 136, 138, 155
chronic illness framework, 40
client-centered care, 14
co-financing mechanism, 173, 175
collaborative and interdisciplinary *family health* care teams, 105–108
  competency levels, 107
  definitions and core concept components, 106
  descriptive analysis of levels of involvement, 108
  disciplinary boundaries, 107
  interprofessional competency frameworks, 109–111
  levels of prevention, 101–102
  mode of collaboration, 106–107
  roles of participants, 107
communicable disease, 65
communication and relationships in health care settings
  active listening, 154
  barriers in person-centered therapeutic communication, 159–160
  cancer care continuum phases, 150
  importance of, 148–149
  mediums of, 151
  model for exchanges of information, 149
  motivational interviewing (MI), 154–155
  one-to-five ethical communication process, 157
  person-centered care, 151–152
  seven Cs of communication, 152–153
  six principles for effective communication, 158
  skills in cultural humility, 152
  SMART goals, 156–157
  soft skills, 151–152
  task-shifting strategies in interprofessional practices, 160
  teaching patient-centered communication skills, 161
community health, 83
community-integrated health system, 171
community- or policy-level strategy, 78
compassionate care and empathy/sympathy, 114
compassionate fatigue, 113
conceptual model of nursing and health policy, 220
conceptual/theoretical frameworks or models, 29
concrete experience, 232
connections, 37, 60, 66, 80, 126, 135, 138, 177, 209, 266
  mind/body/spirit, 13
  to resources and opportunities, 10
context for health development, 10. *See also* 4HEALTH contexts

continuity of health care, 10, 66, 151, 156, 209, 241, 243
  intergenerational continuity, 60
COVID-19 pandemic, 17, 58, 77, 112–114, 177, 199, 221, 243
crisis state, 45–46
cultural shifts, 83

D

Darlington family assessment, 126–127
deficit-based thinking approach to stress and coping, 47
determinants of health, 16–17, 58
Diagnostic and Statistical Manual of Mental Disorders, fifth edition (DSM-5), 32
direct patient care, 77–78, 82–83
disease management, ecological model vs biomedical model, 13–14
dissemination and implementation of evidence, 16
diverse health care settings, 240–241
domains of family practice (DFP) model, 105
Dorothea's self-care concept, 37
double ABCX model, 45
downstream determinants of health, 60

E

ecological map, 138–142
elderly health, 69
emotion-focused coping actions, 47
environmental determinants of health, 58
environment, in *family health* care, 27–28
epidemiology, 64–68
era 3.0 health systems transformation framework, 170–173
Erasmus+ Project, 246–247
European Curriculum for Family and Community Nurses (ENhANCE), 246–247
evidence-based *family health* intervention (FHI), 189–198
  basic assumptions, 190
  efficacy and effectiveness in, 197–198
  hierarchies of evidence, 192–193
  implementation of, 190–197
  intervention effects, 189–190
  levels of evidence, 197
  Melnyk and Morrison-Beedy's progression trajectory, 192
  SORT algorithm, 193–196
  steps in, 191–192
evidence-based practices, 17
  health policies, 199
  informed decision-making (EIDM), 211, 214
  models of payment (reimbursement models), 116
  patient-centered communication, 159
  public health, 177, 199, 219–220
  self-care interventions, 74
experiential learning, 231–232
  family-focused, 233
  forms and structure, 232
experiential pedagogy continuum, 233

F

familial-related health and illness factors, 9
  family roles associated with, 10
family adjustment and adaptation response (FAAR) model, 46
Family APGAR, 129
family assessment and intervention
  Calgary family assessment model (CFAM), 130
  challenges and opportunities within 4HEALTH, 142–143
  circumplex model, 126
  Darlington family assessment, 126–127
  definition, 124–125
  electronic medical record (EMR), 132–133
  ethical considerations in, 138–143
  Family APGAR, 129
  family ecomap (ecological map), 138–142
  family health genogram, 136–138, 139–141
  family health history, 135–136, 140–142
  Family Management Measure (FaMM), 135
  family management style framework (FMSF), 135
  Family Systems Stressors-Strength Inventory (FS3I), 135
  for holistic whole health care, 139
  four areas of family measures, 140–142
  Friedman family assessment model, 135
  general principles, 126
  Gordon's functional health pattern, 132–134
  importance, 124
  in marriage and family therapy, 126
  15-minute family interview, 130–132
  Intervention-Based Family Assessment (IBFA), 127–128
  social determinants of health (SDOH), 138
  tools and models, 125–135
family/families
  based relational and preventative acts, 4
  burden, 80
  definitions, 4, 8–9
  demands, 45
  ecomap (ecological map), 138–142
  health and illness, role in, 210
  healthy child development and caregiving, role in, 175
  identity, 47
  illness beliefs model, 255
  in primary and community health care nursing, 103
  level ecological outcomes, 46
  life education, 246–247
  life stage of life and related tasks, 125–126
  professional development, 273
  reasoning web framework, 140
  relationships, 3–4, 8, 10
  resilience, 9, 46, 48
  science education, 272
  self-efficacy, 10
  service, 273
  shared meanings, 47–48
family-focused collaboration and partnerships, 273
family-focused experiential learning programs, 233
family-focused population-based practice, 12–13
family functions, 9–10
  affection, 63
  economic, 64
  health care, 64
  socialization, 63
family genetics, 58
family health, 36, 60–62, 80–81
  definition, 4
  genogram, 136–138, 140–142
  history, 9, 135–136, 140–142

intersectorial (IA) and multi-sectorial (MSA) approaches in, 175–176
family health and illness cycle models
application, 42
biological perspective, 9
factors considered, 40
life stage constructs, 42–44
limitations, 44
phases of a family's experience, 40
structural perspective, 9
"time thinking" approach, 42
trajectory constructs, 40–41
family health care and family science, 3–4
barriers and facilitators, 17–18
historical context of, 4–8
important milestones, 4–6
in indigenous communities, 5
family health interventions (FHI), 102
affective domain family outcomes, 189
affective focused, 186
behavioral domain family outcomes, 189
benefits, 186–187
Calgary family intervention model (CFIM), 186
challenges and opportunities across 4HEALTH contexts, 198–199
cognitive domain family outcomes, 189
common risks and protective factors, 184–185
effect on interpersonal relationships, 186–187
evidence-based, 189–198
in acute care settings, 182
in critical care, 187
in ICU settings, 187
levels of prevention, 183–184
mechanism of actions and delivery modes, 186–189
points of "intervening,", 182
targets of, 188
ultimate goal of, 185
family health professional portfolio, 270–273
family health teams (FHTs)
21st-century, 270
culturally competent, 239–241
essential competencies for, 241–246
in diverse health care settings, 240–241
in primary care and community-oriented care, 241–243
in private or public health care settings, 241
members' scopes of practice, 241
professional certifications, 241
qualified, 270
WHO self-care competencies, 248–249
family health theories
biomedical perspective, 31–33
biopsychosocial and systems thinking perspective, 33–39
conceptual/theoretical frameworks or models, 29
ecological perspective, 34
family life stage constructs in, 42–44
key constructs in, 41–42
metaparadigms, 26–28
philosophical assumptions, 28–29
reciprocal causations, 34
socioecological framework, 33
stress and coping perspective, 45–48
terminologies in, 26
trajectory models, 40–44
Family Management Measure (FaMM), 135
family management style framework (FMSF), 135
family nursing practice, competencies for, 246
family–provider relationship, 81, 135, 259
family research, 254–255, 272
building, 258–260
criteria for, 256–258
cross-disciplinary perspectives, 257
family-focused recruitment and consenting approach, 256
mixed-method approaches and designs, 256
outcomes model for, 258
settings for, 256
family structures, 9
accounting for family attributes, 9
common, 9
demographic changes, 9
infectious disease considerations, 9
family system, definition, 35
family systems
healthy, 37
nurse interventions at, 104
structural and functional perspectives, 37
Family Systems Stressors-Strength Inventory (FS3I), 135
family systems theory, 35–37
family systems thinking, 13
family vulnerability and regenerative power, 45
family worldview, 47
Feetham's criteria for family research, 257–258
Friedman family assessment model, 135
Friedman's five family functions, 214–215
functional family, definition, 10

G

gender power dynamics, 9
Global Health Observatory, 66
Gordon's functional health pattern, 132–134
grand theories, 30

H

health
care settings, 17
definition, 11
determinants, 11
disparities, 59, 213
equity, 59, 213, 223
indicator, 62, 65–68, 75, 80
in family health care, 27
literate model, 85
outcomes, 4, 8–9, 11–13, 16–17, 28, 46, 58, 60, 62, 74–75, 79, 81, 83, 98, 138, 143–144, 148–149, 160–161, 168–169, 185, 190, 214, 219, 221–222, 240–241
promotion, 11, 16, 26–27, 36–37, 40, 42, 49, 80, 101, 115, 124, 136–137, 140, 209–210, 222–223, 232, 245, 247, 254, 256, 259
health care workforce/providers, 76
burnout and burnout disparities, 112–117
dietitians and nutritionists, 97
diverse family health and whole health care health systems, 98–101
essential health services, 99–101
foreign-born employees, 97
level of family involvement (LFI), 103–105

massage therapists, 97
multidisciplinary *family health* professionals, 100–101
music therapists, 97
occupations, 96
occupation with high concentration of women, 96
physicians and physician assistants, 97
professional involvement and collaboration with families, 101–103
racial differences, 97
risks to mental health, 98
self-employment, 97
trends, 96
United States 2022, 96–97
WHO's global classification, 99
with advanced degrees, 96
4HEALTH contexts, 3–4, 11, 13, 26, 58, 66, 79, 98, 240, 243
barriers to communication, 159–160
ecological constructs in relation to, 34–35
family health assessments within, 142–143
family health intervention (FHI), 198–199
for whole health care workforce, 112–117
social needs within, 68–70
HEALTH21 framework, 241, 244
Health People 2023, objectives and targets, 160–161
health policies
CDC's health policy process, 216–219
conceptual model of nursing and health policy, 220
definition, 208
domains, 216–217
emancipatory methods, 222
evidence-based policy practices, 210–223
family perspective in evidence-based policymaking, 208–209
individual and *family health* level, value determinants at, 222
John Kingdon's model, 215–216
Longest's policy cycle model, 215–216
policy formulation, 216
policy implementation, 216
policy modification, 216
population health level, value determinants at, 222
processes, 215–221
public health family impact (PHFI) checklist, 221
public health level, value determinants at, 222
rational decision-making models, 222
RE-AIM (reach, effectiveness, adoption, implementation, and maintenance) model, 220
triangle framework, 216
Walt and Gilson's policy triangle conceptual framework, 215–216
healthy community characteristics and processes, 64
healthy family system, 37
characteristics, 63–64
Healthy People 2023, 75, 177
Healthy People 2030, 66
high-risk group, 65
holism, 13, 38, 47
human-related illnesses/diseases, 58

I

Ida Jean Orlando's nursing process, 215
Identify, Situation, Background, Assessment and Recommendation (ISBAR) framework, 156
implementation science, 17
incidence and incidence rate, 65
indirect cost of harm, 74
individual health, 79–80
intersectorial (IA) and multisectorial (MSA) approaches in, 175–176
infant mortality rate, 65
Institute for Patient- and Family-Centered Care (IPFCC), 14
International Family Nursing Association (IFNA), 244
internships, 232–233
Interprofessional Education Collaborative (IPEC), 109–110
competencies and sub-competencies, 110–111
Interprofessional Education (IPE) competencies, 109–110
intersectorial (IA) and multisectorial (MSA) approaches, 208
barriers and enablers, 174–177
co-financing or risk-based contracting, 173
definition, 168–169
era 3.0 health systems transformation framework, 170–173
financial mechanisms, 173, 175
in *individual health* and *family health*, 175–176
in *population health*, 176
in public health, 177
role in *family health* care, 169–170
Intervention-Based Family Assessment (IBFA), 127–128

J

John Kingdon's policy streams model, 215–216
Johns Hopkins patient engagement program, 85

K

Kolb's experiential learning cycle, 232

L

length of stay (LoS) predictions, 7–8
level of family involvement (LFI) model, 103–105
benefits in delineating professional roles, 105
descriptive analysis of levels of involvement, 108
in medical education and research, 103–104
levels of involvement, 104–105
model of competency levels, 107–108
level of physician involvement model (LPI), 102–103
Longest's policy cycle model, 215–216

M

Maslow's hierarchy of needs model, 33, 63–64, 66, 68
need for love and belonging, 62
physiological needs, 62
safety needs, 62
sense of esteem needs, 62
Mead, George Herbert, 46
medical family therapy, 6, 35, 241, 247, 273
men health, 67
metaparadigms, 26–27
meta theory, 30
micro-range theory, 30
middle-range theory, 30, 45
midrange theories, 30
midstream determinants of health, 59–60
mind/body/spirit connection, 13

15-minute family interview, 130–132
moral distress and injury, 112–113
morbidity, 65, 259
mortality rate, 65, 259
motivational interviewing (MI), 154–155
    concepts, principles and methods, 155

N

neonate/infant health, 66
Neuman systems model
    physical health of family, 36
    psychosocial-cultural relationships of family, 36
    spiritual influences, 36
noncommunicable diseases (NCDs), 12, 65
non-normative demands, 45
normative demands, 45
nurse-promoted engagement with families, 80
nursing metaparadigm, 28

O

occupational challenges and opportunities, 112–117
one-to-five ethical communication process, 157
oral and written communication messages, attributes, 153

P

paradigm, definition, 31
patient- and family-centered care (PFCC), 4, 14–15, 75, 208
    challenges of implementing, 17
patient and family engagement (PFE), in health care, 76–79, 208
    barriers and facilitators in UK health systems, 82
    civic engagement, 83
    community-level determinant, 83
    community- or policy-level strategy, 78
    conceptual definitions and terminologies, 76
    consultation/information (minimum) level, 77
    direct patient care, 77–78
    examples, 78
    family-level determinant, 80–81
    in clinical and nonclinical settings, 76
    individual-level determinant, 79–80
    involvement level, 77
    organizational-level strategies, 77–78
    partnership/shared leadership level, 77
    population-level determinant, 81–83
    public health, 83–85
    systems-level strategies, 77–78
patient-as-a-person process, 13
patient-centered care, 14, 110, 159, 171, 189, 193
patient–clinician communications and relationship (PCR) processes, 28
patient engagement
    outcomes indicators, 75
    role in quality care and patient safety, 74
    self-care management and, 74
    status of key national *population health* metrics, 75
patient experience, 76, 182
Patient-Reported Outcomes Measurement Information System (PROMIS) roadmap initiative, 143
person(s), in *family health* care, 27
physiological needs, 62, 70
population, 65
    at risk, 12
    health indicators, 66–68
    of interest, 12
population-based public health interventions
    biopsychosocial or ecological health perspective, 13
    community-focused level, 12
    individual/family focus, 12
    systems-focus level, 12
population-focused *family health* care, 11–12, 16
population health, 198
    indicators and outcomes, 62, 66–68, 75
    intersectorial (IA) and multisectorial (MSA) approaches in, 176
    outcomes, 11, 16, 62, 81–83, 143, 169, 219, 221, 239–241, 256
precision medicine (personalized medicine), 9
preconception health, 66
prevalence and prevalence rate, 65
prevention interventions, levels of, 16
primary prevention interventions, 16
problem-focused coping actions, 47
professional associations in family science and health, 265–266
    assessment for joining, 267
    benefits of, 266
    life span of, 266
professional community of practice, 265
    five-stage evolution of, 266
program of family research, 258–260
psychosomatic illness in children, factors contributing, 40
public health, 11, 83–85
    family impact (PHFI) checklist, 221
    intersectorial (IA) and multisectorial (MSA) approaches in, 177
    nursing, 7, 103–104, 241
    patients' engagement IT functionalities and, 84
    surveillance, 65

Q

qualitative research, 256
quantitative research, 256

R

RE-AIM (reach, effectiveness, adoption, implementation, and maintenance) model, 220
real-world data (RWE), 82
reflective observation, 232
relationship-centered care, 14
resilience perspective on *family health*, 9, 46, 48
risk factor, 65

S

safety needs, 62
secondary prevention interventions, 16
self-actualization, 62, 68
self-care concept, 37
    evidence-based self-care interventions, 74
    patient engagement and, 74
self-care roles, 8
self-worth (self-esteem), 62
sense of esteem, 62, 69
service-learning (SL) programs, 232–233
    Barbara Holland's views, 232
    components in, 232–233
    core principles, 233–234
    in family life education, 233
    patient-centered, 232

seven Cs of communication, 152–153
shared theory, 31
sickle cell disease, 58
sick role, 8
simulation, 232
situational meanings, 47
SMART goals, 156–157
  attainable objectives, 157
  measurable objectives, 156
  realistic objectives, 157
  time-phased objectives, 157
  "who" and "what" of clinical–patient communication and interaction activities, 156
social determinants of health (SDoH), 11, 58–60, 138, 143, 208, 214, 233, 240
  epidemiology, 64–68
  major domains, 58–59
  within 4HEALTH context, 68–70
social needs model, 60, 62
soft skills, 151–152
stages of *family health* and levels of prevention, 102
strength-based approaches to stress and coping, 47
strength of recommendation taxonomy (SORT), 193–196
stress and coping theories
  adaptation phase (postcrisis stage), 45
  cognitive appraisal process, 47
  conceptualizing stressful events, 47
  factors theorized in, 45
  family adaptation to stressful events, 46
  family adaptive functions, 47
  family-level ecological outcomes, 46
  family vulnerability and regenerative power, 45
  key constructs in, 48
  limitations, 48
  protective factors or family strengths, 45
  resilience perspective, 46
  strengths-based perspective, 47
  symbolic interaction perspective, 46–47
supportive family relationships, 3–4
symbolic interaction perspectives, 46–47
systems thinking perspective on *family health*, 13, 33–39

T

21st-century health care system, 254
telehealth advice and disease management, 116–117, 151
tertiary prevention interventions, 16
theoretical paradigms, 31
theory/theories
  borrowed or shared, 30–31
  definition, 30
  grand, 30
  meta, 30
  micro-range, 30
  middle-range, 30
  midrange, 30
  phenomena of interest, 30
  theoretical paradigms, 31
timely deaths, 57–58
trajectory models of *family health*, 40–44
  family life course/developmental perspective, 42
  historical contributions, 40
  key constructs in, 40–42
  phases of family's experience, 40
trust, 113–115, 168, 176
  in patient and family engagement, 81–82
  in patient–clinician interactions and communication, 46, 148
  public, in health systems, 82–83, 222
  trusting relationship, 46–47, 81–82, 101, 124, 199, 272

U

universal health care (UHC), 74
upstream determinants of health, 59–60
U.S. health system transformation, 172–173

V

value-based health care (VBHC), 85
value judgments, 221–222
volunteerism, 233

W

Walt and Gilson's policy triangle conceptual framework, 215–216
whole health care, defnition, 84
whole health, definition, 84
whole health systems, definition, 84
women health, 67
workplace violence, 115
World Health Organization (WHO)
  global classification of health care workforce, 99
  HEALTH21 framework, 241, 244
  principles for effective communication, 158
  self-care competencies, 248–249

Y

years of potential life lost, 65

www.ingramcontent.com/pod-product-compliance
Ingram Content Group UK Ltd.
Pitfield, Milton Keynes, MK11 3LW, UK
UKHW050140280726
14058UKWH00006B/754